Practical Psychopharmacology

Practical Psychopharmacology takes the novel approach of writing at three different levels—beginning, intermediate, and advanced—to give the practicing psychopharmacologist a tailored experience. Each chapter focuses on a specific DSM-5 disorder and outlines abbreviated treatment guidelines to help the reader understand where their knowledge base and clinical practice currently resides. At the first level, the book teaches novice prescribers practical diagnostic skills and provides a brief overview of pertinent genetic and neuroimaging findings to increase prescribing confidence. Next, it provides mid-level clinicians with intermediate techniques and guidelines for more difficult cases. The final level provides nuanced guidance for advanced practitioners or those who see the most treatment-resistant patients. This approach allows a clinician to access this book periodically throughout the care of an individual patient and to gradually progress through a series of more advanced psychopharmacological techniques for making accurate and efficient diagnoses. Readers can also visit the book's eResource page to download a bonus chapter on eating disorders, as well as case studies and multiple-choice questions for each chapter.

Thomas L. Schwartz, MD, is a professor and interim chair of psychiatry at SUNY Upstate Medical University in Syracuse, New York. He is co-editor of *Integrating Psychotherapy and Psychopharmacology: A Handbook for Clinicians* and the second edition of *Depression: Treatment Strategies and Management.* He is co-author of *Case Studies: Stahl's Essential Psychopharmacology, Volume 2.* Dr. Schwartz has received the Marc H. Hollander, MD, Psychiatry Award; the SUNY Upstate President's Award; and the SUNY Chancellor's Award for Teaching, as well as the Nancy C.A. Roeske, MD, Certificate and the Irma Bland Award for Excellence in Teaching from the American Psychiatric Association.

Practical Psychopharmacology

Basic to Advanced Principles

Thomas L. Schwartz

Routledge
Taylor & Francis Group
NEW YORK AND LONDON

First published 2017
by Routledge
605 Third Avenue, New York, NY 10017

and by Routledge
4 Park Square, Milton Park, Abingdon, Oxon OX14 4RN

Routledge is an imprint of the Taylor & Francis Group, an informa business

Library of Congress Cataloging-in-Publication Data
A catalog record for this book has been requested

ISBN: 978-1-138-90252-7 (hbk)
ISBN: 978-1-138-90253-4 (pbk)
ISBN: 978-1-315-69738-3 (ebk)

Typeset in Minion Pro
by Apex CoVantage, LLC

Contents

Figures and Tables

Figures

Tables

Series Editor's Foreword

Practical Psychopharmacology: Basic to Advanced Principles is the latest volume in one of Routledge's most popular series, Clinical Topics in Psychology and Psychiatry (CTPP). The overarching goal of CTPP is to provide mental health practitioners with practical information on pharmacological and psychological topics. Each volume is comprehensive but easy to digest and integrate into day-to-day clinical practice. It is multidisciplinary, covering topics relevant to the fields of psychology and psychiatry, and appeals to the student, novice, and senior clinician. Books chosen for the series are authored or edited by national and international experts in their respective areas, and contributors are also highly respected clinicians. The current volume exemplifies the intent, scope, and aims of the CTPP series.

Since identifying the first antidepressants in the 1950s, the practice of clinical psychopharmacology has grown at breakneck speed. It truly began to flourish in the late 1980s after Prozac, the first serotonin reuptake inhibitor, hit the market and became one of the country's all-time bestselling medications. In part, because of Prozac's (and medications with nearly identical chemical structures) popularity and ease of use, psychopharmacology was no longer the sole purview of psychiatry. Nurse practitioners, physician assistants, primary care physicians, and even psychologists with advanced training in psychopharmacology got into the game.

Unfortunately, the field has not seen the same level of proliferation of easy-to-read texts for those interested in learning to practice psychopharmacology. Aside from a few exceptions, available training textbooks are filled with page after page of dense text, much of which is focused on, as the volume's author Thomas Schwartz states in the introduction, "granular molecular fundamentals of psychotropic drugs." Then, there are overly detailed "decision" matrices constructed to help practitioners choose which medication goes with which disorder in which situation. These aides are often so complex and difficult to decipher that they are rendered useless. There is nothing more frustrating than a psychopharmacology text that is either too basic or too advanced in its content. *Practical Psychopharmacology: Basic to Advanced Principles* solves these problems. It is unique in that it is written in advancing levels of knowledge and expertise, so it meets the student or practitioner where they are at in their training and practice.

The reader will find many of this volume's chapters of considerable benefit. Unlike edited books, this authored volume flows seamlessly. Schwartz speaks to you as a colleague and as an educator. The information he provides is based on the latest science, not ideology or conformity to a particular approach. He is, indeed, a gifted practitioner, scholar, and writer.

I am convinced that *Practical Psychopharmacology: Basic to Advanced Principles* will become one of the lead textbooks in training future psychopharmacologists. It will also function as an excellent review for experienced practitioners looking for an easily digestible presentation of the latest science on psychopharmacological practice.

Bret A. Moore, PsyD, ABPP
Series Editor
Clinical Topics in Psychology and Psychiatry

Preface

Psychopharmacology, Psychotherapy, and the Psychosocial Aspects of Prescribing

How many times have you bought a textbook seeking insights into prescribing psychiatric medications only to find it filled with pages and pages of dense text about the granular molecular fundamentals of psychotropic drugs? Or, you find overly detailed tables and circular algorithms that go on for pages. Have you ever bought a psychopharmacology text to find out that it was either too basic, filled with information you already knew, or way too complex and well above your expertise? How about a textbook where the text did not apply to the patients you see because your patients were too comorbid? The concept and design of this clinical handbook is novel in that it is written in advancing levels of practical clinical information. Ideally, the information in this handbook can be used quickly and efficiently by a large variety of prescribers regardless of time in the field or background.

Each chapter will begin with a more simplistic conceptualized approach. Information in Section 1 of each chapter should quickly answer the question: "What do I really need to know right now regarding my psychiatric patient to make a reasonable diagnosis and start a reasonable medication?" Psychiatric screening questions, DSM-5 interviewing criteria, and easy rating scale approaches will be discussed in a way that any variety of clinicians (medical students, primary care and psychiatry residents, primary care physicians and psychiatrists, nurse practitioners, physician assistants, etc.) may make standard of care medical decisions quickly. Approved and clear evidence-based psychiatric medications will be discussed efficiently so that informed consent can be offered to the patient, the drug can be prescribed and the patient monitored, and ideally a good outcome can be obtained. Section 1 is designed to be an initial education for those who provide care to psychiatric disordered patients or as a quick reference guide. It is strongly advised that all readers read through the first ADHD chapter to understand the layout and concept of this book. After this, readers may pick a psychiatric disorder chapter and choose to go the simple route and start with Section 1, or go right to the more advanced Section 2 and onward depending on specific educational and clinical application needs.

Section 2 is designed for prescribers who want to know slightly more about psychopharmacology. These sections go beyond the typical guideline and algorithm approach for patients who have just one psychiatric disorder. Section 2 will educate the reader about some (but not exhaustively) of the basic science and principles behind each psychiatric disorder and its treatment. Less evidence-based, but appropriate second and third line psychopharmacological treatments will be discussed. Prescribing for highly comorbid and treatment resistant patients is covered. Essentially, if your patients are not quite as simple as those in Section 1, or if Section 1 medications have failed to help, then you will need to read Section 2. Section 2 will cover briefly the epidemiology, genetics, and functional neuroanatomy of each disorder. This information gives the prescriber the information needed to explain to their patient who asks, "Why do I have this psychiatric problem?", "Why will this medication make my symptoms go away?", "Why did I get side effects?", etc.

This book is not an exhaustive reference and does not replace a more comprehensive textbook double its size. It is not a full prescriber's guide and will not replace the regulatory information handed down by the FDA. Rather, this book puts a fair amount of knowledge into the prescriber's hands very quickly that ideally translates into better diagnoses, medication selection, and monitoring in clinical practice. It should read like teaching rounds on an academic psychiatry teaching service. All information cannot be covered, but key information should be covered quickly. This book should improve the prescriber's ability to choose a medication, or medications, when initial monotherapy fails to gain a remission. The goal is to have clinicians become more adept and knowledgeably aggressive in managing patients with psychiatric disorders. This book is designed to have an easy learning curve where the reader can choose at which level or density they wish to practice at.

This book is a psychopharmacology handbook but presupposes that the prescriber is adept at employing core psychotherapy skills despite using the medication management or biological model. Outcomes and compliance with treatment regimen likely are enhanced by use of psychopharmacopsychotherapy. In other words, always be mindful and use psychotherapy to your advantage when you are prescribing psychotropics as both skill sets should be paired at all times.

Acknowledgments and Dedication

Dr. Schwartz would like to thank his many mentors who have helped him throughout his career and shaped the way he practices, writes, and teaches. He would like to thank his peers who have provided support, education, and comradery. He would like to thank his residents and students who provide an arena for the imparting of knowledge but also provide an immense sense of satisfaction as they obtain knowledge and become better clinicians through training. It should also be noted that trainees are also excellent teachers! Dr. Jungjin Kim should be commended for his ability to multitask and his tireless effort in his formatting of this book. Dr. Mark Giordano should be commended for his skills as a clinician and gifts as a mentor in writing. Finally, Dr. Schwartz appreciates the balance afforded by a supportive family and supportive psychiatry department leadership at SUNY Upstate Medical University in Syracuse, New York. The latter really is impressive that in an era of productivity-driven educational and clinical models, each successive chair has put effort into the growth of their junior faculty members. Thanks to all.

If you are interested in reading case examples that are designed to further teach and illustrate the information and concepts outlined in this book, you may visit the website: www.routledge.com/9781138902534.

Prologue

Psychopharmacopsychotherapy

What is this term and why is it important for the use of this book? Even though this book is a biological psychopharmacology handbook, it is based on the foundation that the prescriber is generally a good human being who cares about the patient and wants to form a partnership and alliance with the patient in order to get them better. To maximize patient adherence and compliance with medications and to improve visit attendance and session productivity, the core skills of psychotherapy are needed. To maximize the tolerance of known side effects and to diminish the effects of placebo induced side effects (nocebo effects), the core skills of supportive psychotherapy are needed. If the prescriber loses track or does not deploy these skills while prescribing, the author suspects that outcomes will be worse than those advertised.

Supportive psychotherapy can be deployed by any type of provider with any credentials at any time. It is an augmentation strategy and likely creates physiological effects that can be seen and measured in the frontal cortex of the brain. Even though this is a form of psychotherapy, it likely creates electrophysiological brain changes, just like adding medications together. So why not add in this bonus treatment while prescribing? You as the clinician have nothing to lose and likely better outcomes to gain for your patient.

Psychopharmacopsychotherapy essentially means the purposeful combining of psychiatric medication management AND psychotherapy simultaneously.

A model of providing Manualized Psychopharmacopsychotherapy (M-PPPT) might be theorized, learned, and incorporated into clinical practice if the prescriber wishes to pay attention and purposefully deploy these skills. M-PPPT's goal would be to develop a basic psychotherapy treatment for use by psychopharmacologists when employing a *medication management only model* for the treatment of MDD or other psychiatric disorders. The prescriber must be aware and want to maintain the psychotherapeutic stance while in the busy daily practice of providing psychopharmacology to patients. To be realistic, and honest, some prescribers are burned out, never liked training or providing psychotherapy, or find psychotherapy draining when compared to prescribing sessions. Burned out psychopharmacologists may blame their employer or the insurance companies for enforcing the fast medication sessions and split model psychotherapy, but some psychopharmacologists use this as a rationalization because they may not want to admit, or do not want to embrace, psychotherapy as a technique either due to (a) philosophical stance, (b) the sometimes draining nature of psychotherapy, (c) the learning curve of psychotherapy, or (d) the fact that it is often more lucrative to provide a higher volume of shorter medication management visits per day. M-PPPT interventions have an easy learning curve and may be utilized in practice immediately even if a stoic *medications-only approach* is adhered to.

M-PPPT has a goal to increase the prescriber's awareness toward the use of "common factors" mentioned above and felt to be universal to most employed psychotherapies. This simplistic approach often is initially taught in nurse practitioner or psychiatric residency training, or may be used later as a "vocational rehabilitation tool" for the veteran prescriber who becomes burned out or cynical. Using a checklist approach, a psychopharmacology session may be broken down into sections, and both psychopharmacology and psychotherapy may be employed in parallel. Use of a simple checklist should bring M-PPPT approaches to awareness while conducting a session with a patient. A typical M-PPPT checklist might involve the following:

Table P.1 This basic checklist is a manual. It covers the basic processes of a gold standard medication management visit, but at the same time, it works to orient the prescriber to provide core psychotherapy techniques throughout a short session with a patient

M-PPPT CHECKLIST

<u>Psychopharmacology Components:</u>

__Review previous note prior to session
__Check new rating scales prior to session
__Ask about current positive or negative stressors
__Conduct lethality risk assessment
__Review current pivotal target symptoms
__Review medication list
__Review side effects
__Review medical problems
__Check vitals/physical exam/labs if warranted

Provide Informed Consent
__Positive and negative medication effects
__Rationale for psychotherapy as adjunctive treatment

(*Continued*)

Table P.1 (Continued)

Psychotherapy Components:

During Session
__Provide psychoeducation (diagnosis and medication options)
__Provide >3 core psychotherapy skills
__motivation
__empathy
__openness
__collaboration
__warmth
__positive regard
__sincerity
__corrective experience
__catharsis
__establish goals
__establish time limit
__establish patient effort needed

Documentation:

__Compile Note
__Contact collaterals as needed
__Contact other providers as needed
__Contact insurance as needed

In conclusion, prescribing of psychotropics does not occur in a vacuum devoid of interpersonal interaction with your patients. In a busy practice setting, consider consciously employing core therapy skills in each setting to obtain better results for your patient!

Bibliography

Greenberg, R.P. (2012) "Essential ingredients for successful psychotherapy: effect of common factors." In Dewan, Steenbarger, Greenberg (eds.), *The Art and Science of Brief Psychotherapies—A Practitioner's Guide* (15–26). Washington, D.C.: American Psychiatric Publishing.

Liggan, D. Y., & Kay J. (1999) "Some neurobiological aspects of psychotherapy: a review." *The Journal of Psychotherapy Practice and Research*, 8(2), 103.

Stahl, S. M. (2012). "Psychotherapy as an epigenetic 'drug': psychiatric therapeutics target symptoms linked to malfunctioning brain circuits with psychotherapy as well as with drugs." *Journal of Clinical Pharmacy and Therapeutics*, 37(3), 249–253.

CHAPTER 1

Adult Attention Deficit-Hyperactivity Disorder

SECTION 1 Basic Prescribing Practices

Essential Concepts

- ADHD is a heritable illness that is *clinically* diagnosed with a persistent longitudinal pattern of
  - inattention and/or
  - hyperactivity-impulsivity
- Diagnosis should be based on careful history demonstrating impaired functioning in multiple settings (school, home, community) starting before the age of 12.
- Comorbid learning disability and other psychiatric disorders are common in adults.
- Pharmacotherapy is the centerpiece to ADHD treatment.
- First line medications are often stimulants.
- Second line medications are alpha-2 agonists and possibly certain antidepressants.
- Consider using rating scales at baseline and during follow-up sessions.

Phenomenology, Diagnosis, Clinical Interviewing

For any new practitioner in any field, the goal is to be able to make an accurate diagnosis. All of psychiatric prescribing at this beginning level is based on regulatory findings, approvals, and indications that are psychiatric disorder specific. Psychotropics will only deliver the outcomes promised if the patient at hand actually has been accurately identified as having adult ADHD. Inattention, poor concentration, and impaired vigilance are all symptoms that are not unique to adult ADHD. These symptoms are also prevalent in major depressive disorder (MDD), post-traumatic stress disorder (PTSD), and generalized anxiety disorder (GAD). This can make diagnosis complicated but also should alert the reader that one psychotropic may be able to improve inattention regardless of which categorical psychiatric disorder the inattention is being attributed to. Sometimes an antidepressant, like bupropion (Wellbutrin XL/Aplenzin), can treat adult ADHD. Alternatively, an ADHD medication like lisdexamfetamine (Vyvanse) can treat non-ADHD conditions (binge eating disorder [BED]). As this chapter progresses to discuss intermediate and advanced psychopharmacologic prescribing, the use of off-label, less well-studied approaches becomes more apparent. Prescribers need to appreciate that certain discrete psychiatric symptoms can cross the apparent boundaries of categorical diagnostic and regulatory processes. Understanding and appreciating this concept is often needed to treat the more treatment resistant or comorbidly afflicted patient.

Commonly, ADHD in adults is confounded by other psychiatric disorders such as anxiety, substance misuse, depression, and personality disorder. This chapter assumes the reader is comfortable with descriptive, DSM-5 (Diagnostic and Statistical Manual of Mental Disorders) interviewing and diagnostic assessment, or is willing to learn. Furthermore, in the absence of DSM-5 mastery, patient administered rating scales should become more the standard of care. Outside of aiding in diagnosis, routine use of validated scales likely will aid in obtaining outcomes found in regulatory trials which utilize these scales to drive treatment and can motivate the prescriber to address residual symptoms, much like abnormal lab values that prompt action in the primary care setting (ex. monitoring hypertension, hyperglycemia, etc.).

The key to diagnosis is confirming the longitudinal and impairing presence of a combination of (a) inattention, (b) hyperactivity, and/or (c) impulsivity that cannot be explained by another psychiatric disorder, substance misuse, personality disorder, or medical condition. During a routine interview, use of an initial screening question is warranted. If the patient answers positively, this should trigger the use of a full DSM-5 symptom interview or use of a validated, reliable ADHD rating scale.

TIP: Screening Questions

Screening for inattention

- Do you often make careless mistakes at home, work, or school because you aren't paying attention? Do you have difficulty concentrating or focusing more often than not?

Screening for hyperactivity

- Is it hard for you to sit still?

Screening for functional impairment

- What problems do [these behaviors] cause at school, work, or home?

Screening for longitudinal history

- How old were you when you began [these behaviors]?

Remember to screen for other psychiatric illnesses, ex. mood disorder, anxiety disorder, substance use, etc.

The use of the DSM-5 model may seem tedious or effortful in regard to memorization and the implementation of a rigorous systematic, symptom-based approach to adult ADHD diagnosis. Nevertheless, it does promote a very sensitive and specific validated way to make the diagnosis and apply accurate, efficacious treatments. Following this approach should allow the prescriber and patient to obtain the pharmacological outcomes that are reported in the literature. Use of rating scales for each psychiatric disorder will be discussed in later chapters as well. Scales generally allow the clinician to rely less on the DSM-5 clinical interview and more on patient-driven, self-reporting measures. Ideally, both approaches will be used.

DSM-5 Diagnosis

People with ADHD show a persistent pattern of inattention and/or hyperactivity-impulsivity that interferes with functioning or development characterized by (1) and/or (2) (see below) starting before the age of 12.

(1) **Inattention**: Six or more symptoms of inattention for children up to age 16, or five or more for adolescents 17 and older and adults; symptoms of inattention have been present for at least six months and are inappropriate for developmental level:
   - Often fails to give close attention to details or makes careless mistakes in schoolwork, at work, or with other activities.
   - Often has trouble holding attention on tasks or play activities.
   - Often does not seem to listen when spoken to directly.
   - Often does not follow through on instructions and fails to finish schoolwork, chores, or duties in the workplace (e.g., loses focus, gets side-tracked).
   - Often has trouble organizing tasks and activities.
   - Often avoids, dislikes, or is reluctant to do tasks that require mental effort over a long period of time (such as schoolwork or homework).
   - Often loses things necessary for tasks and activities (e.g., school materials, pencils, books, tools, wallets, keys, paperwork, eyeglasses, mobile telephones).

- Is often easily distracted.
- Is often forgetful in daily activities.

(2) **Hyperactivity and Impulsivity:** Six or more symptoms of hyperactivity-impulsivity for children up to age 16, or five or more for adolescents 17 and older and adults; symptoms of hyperactivity-impulsivity have been present for at least six months to an extent that is disruptive and inappropriate for the person's developmental level:

- Often fidgets with or taps hands or feet, or squirms in seat.
- Often leaves seat in situations when remaining seated is expected.
- Often runs about or climbs in situations where it is not appropriate (adolescents or adults may be limited to feeling restless).
- Often unable to play or take part in leisure activities quietly.
- Is often "on the go" acting as if "driven by a motor."
- Often talks excessively.
- Often blurts out an answer before a question has been completed.
- Often has trouble waiting his/her turn.
- Often interrupts or intrudes on others (e.g., butts into conversations or games)

In addition, the following conditions must be met:

- Several inattentive or hyperactive-impulsive symptoms were present before age 12 years.
- Several symptoms are present in two or more settings, (e.g., at home, school, or work; with friends or relatives; in other activities).
- There is clear evidence that the symptoms interfere with, or reduce the quality of, social, school, or work functioning.
- The symptoms do not happen only during the course of schizophrenia or another psychotic disorder. The symptoms are not better explained by another mental disorder (e.g., mood disorder, anxiety disorder, dissociative disorder, or a personality disorder).

Based on the types of symptoms, three kinds (presentations) of ADHD can occur:

- Combined presentation: if enough symptoms of both criteria inattention and hyperactivity-impulsivity were present for the past six months
- Predominantly inattentive presentation: if enough symptoms of inattention, but not hyperactivity-impulsivity, were present for the past six months
- Predominantly hyperactive-impulsive presentation: if enough symptoms of hyperactivity-impulsivity but not inattention were present for the past six months.

Because symptoms can change over time, the presentation may change over time as well.

TIP: Interviewing an ADHD Patient

- Adult practitioners usually find comorbidities, such as ADHD, in their adult patients who present with initial complaints of anxiety, depression, or substance abuse. In this way, ADHD may be a secondary finding.

How to screen for ADHD

- Screening for ADHD often occurs secondarily in the Psychiatric Review of Systems while taking a full psychiatric history, as part of the Social History interview segment, especially when inquiring about psychosocial development from childhood through young adulthood.
- For example: Asking patients how they performed in grade school, middle school, high school, and college is a productive approach. Did the patient do well or have problems in school? Were they labeled or felt like a *bad kid* or *difficult student*? Could they focus and pay attention to the teacher, stay on task, complete assignments, etc.? Were they disruptive to the class, make impulsive decisions that caused problems? Did they often forget to "look before they leaped"? Would their friends, teachers, parents say they were always moving, "hyper," climbing, or fidgeting? Did they day dream or drift off?

Obtain longitudinal history of the symptoms

- If these patterns are found, it is important to identify if they have carried through to adulthood and to clearly delineate if these symptom clusters both appear in multiple spheres of life (home, work, social, etc.) and presently cause psychosocial distress. It is important to determine if ADHD symptoms were present from grade school ages.
- It would be odd for an adult to all of a sudden "develop" or "come down with" ADHD.
- Inattention and poor concentration that develop over several weeks are often related to MDD, GAD, stress, an adjustment disorder, or possibly substance misuse.
- Patients often see a decline in work or school performance and present convinced they have *new onset* ADHD. Longitudinally, it is key to determine whether clear ADHD symptoms predated or were premorbid to the presenting inattentive chief complaint.
- If premorbid ADHD is not detected, then clinicians should treat the current inattentive symptoms as part of another more accurate DSM-5 diagnosis (ex. MDD).
- If premorbid ADHD is detected, then both the ADHD and the new onset DSM-5 disorder should be treated concurrently.

Pay particular attention to inattentivity when diagnosing adult ADHD

- Adult ADHD diagnosis may be difficult to detect as one expects the adult to have the classic triad of inattention, hyperactivity, and impulsivity.
- In fact, as a patient ages with ADHD, it is common for the hyperactivity and impulsivity symptoms to lessen, while the inattentive ones continue.
- More often, adult patients appear to have inattentive ADHD rather than hyperactive/impulsive type.

Confirm history with collateral information

- Clinicians can improve diagnostic accuracy for adult ADHD by interviewing a significant other (parent, sibling, etc.) for a few minutes to confirm the longitudinal presence of ADHD symptoms from a younger age. Use of rating scales may also help.

Rating Scales

Adult ADHD Self-Report Scale (ASRSv1.1)

- This scale was adapted and validated from the well accepted version utilized for childhood ADHD called the ASRS.V1. It is in the public domain and simple to use. It takes approximately 1–2 minutes for the patient to complete and several seconds to score.
- Scoring suggests that a positive score of any kind in four or more shaded areas of *Section A* is suggestive of an ADHD diagnosis. Scores may be followed sequentially over time to track treatment outcomes.
- To obtain this public domain scale please refer to Adler, Lenard, et al. (2006) "Validity of Pilot Adult ADHD Self-Report Scale (ASRS) to rate adult ADHD symptoms." *Annals of Clinical Psychiatry* 18.3, 145–148; Kessler, R.C., Adler, L., Ames, M., (2005) "The World Health Organization adult ADHD self-report scale (ASRS): a short screening scale for use in the general population." *Psychological Medicine* 35, *245–56*; Hines, J.L., King, T.S., & Curry, W.J. (2012) "The adult ADHD self-report scale for screening for adult attention deficit–hyperactivity disorder (ADHD)." *The Journal of the American Board of Family Medicine* 25.6, 847–853. www.hcp.med.harvard.edu/ncs/asrs.php. It is free and copyrighted by the World Health Organization.

Table 1.1 The ASRS-V1.1 for Use in Adult ADHD

Adult ADHD Self-Report Scale (ASRS-V1.1) Symptom Checklist					
Patient Name:	Today's Date:				
Please answer the questions below, rating yourself on each of the criteria shown using the scale on the right side of the page. As you answer each question, place an X in the box that best describes how you have felt and conducted yourself over the past six months. Please give this completed checklist to your healthcare professional to discuss during today's appointment.	Never	Rarely	Sometimes	Often	Very Often
1. How often do you have trouble wrapping up the final details of a project, once the challenging parts have been done?					
2. How often do you have difficulty getting things in order when you have to do a task that requires organization?					
3. How often do you have problems remembering appointments or obligations?					
4. When you gave a task that requires a lot of thought, how often do you avoid or delay getting started?					
5. How often do you fidget or squirm with your hands or feet when you have to sit down for a long time?					
6. How often do you feel overly active and compelled to do things, like you were driven by a motor?					
					Part A
7. How often do you make careless mistakes when you have to work on a boring or difficult project?					
8. How often do you have difficulty keeping your attention when you are doing boring or repetitive work?					
9. How often do you have difficulty concentrating on what people say to you, even when they are speaking to you directly?					
10. How often do you misplace or have difficulty finding things at home or work?					
11. How often are you distracted by activity or noise around you?					
12. How often do you leave your seat in meetings or other situations in which you are expected to remain seated?					
13. How often do you feel restless or fidgety?					
14. How often do you have difficulty unwinding or relaxing when you have time to yourself?					
15. How often do you find yourself talking too much when you are in social situations?					
16. When you're in a conversation, how often do you find yourself finishing the sentences of the people you are talking to, before they can finish them themselves?					
17. How often do you have difficulty waiting your turn in situations when turn taking is required?					
18. How often do you interrupt others when they are busy?					
					Part B

TIP: Commentary on Rating Scales in Psychiatric Practice

Rating scales should not replace but rather supplement a good clinical interview

- Rating scales cannot bring about the development of rapport and improvement of medication compliance that a responsive, professional clinical interview provides.
- Rating scales that are completed by the patient on paper, electronically, or otherwise should be considered equivalent to the use of sphygmomanometry in treating hypertensives or blood glucose readings in treating diabetics.
- Rating scales ask the same questions, the same way, at each encounter. Only the patient's answers change. The clinician obtains a reliable measure, or score, that is normal, abnormal, better, worse, or the same.
- Abnormal findings prompt the clinician to act to optimize current treatment or abandon treatment that is ineffective.
- This approach can lead to better outcomes as clinicians receive evidence in real time that their medication choices are sub-optimally performing.

Common Myth 1: Scales are copyrighted, expensive, and unwieldly

- A common myth suggests that all rating scales are copyrighted, must be purchased, are long, impair patient flow and throughput, are disliked by patient and prescriber alike, etc.
- There are expensive and copyrighted scales, but for each DSM-5 disorder there are available free, public domain scales for use. Additionally, some scales are free, and you must email the author for permission to use.
- Some scales are very short *and* very valid. They often take a few minutes for the patient to complete and several seconds for the clinician to score. This book will provide information on short, free, easy to score rating scales when possible.
- Scales can be completed via the web by the patient at home, in the waiting room at a computer kiosk, or on a tablet or phone.

Common Myth 2: Scales are time consuming

- There is a myth that scales will take too long or cost the clinician valuable time. Contrary to this, a rating scale that is completed prior to the patient's being seen costs the clinician no additional time.

- Deploying written rating scales in the waiting room is "low tech" but does create a work flow routine in the outpatient office setting.
- For example: when a clinician is finished seeing a patient (prior to writing their progress note), he or she can walk to the waiting room and hand out the paper version of the rating scale to the next patient. After the first session, patients rarely need reorientation or explanation on how to complete them. The clinician can return to his or her office and in the time it takes to type a progress note, the patient completes his or her scale. The clinician can gather the patient from the waiting area and calculate the score while walking the patient back to the office to start the session.
- Alternatively, an assistant could be trained to hand out and score the scales. Rating scale scores can be tracked in almost any chart similar to tracking blood pressures. Often they can be graphed out by electronic record systems.
- The rating scale can ask many questions quickly and allows the clinician to avoid asking symptomatic DSM questions where the patient has already acknowledged NO to experiencing the symptom and to focus on key symptoms that were responded to as YES.
- This often allows a faster, more focused psychopharmacologic follow-up session. It allows more time for the prescriber to conduct a lethality assessment, engage in safety planning, or use those core psychotherapy techniques, as less time was actually spent determining that several symptoms were resolved and essentially did not need to be addressed.
- Therefore, efficient, simplistic deployment of rating scales in psychopharmacology practice should be equated to vital sign testing and be done as routinely as possible. A short, free, easy to administer and score scale should be selected and worked into the work flow of the clinical practice.

Benefits of using rating scales

- The benefits include better patient outcomes, greater remission rates, and in practice allow more efficient and effective use of time for rapport and compliance building, informed consent, lethality assessment, and improved documentation.

Treatment Guidelines

For the novice prescriber who attempts to treat an adult with ADHD, it is essential to know the basics of the available guidelines which help provide a high level of care. Next, a prescriber must know what psychotropics are specifically approved for adult ADHD. This is the medico-legally sound way to prescribe and ideally obtain the outcomes desired for the patient. It is important to disclose to the patient that the approach being used is approved by the FDA (U.S. Food and Drug Administration). The prescriber and patient can find some reassurance knowing that at least two or more large-scale clinical trials exist where the drug was able to outperform a placebo and have a distinct safety profile. Imparting this information is the basis for informed consent and helps increase patient acceptance of the medication. A higher level technique discussed in the next section for the more *Advanced Prescriber* would be to explain the biological basis of ADHD and how the prescribed medication functions to lower ADHD symptoms. This is similar to the way a primary care clinician explains high blood sugars and insulin receptor insensitivity to a diabetic patient so that they can understand their illness and why taking insulin will help. It provides a story the patient can understand and assigns a tangible reason to why the medicine must ultimately be taken. These approaches induce patient confidence in the medication and the prescriber. Compliance rates, the ability to tolerate side effects, and perception of the prescriber's competence and thoroughness all should increase as well. These are the qualities of care that make for better outcomes.

After an accurate DSM-5 diagnosis is established, the prescriber should choose from one of the FDA approved adult ADHD indicated medications that are available. (**See Prescribing Table.**) Generally, the slow-release, once-daily products are chosen over divided dose immediate-release ones. Once a day use improves compliance and theoretically lowers addiction risk. Generally, the slower an addictive drug is absorbed, the more consistent its blood levels over time, and the more gradually it is metabolized. This allows for a gradual clinical effect and minimal intoxicating effects. The patient should feel less of an energy/mood boost at onset which lessens its reward and addictive potential. Stimulant medications are considered first line as they work more often and more completely in the average adult ADHD patient. These drugs should be considered second or third line in patients with addiction histories, cardiac histories, or anorexia histories as stimulants can create addiction, arrhythmia, and weight loss. Furthermore, adolescents and young adults have a greater likelihood of abusing these medications, and also may divert or share these drugs with peers. The clinician must weigh the superior effectiveness and available evidence-base supporting the use of stimulants as initial treatment versus using a less effective but less addictive product.

Table 1.2 Prescribing Table for ADHD Medications

Drugs listed in **BOLD** are approved agents for Adult ADHD. Dosing is based upon clinical application. Approved dosing guidelines should be further referenced by the prescriber.						
1. Stimulants						
Brand	Generic	Indication (Bold for FDA Indication)	Drug Mechanism	Dosing Tips	Monitoring Tips	Medicolegal Tips
Amphetamine Stimulant Products (Slow Release)						
Adderall XR	**d/l-mixed amphetamine extended release**	• **ADHD**	• **Both amphetamine and methylphenidate stimulants block dopamine and norepinephrine neuronal reuptake** • **Amphetamine class differs from methylphenidate class in that it blocks and then reverses dopamine reuptake pumps causing greater amounts of dopamine release** • **Amphetamines may release dopamine from nerve terminals via VMAT2 transport**	• **Usual dosing is 5–60mg/day** • **Increase by 5–10mg every week** • **Lasts several hours**	• **Common side effects include anxiety, insomnia, weight loss, nausea, palpitations, dry mouth, or diaphoresis** • **Serious side effects include psychosis, seizures, hypertension, activation of (hypo) mania and suicidal ideation, addiction, hypertension, and cardiovascular events** • **Monitor vital signs and consider urine drug screening**	• **Stimulants carry classic warnings of drug dependency and in younger adults activation of suicidal ideation** • **Avoid stimulants in those with cardiac structural abnormalities, arrhythmia, history of myocardial infarction**
Vyvanse	**lisdexamfetamine**	• **ADHD** • **BED (Binge Eating Disorder)**	• **Same as above**	• **Usual dosing is 10–70mg/day** • **Increase by 10–20mg every week** • **Lasts more than several hours**	• **Same as above**	• **Same as above**

(Continued)

Table 1.2 (Continued)

Amphetamine Stimulant Products (Immediate Release)						
Dexedrine/ Dextrostat	d-amphetamine	• ADHD • Narcolepsy	• Same as above	• Usual dosing is 5–60mg/day • Increase by 5mg every week • Lasts a few hours	• Same as above	• Same as above
Adderall	d/l-mixed amphetamine	• ADHD • Narcolepsy	• Same as above	• Usual dosing is 5–60mg/day • Increase by 5mg every week • Lasts few hours	• Same as above	• Same as above
Methylphenidate Stimulant Products (Slow Release)						
Concerta	**methylphenidate OROS extended release**	• **ADHD** • **Narcolepsy**	• **Same as above**	• **Usual dosing is 18–72mg/day** • **Up to 12 hours of duration** • **Increase by 18mg every week**	• **Same as above**	• **Same as above**
Focalin XR	**d-methylphenidate extended release**	• **Same as above**	• **Same as above**	• **Usual dosing is 5–40mg/day** • **Increase by 10mg every week** • **Lasts several hours**	• **Same as above**	• **Same as above**
Metadate ER/ CD, Ritalin SR/LA	methylphenidate	• Same as above	• Same as above	• Usual dosing is 10–60mg/day • Increase by 10mg every week • Lasts a few to several hours	• Same as above	• Same as above

Daytrana Patch	methylphenidate transdermal patch	• Same as above	• Same as above	• Initial 10mg patch applied for 9 hours; increase by 5mg/9 hours every week; maximum dose is 30mg/9 hours • Apply patch 2 hours prior to when effect is needed and wear for 9 hours • Lasts several hours	• Same as above except watch for skin irritation	• Same as above
Quillivant Liquid/Chews	methylphenidate liquid	• Same as above	• Same as above	• Usual dosing is 10–60mg/day • Increase by 5–10mg every week • Lasts several hours	• Same as above	• Same as above
Methylphenidate Stimulant Products (Immediate Release)						
Methylin tabs/liquid/chewable	Methylphenidate	• Same as above	• Same as above	• Dosing is 5–30mg twice daily • Increase by 10mg every week • Lasts few hours	• Same as above	• Same as above
Ritalin	Methylphenidate	• Same as above	• Same as above	• Same as above • Lasts few hours	• Same as above	• Same as above
Focalin	**d-methylphenidate**	• **Same as above**	• **Same as above**	• **Dosing is 2.5–10 twice daily** • **Increase by 2.5–5mg every week** • **Lasts few hours**	• **Same as above**	• **Same as above**

(Continued)

Table 1.2 (Continued)

2. Non-stimulant Products

Brand	Generic	Indication (Bold for FDA Approved)	Drug Mechanism	Dosing Tips	Monitoring Tips	Medicolegal Tips
The Norepinephrine Reuptake Inhibitors						
Strattera	**Atomoxetine**	• **ADHD**	• **Not a stimulant and works through norepinephrine reuptake inhibition** • **This usually takes longer to achieve therapeutic effect**	• **Usual dose is 40–100mg/day in adults** • **Increase to 80mg/day after 1 week** • **Increase to 100mg/day (maximum daily dose) if no effect prior** • **Should be maintained on dose for 2–4 weeks or even longer to observe a more gradual onset of efficacy over time**	• **Common side effects include sedation and nausea** • **Less common side effects include dry mouth, headache, palpitations, blood pressure increase, tremor, insomnia** • **Monitor vital signs**	• **Benefit of this medication is no clear long-term, end-organ, or addiction side effects** • **Use caution with patients with cardiovascular disease and hypertension** • **Lower dose in p4502D6 deficient patients**
Wellbutrin, SR/XL/ Aplenzin	Bupropion	• MDD • Seasonal affective disorder • Smoking cessation • ADHD (off-label)	• Norepinephrine and dopamine reuptake inhibitor (NDRI)	• Usual dose is 200–450mg/day in divided doses for SR & 150–450mg/day in single dose for XL • For SR titrate up to target dose from standard starting dose of 100mg twice daily • Increase to 150mg twice daily after 4 days and wait for 4 weeks before increasing dose to 400mg/d maximum • For XL titrate up to target dose from standard starting dose of 150mg once daily • Increase to 300mg once daily as early as 4 days and wait for 4 weeks before increasing to maximum daily dose of	• Common initial side effects include dry mouth, insomnia, headache, anxiety • Serious side effects include rare seizures, (hypo)mania, and increased suicidal ideation	• *Inform risk of rare seizures, (hypo)mania, and increased suicidal ideation* • *Do not use if history of seizures or eating disorder*

Norpramin, Pamelor, Vivactil	Desipramine, Nortriptyline, Protriptyline	• Depression • ADHD (off-label)	• All are older TCA antidepressants with prominent norepinephrine reuptake inhibitor properties	• Desipramine: usual dose is 50–200mg/day • Titrate up to target dose from standard starting dose of 25mg at bedtime and increase by 25mg every 3-7 days • Nortriptyline: usual dose is 25–150mg/day • Titrate up to target dose from standard starting dose of 25mg at bedtime and increase by 25mg every 3–7 days to maximum daily dose of 150mg/day • Protriptyline: usual dose is 5mg three times daily • Increase dose as needed to maximum daily dose of 60mg/day • Most TCA have measurable blood levels and should be titrated to within the therapeutic range	• Common side effects include anticholinergic side effects (sedation, dry mouth, weight gain, constipation, blurred vision), and nausea, anxiety, insomnia • Serious side effects include activation of (hypo)mania, suicidal ideation, cardiac conduction anomalies • Monitor EKGs through blood levels, weight, and BMI	• Do NOT use in suicidal patients as overdose can be fatal due to cardiac arrhythmia • Side effect burden quite high compared to other treatments • Should use lower doses in those who are p4502D6 deficient

(*Continued*)

Table 1.2 (Continued)

Brand	Generic	Indication (Bold for FDA Approved)	Drug Mechanism	Dosing Tips	Monitoring Tips	Medicolegal Tips
Savella/ Fetzima	Milnacipran/ Levomilnacipran	• Fibromyalgia (for milnacipran only) • Depression (for levomilnacipran only) • ADHD (off-label)	• Norepinephrine and serotonin reuptake inhibitor (SNRI)	• Milnacipran: usual dose is 12.5–100mg twice daily. Generally it is started as a low morning dose only • Titrate up to target dose from standard starting dose of 12.5mg once daily; increase to 25mg/day in 2 divided doses on day 2; increase to 50mg/day in 2 divided dose on day 4; increase to 100mg/day in 2 divided doses on day 7; maximum daily dose is 200mg/day • Levomilnacipran: usual dose is 20–120mg once daily • Titrate up to target dose from standard starting dose of 20mg once daily for 2 days; increase to 40mg/day then increase by 40mg every 2-3 days	• Common side effects include nausea, sweating, urinary hesitancy, anxiety, insomnia, palpitations • Serious side effects include induction of (hypo)mania and suicidal ideation, hypertension • Monitor for vital signs, especially blood pressure	• Caution with patients who have poorly controlled hypertension • Lower dose in those who are p4503A4 deficient

Seroquel XR	Quetiapine	• Schizophrenia • Acute mania • Bipolar maintenance • Bipolar depression • Depression • ADHD (off-label)	• Blocks dopamine-2 receptors leading to stabilization of psychosis and affective instability • Blocks serotonin-2A receptors improving cognitive and affective symptoms • Norepinephrine reuptake inhibitor may help ADHD	• Usual dose is 400–800mg/day for schizophrenia and bipolar mania and 300–600mg/day for bipolar depression • Titrate up to target dose from standard starting dose of 25mg at nighttime; increase by 25–50mg daily; maximum daily dose is 800mg/day	• Common side effects include dizziness, sedation, dry mouth, orthostatic hypotension • Serious side effects include risk of cardiometabolic complication (weight gain, diabetes, and dyslipidemia), rare neuroleptic malignant syndrome, increased risk of mortality in demented elderly due to stroke, Parkinsonism, Dystonia, and tardive dyskinesia • Monitor for vital signs, abnormal movements, metabolic labs, and cell counts for agranulocytosis	• Side effect burden is high compared to other options • Must follow and document monitoring to prevent long-term serious side effects

(Continued)

Table 1.2 (Continued)

The Alpha-2 Noradrenergic Receptor Agonists						
Tenex/ Intuniv	Guanfacine/ guanfacine extended release	• Hypertension • ADHD (children)	• Stimulates central action of alpha-2A norepinephrine receptors in the prefrontal cortex leading to enhanced cognition and attention through glutamate facilitation	• Usual dose is 1–3mg/day for immediate release and 1–4mg/day for extended release • Immediate release: titrate up to target dose from standard starting dose of 1mg/day at bedtime; increase to 2mg/ day after 3–4 weeks • Extended release: titrate up to target dose from standard starting dose of 1mg/d; increase by 1mg per week; maximum daily dose is 4mg	• Common side effects include sedation and hypotension • Serious side effects include sinus bradycardia and hypotension	• Relatively safe medication with no abuse potential • *Taper upon cessation*
Catapres/ Catapres-TTS/Kapvay	Clonidine/ extended releases/ transdermal patch	• Hypertension • ADHD (only for Kapvay)	• Same as above	• Usual dose is 0.1–2.4mg/d in divided doses • Oral: titrate up to target dose from standard starting dose of 0.1mg at bedtime; increase by 0.1mg per week up to maximum dose of 2.4mg/day • Slow release (Kapvay) is approved to 0.4mg/day in children	• Common side effects include dry mouth, dizziness • Serious side effects include sinus bradycardia, AV block, and rare withdrawal hypertensive crisis • Monitor vital signs	• Abrupt discontinuation may lead to rare hypertensive crisis, encephalopathy, stroke, and death • Taper over 2–4 days or longer to avoid rebound in blood pressure

3. Wakefulness Promoting Agents

Brand	Generic	Indication (Bold for FDA Approved)	Drug Mechanism	Dosing Tips	Monitoring Tips	Medicolegal Tips
Wakefulness Promoting Agents						
Provigil	Modafinil	• Hypersomnia in narcolepsy, shiftwork sleep disorder, and obstructive sleep apnea • ADHD (off-label)	• Unknown but different from amphetamine or methylphenidate products • Requires presence of functional dopamine transporter (DAT) but unclear if DA reuptake inhibition occurs • Activates norepinephrine receptors • Increases orexin and histamine activity both of which are known to improve wakefulness and alertness in the frontal cortex	• Usual dose is 50–400mg/day in the morning • Titrate up or down to target dose from standard starting dose of 100mg/day	• Common initial side effects include headache, hyperarousal, insomnia, anxiety, nausea, tremors • Serious side effects include rare activation of (hypo)mania, psychosis, Stevens-Johnson syndrome reported in children, and addiction • Monitor vital signs, skin rashes, and for addiction. This is a class IV drug compared to the Class II stimulants	• Consider urine drug screens • May be less addictive than true stimulants • Very good evidence base for ADHD use but less robust effects (may be better for inattentive symptoms) • CYP3A4 inducer may lower effectiveness of birth control and other medications
Nuvigil	Armodafinil	• Same as modafinil	• Same as modafinil • Armodafinil is a longer duration right hand isomer of modafinil	• Usual dose is 50–250mg/day • Titrate up or down to target dose from standard starting dose of 50mg/day • Like modafinil, higher dose is better than lower dose for excessive sleepiness and lower dose is better for ADHD and fatigue	• Similar to modafinil, though less CYP3A4 activity	• Same as above, though has less ADHD evidence base

TIP: Psychopharmacology

- Initiate all at the lowest possible dose (even lower than FDA suggested).
- Full prescribing information is readily available electronically and in print from a myriad of resources.
- Stimulants allow for therapeutic effects within a single dose that can be measured over a few days. The dose may be systematically titrated upward every several days until ADHD symptoms resolve or side effects occur.
- The maximum dose of each stimulant should be used for an appropriate duration before drug treatment can be deemed a failure.
- During upward titration, if side effects occur, the dose can be lowered and titration slowed.
- Atomoxetine is not a stimulant and works through norepinephrine reuptake inhibition. This process takes longer to deliver a therapeutic effect.
- For the first few days, start with a low dose, then increase for effectiveness. This is a general strategy for all psychotropic use.
- The patient should be maintained on dose for 2–4 weeks, or even longer, to observe for gradual onset of efficacy over time.
- Regarding medication switch protocols, an abrupt switch occurs when drug 1 is stopped and drug 2 is started the next day. This may allow for withdrawal side effects of drug 1 and acute onset side effects of drug 2 to occur simultaneously.
- Alternatively, a true cross-titration occurs when drug 1 is lowered equally while drug 2 is raised equally. This generally is the standard when switching psychotropics as it lends toward better tolerability. However, when using stimulants, given their short half-lives, an abrupt switch may be considered.

Summary

Basic levels of ADHD management suggest:

- Screen first and routinely for ADHD.
- Make an accurate diagnosis using DSM-5 or a rating scale.
- If ADHD is the sole diagnosis and there is minimal comorbidity, start a stimulant.
- Monitor by rechecking DSM-5 symptoms at each visit or use a rating scale.
- Titrate medication until there is full symptom remission or side effects.
- If a methylphenidate product fails, use an amphetamine product.

- If there is an addiction risk, or psychiatric or medical comorbidity risk to stimulant use, atomoxetine should be used.
- Other ADHD treatments are not FDA approved but may help. Items listed in **BOLD** in the **PRESCRIBING TABLE** are approved and considered front line due to clear efficacy and safety data. Items in regular text may be riskier or less well-proven by current data.

SECTION 2 Advanced Prescribing Practices

Introduction

In Section 1, the premise was to convince the reader that they must make an accurate diagnosis and pick an approved agent with well-defined dosing guidelines and expected clinical outcomes. This approach is largely one of pattern recognition and ideally becomes a stimulus-response phenomenon for the prescriber. Essentially, one has to make a diagnosis and reflexively choose from a well-defined, limited set of approved medications. The therapeutic approach regardless of diagnosis would be to: (1) identify the pattern of apparent phenotypic symptoms, (2) choose from a finite list of available, proven effective drugs, (3) start dosing low and escalate through an approved dosing range, (4) assess for effectiveness, and (5) continue medication if effective and cross-titrate to a new drug if ineffective or not tolerated. This methodical and mathematical approach can improve the standard of care and, ideally, patient outcomes when treated by the novice psychopharmacologist. This approach should be used for any assumed DSM-5 psychiatric disorder.

Section 2 is designed to provide a greater depth of neuroscience and pharmacodynamic knowledge to the reader. The basis for this is two-fold. First, understanding the way a drug works may help the prescriber choose among a variety of drugs that regulatory bodies consider completely equal in their ability to treat adult ADHD. Second, understanding the science of the psychiatric symptoms at hand can increase prescriber self-confidence which, in turn, can increase the patient's perception of the prescriber's knowledge, competence, and thoroughness. These qualities are known to improve placebo effects, lower nocebo (placebo induced side effects) effects, and improve medication adherence and visit compliance. This neuroscientific approach turns the clinician into a teacher who uses supportive and psychoeducational therapeutic techniques to build a partnering relationship with the patient.

Explaining to patients the possible etiology of their symptoms and how drugs work mechanistically to improve their brain neurochemistry or neuroanatomical function lends a value to the care the prescriber provides and allows the patient to develop a story they can internalize regarding why the medicine needs to be taken consistently. For example, simply telling the patient that your interview indicated ADHD, that the FDA says to take a stimulant, prescribing the stimulant, and sending them home is a minimal level of education and informed consent. In research trials, this is commonly found when providers emphasize the details of illness and treatment over establishing patient rapport. In research trials, this is common where there is less patient rapport built and more attention is paid to the facts of the illness and its treatment. Often nocebo effects may increase as a result. Building rapport together with discussing the disease and its treatment using a systematic teaching model may lower nocebo effects and improve compliance.

TIP: Clinical Practice

- Spending a few more minutes to explain the neurobiology of ADHD and mechanism of medications may be helpful in building patient confidence, trust, and rapport.
- This clinical approach can be applied to any psychiatric disorder.

Taking the extra time with the patient allows physicians to explain that ADHD often involves underfunctioning brain areas with low dopamine activity which stimulants can restore to proper activity. This should remove inattention symptoms and supply additional context and meaning regarding WHY the medication should be taken. It is one thing to tell a patient the FDA says to use a stimulant and something more meaningful to explain why the drug most likely works to improve the patient's symptoms. This imparting of factual regulatory knowledge paired with a theoretical explanation, or story, makes the clinician a de facto teacher and educator. This approach helps develop an alliance with the patient. This becomes a partnership of exploring different medications that are available and understanding what is approved and how the available choices differ. This also makes clear the link between the illness and the treatment. This multi-level informed consent process creates a partnership that is patient-centered, improving rapport, compliance, and likely outcomes. Research indicates that prescribers who communicate well and are definitive in explaining an illness and its treatment will increase patient satisfaction overall. This actually has a greater effect than patient-doctor partnership and decision making when it comes to patient perception of their prescriber. In short, the benefits of making the effort to explain the details of disease and its approved treatments, adding a little background neuroscience education, may go a long way in improving the doctor-patient relationship, your patient's willingness to take a medication, and acceptance of mild side effects, all of which should allow for outcomes in keeping with those noted in research trials where patients stay on the right dose of drug for the right duration. Being a dedicated teacher of your patients makes the clinician an effective model of providing informed consent, improving compliance, and achieving patient satisfaction.

Section 2 is written for prescribers who are knowledgeable and competent in those skills outlined in Section 1 (initial diagnosis and prescribing). Section 2 is also more academic, as it will describe epidemiology, genetic findings, and neuroanatomic evidence that are suited for those with a greater interest in understanding the basis of psychiatric disorder development. It is also written for those clinicians treating patients who fail to respond to first level treatments (treatment resistance). This means that the adult ADHD patient has failed to respond to stimulant monotherapy and also an approved non-stimulant (atomoxetine) monotherapy. Off-label prescribing will be discussed here. Section 2 will also teach more about ADHD psychopharmacology when treatment is complicated by patients who suffer from comorbid conditions.

Finally, this section will address appropriate combinations and augmentations of medications which are usually reserved for those patients who have failed basic pharmacological approaches. A *combination* occurs when a prescriber adds one approved ADHD medication to a second approved ADHD medication in the hope of gaining additive effects and further reducing ADHD symptoms when monotherapy has failed. An *augmentation* occurs when a non-approved, or off-label, medication is added to an approved ADHD medication that failed to allow a full remission of symptoms. Off-label prescribing is not *experimental, nor illegal.* These medications are often approved for other medical disorders (hypertension, sleep apnea, etc.) and have efficacy and safety data available in the literature for these indicated conditions, but are repurposed for use in adult ADHD. Augmentations have a wide variety of data available in the evidence base. In Section 2, the drugs reviewed are recognized as having at least a moderate amount of effectiveness and safety data to support their use in adult ADHD, have solid neuroscience and pharmacodynamic theory to support their use, and are thought to be commonly deployed in clinical practice and considered within the standard of care in treating adults with ADHD. It can also be documented that there may be evidence to support this practice. Off-label prescribing is valid and often necessary to get patients better. It is also imperative to document in your medical chart why you are choosing to go this route clinically (ex. approved treatments have failed and that the rationale to use a combination or augmentation is warranted due to the ADHD's resistance to treatment).

TIP: Clinical Practice

- Off-label prescribing is not experimental. It is a valid and necessary treatment strategy to get certain patients better.
- This practice is generally applied to patients with more treatment resistant symptoms.
- Clinicians should be ready to justify its use for the condition being treated.

Epidemiology

- ADHD is often thought to be a childhood disorder but clearly carries through into adulthood with a 4.4% prevalence rate.
- Comparatively, that makes adult ADHD more common than schizophrenia and bipolar disorder, but less common than major depressive disorder (MDD).

Genetics

- Heritability within ADHD families has been found to be 60–90%, in twin studies 80%, and there is a 5- to 10-fold risk if a parent or sibling has ADHD.
- Dopamine-4 receptor genes (DRD4) and dopamine transporter (reuptake pump) genes (DAT1) appear to be the most consistent abnormal findings. Further dopamine and norepinephrine receptor and transporter gene abnormalities are noted as well.
- It should be made clear that there is no single gene that causes ADHD. More likely, many genes code for several central nervous system (CNS) proteins that when mutated create a subtle risk for the development of certain ADHD symptoms, i.e., inattention vs. impulsivity. As genetic risks build, more brain neurocircuitry malfunction occurs and more phenotypic, externally noticeable symptoms may develop.
- Theoretically, a patient inherits genes from both parents: *a **genotype.*** If a gene is mutated, it often yields an abnormal protein.
- These proteins might be enzymes, receptors, ion channels, etc. If enough of these function improperly in the brain, it may cause hyperfunctioning or hypofunctioning within or between certain brain areas that may be able to be detected with neuroimaging: *an **endophenotype.***
- This alteration in brain neurocircuitry function may lead to specific psychiatric symptoms (inattention, poor concentration, and loss of vigilance) that can be detected by interviewing. These outward symptoms that the DSM-5 is based upon are considered the patient's ***phenotype.***
- This concept can be applied to all DSM-5 psychiatric disorders.

Neuroanatomy

- Some patients with ADHD will have an endophenotype notable on fMRI (brain functional) images where their anterior cingulate cortices (ACC) and dorsolateral prefrontal cortices (DLPFC) are underactive and accessory areas (insular cortices) may be overactive.
- This would suggest that certain ADHD patients are under-utilizing the brain areas designed specifically for alertness, attention, and vigilance, and over-utilizing less efficient and improper areas of the brain in order to pay attention to tasks at hand.
- Use of stimulant medication has also been shown to normalize or partially reverse these brain abnormality findings.
- The mark of a good biological psychiatric intervention ideally would be to detect an abnormal genotype, endophenotype, and phenotype through genetic testing, functional neuroimaging, and clinical interviewing and then prescribe a treatment that can change the endophenotype and phenotype despite the genetic precursors remaining the same.

Neuroscientific Background and Rationale for Medication Use

In treating ADHD, there are four families of medications that are most often utilized (**See Prescribing Table**):

1) Stimulants

MECHANISM OF ACTION

Methylphenidate (Ritalin, Concerta, Metadate, Focalin), amphetamines (Adderall, Vyvanse)

- Both methylphenidate and amphetamine based stimulants block the dopamine transporter (DAT). This increases dopamine available for neuronal firing which improves vigilance, alertness, and motivation.
- Both methylphenidate and amphetamine based stimulants block the norepinephrine transporter (NET). This increases norepinephrine available for increased alertness.
- Amphetamines differ from methylphenidate in that they block and then reverse the DAT function which can result in greater amounts of dopamine to be available for neuronal firing.
- Amphetamines may also affect the vesicular monoamine transport system (VMAT2) causing vesicles to release excess dopamine into the synapse as well.

2) Wakefulness Promoting Agents

MECHANISM OF ACTION

Modafinil (Provigil), armodafinil (Nuvigil)

- No clear chemical relation to amphetamines or methylphenidate products.
- They do require that functioning DATs exist but it is unclear if DA reuptake inhibition is a major factor.
- These drugs may actually activate norepinephrine receptors.
- These drugs may increase orexin activity and histamine activity, both of which are known to improve wakefulness and alertness by stimulating fronto-cortical areas of the brain.
- These drugs are approved in the treatment of narcolepsy, sleep apnea, and shiftwork sleep disorder.
- They may be used off-label in ADHD if there is greater risk of cardiovascular compromise or addiction history.

3) The Norepinephrine Reuptake Inhibitors (NRIs)

MECHANISM OF ACTION

Atomoxetine (Strattera) and antidepressants

- These increase norepinephrine available in the frontal cortex contributing to enhanced alertness.
- Examples include atomoxetine, off-label tricyclic (TCA) antidepressants, SNRI antidepressants, an NDRI antidepressant, and the antipsychotic quetiapine.
- Atomoxetine is the only FDA approved medication for ADHD in this class. (See Section 1.) The list of drugs that follow also possess norepinephrine reuptake inhibition (NRI) properties and also block NETs to ideally improve concentration.
- TCAs that are primarily NRI may help ADHD (desipramine [Norpramin], nortriptyline [Pamelor], protriptyline [Vivactil]) and could be considered especially with comorbid major depressive disorder [MDD]).
- SNRIs (venlafaxine [Effexor XR], desvenlafaxine [Pristiq], duloxetine [Cymbalta], levomilnacipran [Fetzima/Savella]) should be considered with comorbid major depressive disorder (MDD), anxiety disorders, fibromyalgia, and neuropathic pain.
- NDRI (bupropion [Wellbutrin/Aplenzin]) should be considered with comorbid seasonal depressive disorders and for smoking cessation.

- Quetiapine (Seroquel XR) should be considered with comorbid schizophrenia or bipolar disorder.
- These are all non-addicting and often considered safer for use in adult patients who are more likely to have comorbid psychiatric conditions.

4) The Alpha-2 Receptor Agonists

MECHANISM OF ACTION

Clonidine (Catapres), guanfacine (Tenex)

- These stimulate alpha-2 receptors residing on glutamate neurons in the frontal cortex leading to improved alertness and focus.
- Overall lowers NE tone while enhancing glutamatergic efficacy.
- May be beneficial for insomnia, anxiety, and hyperarousal as sedation is a side effect.
- These are all non-addicting and often considered safer for use in adult patients who are more likely to have comorbid psychiatric conditions.
- These agents may lower activating (anxiety, insomnia) side effects if combined with initial stimulant use.
- Sometimes combining medications further lowers symptoms while trying to achieve remission.
- Sometimes combining medications lowers side effect burden as side effects may cancel each other out.

Advanced Practical Applications to Consider

Good and Bad Polypharmacy

DO

- Start low dose to minimize side effects.
- Escalate dosing within full range for optimal effectiveness.
- Consider using non-addictive medications first despite less effectiveness or less evidence base to avoid diversion and addiction.
- Monitor for weight loss, abuse, vital sign elevation.
- Add alpha-2 agonist antihypertensives to stimulants for more treatment resistant cases or to combat stimulant side effects of hypertension, hyperarousal, anxiety, or insomnia.
- These may also be added to antidepressant NRI type medications.

DON'T

- Add two stimulants together.
- Unless . . . it is okay to add a low dose, immediate-release stimulant to a slow-release stimulant if there is a loss of effect later in the day or if a boost in effect is needed late in the day for studying, focusing on the job, etc.
- Add two NRIs together.
- Add two alpha-2 agonist antihypertensives together.
- Use stimulants in those who are highly anxious or have remarkable insomnia.
- Use stimulant or wakefulness agents in those who are at cardiovascular risk.
- Use stimulant or wakefulness agents in those who are at risk for addiction or suffer from borderline personality where affective dyscontrol is common.

Good Polypharmacy for Comorbid Patients

ADHD + Major Depressive Disorder

- Use of NDRI: bupropion (Wellbutrin XL) monotherapy.
- Use of SNRI: venlafaxine XR, duloxetine, desvenlafaxine, levomilnacipran monotherapy.
- Use norepinephrine based TCA: desipramine, nortriptyline, protriptyline
- Use MAOI: selegiline transdermal patch (actually has amphetamine derivatives) (EMSAM).
- Use second-generation antipsychotic (SGA) augmentation: aripiprazole (Abilify), brexpiprazole (Rexulti), cariprazine (Vraylar) as all have partial dopamine receptor 2/3 (agonism), quetiapine (Seroquel) XR (has potent NRI).
- For all of the above, increasing dopamine or noradrenergic tone may lower symptoms from both disorders.

ADHD + Anxiety Disorder

- Use of SNRI: venlafaxine XR, duloxetine, desvenlafaxine monotherapy.
- Use serotonergic based TCA: imipramine (Tofranil), amitriptyline (elavil), clomipramine (Anafranil) as all have serotonin reuptake inhibition initially and also have norepinephrine reuptake inhibiting metabolites secondarily.

- Use alpha-2 agonists: guanfacine (Tenex), clonidine (Catapres) as they often dampen agitation.
- Most of these increase norepinephrine which may help both disorders and help lower the non-ADHD symptoms.
- Avoid benzodiazepines (BZ) as they may create cognitive side effects increasing inattention and fatigue.

ADHD + Bipolar Disorder

- Use second-generation antipsychotic (SGA) augmentation: aripiprazole (Abilify), cariprazine (Vraylar), quetiapine (Seroquel XR).
- These agents may increase dopamine or norepinephrine to help ADHD and depression but also dampen dopamine to avoid mania.
- Interestingly, the stimulants likely carry less risk of inducing mania or mixed features when compared to antidepressants.

ADHD + Schizophrenia

- Use second-generation antipsychotic (SGA) augmentation: aripiprazole (Abilify), cariprazine (Vraylar), brexpiprazole (Rexulti), quetiapine (Seroquel XR).
- These agents may increase dopamine or norepinephrine to help ADHD and depression but also dampen dopamine to avoid psychosis.

ADHD + Substance Abuse

- Use alpha-2 agonists: guanfacine, clonidine (as non-addictive).
- Use atomoxetine ([Strattera] NRI [as non-addictive] or bupropion [Wellbutrin/Aplenzin] [NDRI]).
- These may be used to treat ADHD and avoid substance use.

ADHD + Borderline Personality

- Use second-generation antipsychotic (SGA) augmentation: similar to those listed for bipolar disorder or schizophrenia.

In conclusion, when faced with patients who are more straightforward and solely have ADHD, it makes sense to follow well-known guidelines and use approved and indicated treatments. Usually, this starts with long acting stimulant medications. As treatment resistance to the stimulants mounts or if the patient has relative comorbidities that make stimulants more risky, the off-label medications and rational polypharmacy approaches become even more warranted in hopes of gaining symptom remission. Sometimes, side effects must be managed by altering doses, titration schedules, or, frankly, by adding other medications to combat the side effects while maintaining remission.

Bibliography

American Psychiatric Association. (2013) *Diagnostic and Statistical Manual of Mental Disorders: DSM-5*. Washington, D.C.: American Psychiatric Association.

Balint, J., & Shelton, W. (1996) "Regaining the initiative: forging a new model of the patient-physician relationship." *JAMA* 275(11), 887–891.

Colloca, L., & Miller, F. G. (2011) "The nocebo effect and its relevance for clinical practice." *Psychosomatic Medicine* 73(7), 598.

del Campo, N., Müller, U., & Sahakian, B. J. (2012) "Neural and behavioral endophenotypes in ADHD." In C. S. Carter and J. W. Dalley (eds.). *Brain Imaging in Behavioral Neuroscience*. Berlin: Springer-Verlag Berlin Heidelberg, 65–91.

Heisler, M., et al. (2002) "The relative importance of physician communication, participatory decision making, and patient understanding in diabetes self-management." *Journal of General Internal Medicine* 17(4), 243–252.

Kessler, R. C., et al. (2006) "The prevalence and correlates of adult ADHD in the United States: results from the National Comorbidity Survey Replication." *The American Journal of Psychiatry* 163(4), 716–723.

Kooij, S. J., et al. (2010) "European consensus statement on diagnosis and treatment of adult ADHD: The European Network Adult ADHD." *BMC Psychiatry* 10(1), 1.

Little, P., et al. (2001) "Observational study of effect of patient centredness and positive approach on outcomes of general practice consultations." *The BMJ* 32, 908–911.

Rajagopal, S. (2006) "The placebo effect." *Psychiatric Bulletin* 30(5), 185–188.

Reas, D. L., & Grilo, C M. (2014) "Current and emerging drug treatments for binge eating disorder." *Expert Opinion on Emerging Drugs* 19(1), 99–142.

Stahl, S. M. (2003) "Deconstructing psychiatric disorders, part 1: genotypes, symptom phenotypes, and endophenotypes." *Journal of Clinical Psychiatry* 64(9), 982–983.

Stahl, S. M. (2003) "Deconstructing psychiatric disorders, part 2: an emerging, neurobiologically based therapeutic strategy for the modern psychopharmacologist." *Journal of Clinical Psychiatry* 64(10), 1145–1152.

Stahl, S. M. (2013) *Stahl's Essential Psychopharmacology: Neuroscientific Basis and Practical Applications*. Cambridge, UK: Cambridge University Press.

Theis, S. L., & Johnson, J. H. (1995) "Strategies for teaching patients: a meta-analysis." *Clinical Nurse Specialist* 9(2), 100–105.

Vermeire, E., et al. (2001) "Patient adherence to treatment: three decades of research: a comprehensive review." *Journal of Clinical Pharmacy and Therapeutics* 26(5), 331–342.

Wilens, T. E., et al. (2001) "A controlled clinical trial of bupropion for attention deficit hyperactivity disorder in adults." *American Journal of Psychiatry* 158(2), 282–288.

Zimmerman, M. (2013) *Interview Guide for Evaluating DSM-5 Psychiatric Disorders and the Mental Status Examination*. East Greenwich, RI: Psych Products Press.

CHAPTER 2

Anxiety Disorders: Panic, Social, Obsessive-Compulsive, Generalized, and Post-Traumatic Anxiety

SECTION 1 Basic Prescribing Practices

Essential Concepts

- Anxiety is a generic term and may be considered a normal reaction to stress.
- Pathologic anxiety is abnormal and occurs when symptoms are in great excess or out of proportion to the stressor OR when it interferes with psychosocial functioning.
- There are five major anxiety disorders:
  - Generalized anxiety disorder (GAD) is excessive, unremitting, diffuse, multifocal worrying.
  - Social anxiety disorder (SAD) is characterized by an intense, phobic fear about being the center of attention or being scrutinized.
  - Panic disorder (PD) is the acute experience of hyperautonomic and psychological distress symptoms without clear triggering events on a repeated basis.
  - Post-traumatic stress disorder (PTSD) occurs after a person is traumatized, and, despite being safe, continues to have disruptive recollections, phobic avoidance, emotional changes, and hyperarousal.
  - Obsessive-compulsive disorder (OCD) occurs when people experience intrusive thoughts or images and have compelling urges to repeat behaviors in order to feel less anxious.
- Comorbid major depressive disorder (MDD) and substance use disorder (SUD) are common as patients tend to self-medicate.
- Patients who suffer from personality disorder have maladaptive coping skills and often experience excesses of anxiety.
- Psychotherapy, pharmacotherapy, or their combination—psychopharmacopsychotherapy (PPPT)—are warranted.

Phenomenology, Diagnosis, and Clinical Interviewing

For any new practitioner in any field, the goal is to be able to make an accurate diagnosis. All of psychiatric prescribing at this beginning level is based on regulatory findings, approvals, and indications that are psychiatric disorder specific. Psychotropics will only deliver the outcomes promised if the patient actually has been accurately identified as having a bona fide DSM-5 anxiety disorder. The reader should appreciate the commonalities of the genetic heritability and brain functional abnormalities that appear to be common across the DSM-5 anxiety disorders and should also understand there may be significant symptom overlap. For example, most anxiety disorders have a physical component (agitation, insomnia, etc.) and a mental component (worry, avoidance, etc.). The key is in the details of the symptom (phenotypic) presentation and, frankly, in the *laundry list effect* provided by the DSM-5 system. Particular attention to details leads to better diagnosis, treatment selection, and outcome. In other words, it is important to be precise in order to most accurately determine the type of anxiety experienced by the patient in front of you. Some comfort may also rest, on the contrary, that even if the clinician misses the diagnosis, providing a serotonergic treatment is likely to help to some degree! As this chapter progresses into intermediate and advanced psychopharmacologic prescribing, it is vital to appreciate that certain psychiatric symptoms can cross the barriers of categorical diagnostic and regulatory processes. Understanding and appreciating this concept encourages the use of off-label approaches in the more treatment resistant or comorbidly afflicted patient. In fact, anxiety disorder in adults is confounded by other psychiatric conditions, such as the existence of a second anxiety disorder, substance misuse, depression, bipolarity, or personality disorder.

Proper diagnosis is often confounded as patients present often initially with MDD or SUD. In these situations, the anxiety disorder creates enough social distress (loss of work, family, finances, etc.) that MDD or SUD ensues secondarily. When MDD is detected, good clinicians should always screen for anxiety disorders as well. Alternatively, MDD may generate anxiety symptoms. Many MDD patients are generally anxious, ruminate, or even obsess. There is often psychomotor agitation as well. A clinical convention exists where if the anxiety disorder was premorbid to the depressive disorder, then the patient carries two diagnoses: a depressive one and an anxious one. If the MDD is premorbid and the anxiety only occurs while depressed, then the patient just carries the single MDD diagnosis and all anxiety falls under the rubric of the patient having *psychomotor agitation*. Finally, if a patient carries both an anxiety disorder and MDD simultaneously, failure to gain remission in one disorder creates greater likelihood of recurrence in the other. Therefore, both must be treated aggressively and simultaneously.

TIP: Screening Questions

Screening for GAD

- Do you worry? Do you worry nonstop, all day, all the time more often than not? Do you find it hard to control the worry, feel tense, restless, or have insomnia?

Screening for SAD

- Do you fear being the center of attention or being scrutinized where you feel you will be totally embarrassed all the time? Do you avoid life events due to this?

Screening for PD

- Do you have panic attacks where you get sweaty, shaky, or jittery with palpitations for no apparent reason?

Screening for PTSD

- Have you been in a traumatic event such as a mugging, assault, car crash, tornado, etc. where even though you were safe, months later you still had nightmares or flashbacks about it?

Screening for OCD

- Do you have repetitive thoughts that are difficult/horrible and impossible to dismiss? Do you have repetitive behaviors like hand washing, checking things, etc. that you feel you cannot stop doing?

DSM-5 Diagnosis

People with GAD experience persistent, hard to control, multi-focal worries more often than not. These worries are in excess to what the average person might experience or perceive. These worries are accompanied by physical and mental anxiety symptoms. More formal diagnosis is as follows:

Generalized Anxiety Disorder

A. Excessive anxiety and worry (apprehensive expectation) occurring more days than not for at least six months about a number of events or activities.
B. Difficulty controlling the worry.

C. Anxiety and worry are associated with three (or more) of the following six symptoms (with at least some symptoms having been present for more days than not for the past six months):
   - Restlessness or feeling keyed up or on edge
   - Being easily fatigued
   - Difficulty concentrating or mind going blank
   - Irritability
   - Muscle tension
   - Sleep disturbance (difficulty falling or staying asleep or restless, unsatisfying sleep)

D. The anxiety, worry, or physical symptoms cause clinically significant distress or impairment in social, occupational, or other important areas of functioning.*

E. The disturbance is not attributable to the physiological effects of a substance (e.g., a drug of abuse, a medication) or another medical condition (e.g., hyperthyroidism).*

F. The disturbance is not better explained by another mental disorder.*

***NOTE: These final psychosocial distress and comorbidity criteria are uniform throughout the DSM-5.**

People with SAD experience an acute level of distress upon experiencing real or perceived negative attention from others. This may be specific performance anxiety (giving a speech or presentation) or more generalized (speaking to peers, going on a date, ordering food, walking to the office or in a mall). These patients become challenged by anxiety in social situations or when anticipating an upcoming social event. They are not anxious in other areas or situations. This anxiety is in excess to what the average person might experience or perceive, may be accompanied by physical symptoms, including panic attacks, that are triggered and expected to result from exposure to social situation. DSM-5 diagnosis is as follows:

Social Anxiety Disorder

A. A persistent fear of one or more social or performance situations in which the person is exposed to unfamiliar people or to possible scrutiny by others. The individual fears that he or she will act in a way (or show anxiety symptoms) that will be embarrassing and humiliating.

B. Exposure to the feared situation almost invariably provokes anxiety, which may take the form of a situationally bound or situationally predisposed panic attack.

C. The person recognizes that this fear is unreasonable or excessive.

D. The feared social situations are avoided or else are endured with intense anxiety and distress.

People with PD, by definition, do not experience generalized worrying, nor are they solely triggered into panic attacks by social situations or reminders of traumatic events (PTSD). Instead they experience abrupt, intense physical anxiety without a clear trigger. The hallmark is recurrent and unexpected panic attacks. Over time, patients will associate panic attacks with certain locations (shopping malls, work, classrooms, etc.) and will begin avoiding these places (agoraphobia) due to the apprehension and expectation that these places will cause panic attacks again. When asking about the first few panic attacks, clinicians often find no rhyme or reason for why the attacks started. Attacks are in excess to what the average person might experience in a similar setting. They are often accompanied by psychological symptoms (fear of death/dying, losing control, avoidance, etc.). DSM-5 diagnosis is as follows:

Panic Disorder

A. Recurrent unexpected panic attacks. A panic attack is an abrupt surge of intense fear or intense discomfort that reaches a peak within minutes, and during which time four (or more) of the following symptoms occur:
   - Palpitations, pounding heart, or accelerated heart rate
   - Sweating
   - Trembling or shaking
   - Sense of shortness of breath or smothering
   - Feeling of choking
   - Chest pain or discomfort
   - Nausea or abdominal distress
   - Feeling dizzy, unsteady, lightheaded, or faint
   - Derealization or depersonalization (feeling detached from oneself)
   - Fear of losing control or going crazy
   - Fear of dying
   - Numbness or tingling sensations
   - Chills or hot flashes

B. At least one of the attacks has been followed by one month (or more) of one or both of the following:
   1. Persistent concern or worry about additional panic attacks or their consequences (e.g., losing control, having a heart attack, "going crazy").
   2. A significant maladaptive change in behavior related to the attacks (e.g., behaviors designed to avoid having panic attacks, such as avoidance of exercise or unfamiliar situations).

During a panic episode, patients may have the urge to flee or escape and have a sense of impending doom, as though they are dying from a heart attack or suffocation. Furthermore, with the full development of PD these episodes are compounded by the anticipatory fear of reoccurrence with resultant behavioral changes (avoidance and agoraphobia) and worry about the implications or consequences of these attacks (losing control, "going crazy," dying).

People with PTSD have experienced a trauma in person or vicariously. Traumas may include accidents, assaults, combat, job exposure, natural disasters, etc. Hearing about or seeing a trauma remotely (receiving a phone call about the death of a loved one, etc.) may instigate the onset of PTSD, particularly (but not necessarily) if the patient suffers an extreme panic attack response at the time. PTSD patients can have panic attacks, but they are triggered only by cues that remind them of their specific trauma. Patients will experience reliving events (nightmares, flashbacks, etc.), avoid remembering or cues of the event, may experience emotional change (depression, irritability, etc.), feel tense, be insomnic, and become easily startled as key clinical symptom clusters. DSM-5 diagnosis is as follows:

Post-Traumatic Stress Disorder

A. **Traumatic events (one or more required)**

Trauma survivors must have been exposed to actual or threatened:

- Death
- Serious injury
- Sexual violence

The exposure can be:

- Direct
- Witnessed
- Indirect, by hearing of a relative or close friend who has experienced the event—indirectly experienced death must be accidental or violent
- Repeated or extreme indirect exposure to traumatic events, usually by professionals in the line of duty or work

B. **Intrusion or re-experiencing (one required)**
- Intrusive thoughts or memories
- Nightmares related to the traumatic event
- Flashbacks or dissociative events, feeling like the event is happening again
- Psychological and physical reactivity/distress to reminders of the traumatic event, such as an anniversary or environmental cues

C. **Avoidant symptoms (one required)**
- Avoiding thoughts or feelings connected to the traumatic event
- Avoiding people or situations connected to the traumatic event

D. **Negative alterations in mood or cognitions (two required)**
- Memory problems and inability to remember key parts of the trauma
- Negative thoughts or beliefs about one's self or the world
- Distorted sense of blame for one's self or others related to the event
- Being stuck in severe emotions related to the trauma (e.g., horror, shame, sadness)
- Severely reduced interest in pre-trauma activities
- Feeling detached, isolated, or disconnected from other people

E. **Increased arousal symptoms (two required)**
- Difficulty concentrating
- Irritability, increased temper or anger
- Difficulty falling or staying asleep
- Hypervigilance
- Being easily startled

People with OCD experience very specific and recurrent intrusive/distressing images or thoughts (seeing themselves killing other people, hurting their own children, thoughts that harm will befall themselves or a loved one, etc.) and/or experience repetitive behaviors that they cannot stop themselves from re-enacting (hand washing, checking locks, counting numbers or events, etc.). These thoughts and behaviors are inappropriate, or in excess to, what the average person might experience in a more fleeting and situation-specific manner. These repetitions take an inordinate amount of time and often significantly interfere with a patient's life psychosocially speaking. DSM-5 diagnosis is as follows:

Obsessive-Compulsive Disorder

A. Presence of obsessions, compulsions, or both:
- Obsessions are defined by (1) and (2):
  1. Recurrent and persistent thoughts, urges, or impulses that are experienced at some time during the disturbance as intrusive and unwanted, and that in most individuals cause marked anxiety or distress.
  2. The individual attempts to ignore or suppress such thoughts, urges, or images, or to neutralize them with some other thought or action (i.e., by performing a compulsion).
- Compulsions are defined by (1) and (2):
  1. Repetitive behaviors (e.g., hand washing, ordering, checking) or mental acts (e.g., praying, counting, repeating words

silently) that the individual feels driven to perform in response to an obsession or according to rules that must be applied rigidly.

2. The behaviors or mental acts are aimed at preventing or reducing anxiety or distress, or preventing some dreaded event or situation; however, these behaviors or mental acts are not connected in a realistic way with what they are designed to neutralize or prevent, or are clearly excessive.

B. The obsessions or compulsions are time-consuming (e.g., take more than one hour per day) or cause clinically significant distress or impairment in social, occupational, or other important areas of functioning.

Rating Scales

Generalized Anxiety Disorder-7 (GAD-7)

- This scale was adapted and validated using a DSM-based GAD symptom checklist structure. It is public domain and offered free of charge, and it is short and easy for patients to complete in office-based settings.
- A positive score of 10 or greater is indicative of moderate anxiety-driven distress and specifically may indicate GAD.
- Positive scores may also help to detect other anxiety disorders due to symptom overlap.
- It can be found online at: www.phqscreeners.com/pdfs/03_GAD-7/English.pdf.

Table 2.1 The GAD-7 Scale for Generalized Anxiety Disorder

GAD-7				
Over the last two weeks, how often have you been bothered by the following problems? (Use "✓" to indicate your answer)	**Not at all**	**Several days**	**More than half the days**	**Nearly every day**
1. Feeling nervous, anxious, or on edge	0	1	2	3
2. Not being able to stop or control worrying	0	1	2	3
3. Worrying too much about different things	0	1	2	3
4. Trouble relaxing	0	1	2	3
5. Being so restless that it is hard to sit still	0	1	2	3
6. Becoming easily annoyed or irritable	0	1	2	3
7. Feeling afraid as if something awful might happen	0	1	2	3
(For office coding: Total Score T__ = __+__+__)				

Social Anxiety Questionnaire for Adults (SAQ)

- This scale was adapted and validated using a DSM-based SAD symptom checklist structure. It is easily obtainable online, is free for use in clinical practice if it is not modified or changed, and is easy for patients to complete in office-based settings.
- A positive score of 89 for men or 98 for women is indicative of SAD.
- To obtain this scale, please refer to: http://www.midss.org/content/social-anxiety-questionnaire-adults-saq-a30.
- Copyright by Fundacion VECA. Reprinted with permission Caballo, V. E., Salazar, I. C., Arias, B., Irurtia, M. J., Calderero, M., and the CISO-A Research Team Spain. (2010) "Validation of the Social Anxiety Questionnaire for Adults (SAQ-A30) with Spanish university students: Similarities and differences among degree subjects and regions." *Behavioral Psychology/Psicologia Conductual* 18, 5–34.

Table 2.2 The Social Anxiety Questionnaire for Use in Adults with Social Anxiety Disorder

Social Anxiety Questionnaire for Adults (SAQ-A30)
(Caballo, Salazar, Inaria, Arias, and CISO-A Research Team, 2010)

Below are a series of social situations that may or may not cause you UNEASE, STRESS, or NERVOUSNESS. Please place and "X" on the number next to each social situation that best reflects your reaction where "1" represents no unease, stress, or nervousness and "5" represents very high or extreme unease, stress, or nervousness.

If you have never experienced the situation described, please **imagine** what your level of UNEASE, STRESS, or NERVOUSNESS might be if you were in that situation and rate how you imagine you would feel by placing an "X" on the corresponding number.

Please rate all items and do so **honestly**. Do not worry about your answer because there are no right or wrong ones. Thank you very much for your collaboration.

Level of Unease, Stress, or Nervousness

Not at all or very slight 1	Slight 2	Moderate 3	High 4	Very or extremely high 5

1. Greeting someone and being ignored	1	2	3	4	5
2. Having to ask a neighbor to stop making noise	1	2	3	4	5
3. Speaking in public	1	2	3	4	5
4. Asking someone attractive of the opposite sex for a date	1	2	3	4	5
5. Complaining to the waiter about my food	1	2	3	4	5
6. Feeling watched by people of the opposite sex	1	2	3	4	5
7. Participating in a meeting with people in authority	1	2	3	4	5
8. Talking to someone who isn't paying attention to what I am saying	1	2	3	4	5
9. Refusing when asked to do something I don't like doing	1	2	3	4	5

(*Continued*)

Table 2.2 (Continued)

10. Making new friends	1	2	3	4	5
11. Telling someone that they have hurt your feelings	1	2	3	4	5
12. Having to speak in class, at work, or in a meeting	1	2	3	4	5
13. Maintaining a conversation with someone I've just met	1	2	3	4	5
14. Expressing my annoyance to someone that is picking on me	1	2	3	4	5
15. Greeting each person at a social meeting when I don't know most of them	1	2	3	4	5
16. Being teased in public	1	2	3	4	5
17. Talking to people I don't know at a party or a meeting	1	2	3	4	5
18. Being asked a question in class by the teacher or by a superior in a meeting	1	2	3	4	5
19. Looking into the eyes of someone I have just met while they are talking	1	2	3	4	5
20. Being asked out by the person I am attracted to	1	2	3	4	5
21. Making a mistake in front of other people	1	2	3	4	5
22. Attending a social event where I know only one person	1	2	3	4	5
23. Starting a conversation with someone of the opposite sex that I like	1	2	3	4	5
24. Being reprimanded about something I have done wrong	1	2	3	4	5
25. While having dinner with colleagues, classmates, or workmates, being asked to speak on behalf of the entire group	1	2	3	4	5
26. Telling someone that their behavior bothers me and asking them to stop	1	2	3	4	5
27. Asking someone I find attractive to dance	1	2	3	4	5
28. Being criticized	1	2	3	4	5
29. Talking to a superior or a person in authority	1	2	3	4	5
30. Telling someone I am attracted to that I would like to get to know them better	1	2	3	4	5

Severity Measure for Panic Disorder

- The American Psychiatric Association developed this scale specifically for use with DSM-5 panic disorder criteria. It is an experimental measure in the public domain and free for use without permission.
- Scoring currently is not established as to a definitive cut off for diagnosing PD, but this scale is effective to aid in diagnosis and clearly can track treatment response.
- It can be found via Internet search engine for "Severity Measure for Panic Disorder" in PDF form to download or at https://www.psychiatry.org/psychiatrists/practice/dsm/dsm-5/online-assessment-measures.

Table 2.3 The Severity Measure for Panic Disorder for Use in Adults with Panic Disorder

Instructions: The following questions ask about thoughts, feelings, and behaviors about panic attacks. A panic attack is an episode of intense fear that sometimes comes out of the blue (for no apparent reason). The symptoms of a panic attack include a racing heart, shortness of breath, dizziness, sweating, and fear of losing control or dying. **Please respond to each item by marking (✓ or x) one box per row.**							
							Clinician Use
	During the **PAST 7 DAYS** I have…	Never	Occasionally	Half of the time	Most of the time	All of the time	Item score
1.	felt moments of sudden terror, fear, or fright, sometimes out of the blue (i.e., a panic attack)	☐ 0	☐ 1	☐ 2	☐ 3	☐ 4	
2.	felt anxious, worried, or nervous about having more panic attacks	☐ 0	☐ 1	☐ 2	☐ 3	☐ 4	
3.	had thoughts of losing control, dying, going crazy, or other bad things happening because of panic attacks	☐ 0	☐ 1	☐ 2	☐ 3	☐ 4	
4.	felt a racing heart, sweaty, trouble breathing, faint, or shaky	☐ 0	☐ 1	☐ 2	☐ 3	☐ 4	
5.	felt tense muscles, felt on edge or restless, or had trouble relaxing or trouble sleeping	☐ 0	☐ 1	☐ 2	☐ 3	☐ 4	
6.	avoided, or did not approach or enter, situations in which panic attacks might occur	☐ 0	☐ 1	☐ 2	☐ 3	☐ 4	
7.	left situations early, or participated only minimally, because of panic attacks	☐ 0	☐ 1	☐ 2	☐ 3	☐ 4	
8.	spent a lot of time preparing for, or procrastinating (putting off), situations in which panic attacks might occur	☐ 0	☐ 1	☐ 2	☐ 3	☐ 4	
9.	distracted myself to avoid thinking about panic attacks	☐ 0	☐ 1	☐ 2	☐ 3	☐ 4	
10.	needed help to cope with panic attacks (e.g., alcohol or medication, superstitious objects, other people)	☐ 0	☐ 1	☐ 2	☐ 3	☐ 4	
						Total/Partial Raw Score:	
						Prorated Total Raw Score (If 1–2 items left unanswered):	
						Average Total Score:	

PTSD Civilian Checklist (PCL-5)

- This scale was adapted and validated using DSM-5 specific language and was created by the U.S. Veterans Administration. It can be downloaded for free.
- It is 20 items and easy for patients to complete in office-based settings.
- A positive score of 38 or greater is indicative of PTSD.
- To obtain this scale, please refer to www.ptsd.va.gov/professional/assessment/adult-sr/ptsd-checklist.asp.

Table 2.4 The PTSD Civilian Checklist for Patients with Post-Traumatic Stress Disorder

PCL-5

Instructions: Below is a list of problems that people sometimes have in response to a very stressful experience. Please read each problem carefully and then circle one of the numbers to the right to indicate how much you have been bothered by that problem **in the past month**.

In the past month, how much were you bothered by:	Not at all	A little bit	Moderately	Quite a bit	Extremely
1. Repeated, disturbing, and unwanted memories of the stressful experience?	0	1	2	3	4
2. Repeated, disturbing dreams of the experience?	0	1	2	3	4
3. Suddenly feeling or acting as if the stressful experience were actually happening again (as if you were actually back there reliving it)?	0	1	2	3	4
4. Feeling very upset when something reminded you of the stressful experience?	0	1	2	3	4
5. Having strong physical reactions when something reminded you of the stressful experience (for example, heart pounding, trouble breathing, sweating)?	0	1	2	3	4
6. Avoiding memories, thoughts, or feelings related to the stressful experience?	0	1	2	3	4
7. Avoiding external reminders of the stressful experience (for example, people, places, conversations, activities, objects, or situations)?	0	1	2	3	4
8. Trouble remembering important parts of the stressful experience?	0	1	2	3	4

9. Having strong negative beliefs about yourself, other people, or the world (for example, having thoughts such as: I am bad, there is something seriously wrong with me, no one can be trusted, the world is completely dangerous)?	0	1	2	3	4
10. Blaming yourself or someone else for the stressful experience or what happened after it?	0	1	2	3	4
11. Having strong negative feelings such as fear, horror, anger, guilt, or shame?	0	1	2	3	4
12. Loss of interest in activities you used to enjoy?	0	1	2	3	4
13. Feeling distant or cut off from other people?	0	1	2	3	4
14. Trouble experiencing positive feelings (for example, being unable to feel happiness or having loving feelings for people close to you)?	0	1	2	3	4
15. Irritable behavior, angry outbursts, or acting aggressively?	0	1	2	3	4
16. Taking too many risks or doing things that could cause you harm?	0	1	2	3	4
17. Being "super-alert" or watchful or on guard?	0	1	2	3	4
18. Feeling jumpy or easily startled?	0	1	2	3	4
19. Having difficulty concentrating?	0	1	2	3	4
20. Trouble falling or staying asleep?	0	1	2	3	4

Obsessive-Compulsive Inventory (OCI-R)

- This scale was adapted and validated using DSM specific language for OCD. It can be obtained with permission by contacting the author.
- It is 18 items and easy for patients to complete in office-based settings.
- A score of 21 or greater is indicative of OCD.
- To obtain this scale via permission, please refer to: http://www.caleblack.com/psy5960_files/OCI-R.pdf.
- See Table 2.5 on the next page.

Treatment Guidelines

For the novice prescriber who attempts to treat an adult with anxiety, it is essential to know the basics of the available guidelines which help provide a high level of care. Next, a prescriber must know what psychotropics are specifically approved for each anxiety disorder. This is the medico-legally sound way to prescribe and

Table 2.5 The Obsessive-Compulsive Inventory for Patients with Obsessive-Compulsive Disorder

The following statements refer to experiences that many people have in their everyday lives. Circle the number that best describes **HOW MUCH** that experience has **DISTRESSED** or **BOTHERED** you during the **PAST MONTH**. The numbers refer to the following verbal labels:

0 Not at all	1 A little	2 Moderately	3 A lot	4 Extremely

1.	I have saved up so many things that they get in the way.	0	1	2	3	4
2.	I check things more often than necessary.	0	1	2	3	4
3.	I get upset if objects are not arranged properly.	0	1	2	3	4
4.	I feel compelled to count while I am doing things.	0	1	2	3	4
5.	I find it difficult to touch an object when I know it has been touched by strangers or certain people.	0	1	2	3	4
6.	I find it difficult to control my own thoughts.	0	1	2	3	4
7.	I collect things I don't need.	0	1	2	3	4
8.	I repeatedly check doors, windows, drawers, etc.	0	1	2	3	4
9.	I get upset if others change the way I have arranged things.	0	1	2	3	4
10.	I feel I have to repeat certain numbers.	0	1	2	3	4
11.	I sometimes have to wash or clean myself simply because I feel contaminated.	0	1	2	3	4
12.	I am upset by unpleasant thoughts that come into my mind against my will.	0	1	2	3	4
13.	I avoid throwing things away because I am afraid I might need them later.	0	1	2	3	4
14.	I repeatedly check gas and water taps and light switches after turning them off.	0	1	2	3	4
15.	I need things to be arranged a particular way.	0	1	2	3	4
16.	I feel that there are good and bad numbers.	0	1	2	3	4
17.	I wash my hands more often and longer than necessary.	0	1	2	3	4
18.	I frequently get nasty thoughts and have difficulty getting rid of them.	0	1	2	3	4

ideally obtain the outcomes desired for the patient. It is important to disclose to the patient that the approach being used is approved by the FDA (U.S. Food and Drug Administration).

Each DSM-5 anxiety disorder will have essentially the same approach to guideline-based treatment. The safer serotonergic drugs (selective serotonin reuptake inhibitors (SSRIs), such as fluoxetine (Prozac), sertraline (Zoloft), paroxetine (Paxil), citalopram (Celexa), escitalopram (Lexapro), and fluvoxamine (Luvox), are always preferred as a first intervention. Next, serotonin-norepinephrine reuptake inhibitors (SNRIs), such as venlafaxine (Effexor XR), duloxetine (Cymbalta) may be used. Next, the clinician must weigh using a benzodiazepine (BZ) sedative-anxiolytic (alprazolam [Xanax], clonazepam [Klonopin], diazepam [Valium], etc.) with their significant addiction and psychomotor impairment risks versus use of a tricyclic antidepressant (TCA) or even a monoamine oxidase inhibitor (MAOI) antidepressant. These latter two classes do not carry an addiction risk but have greater cardiac, overdose, drug, and dietary interaction concerns. It is in these later subtle yet pivotal decision-making areas that nuances among the anxiety disorder guidelines arise.

TIP: Guidelines

- Establish therapeutic alliance.
- Perform psychiatric history.
- Rule out medical and other causes.
- Educate and inform patient about diagnosis and treatment options.
- Coordinate care with providers.
- Enhance treatment compliance.
- Monitor for response, remission, and future relapse.
- Use successive, maximally dosed monotherapies for substantial durations when possible.
- Choose among psychotherapy, SSRI, or an SNRI as initial treatment.

Note: The first 7 items apply to every psychiatric disorder.

After making an accurate diagnosis, a clinician should ideally choose an FDA approved initial treatment. Below are summaries of the FDA approved medications for each anxiety disorder. For further details, the reader is referred to the quick reference **Prescribing Table**.

TIP: GAD Approved Medications

Serotonin (5HT)-1a Receptor Partial Agonist:

Buspirone (BuSpar)

SSRIs:

Escitalopram (Lexapro)
Paroxetine (Paxil and Paxil CR)

SNRIs:

Duloxetine (Cymbalta)
Venlafaxine XR (Effexor XR)

TIP: GAD Prescribing

- Clinicians will often start with buspirone (BuSpar) as it typically has the least side effect burden. It is only approved to treat GAD, so this approach becomes less effective and appropriate as a first line treatment if the patient is concurrently depressed or suffers from another anxiety disorder.
- Alternatively, an SSRI is generally started at a very low dose for a few days and then titrated to the approved minimum therapeutic dose. After a few weeks if there is full remission, the drug is continued for several months and then a slow discontinuation may be considered.
- If the GAD is more severe, recurrent, or refractory in nature, the SSRI may be continued longer term.
- If the patient does not respond to the initial low therapeutic dose, increase to the middle of the dose range for another few weeks of treatment. If this fails, the full dose should be used for several weeks and, if no remission is obtained, then the drug can be considered a therapeutic failure.
- This strategy of initial very low dose, low therapeutic dose, moderate therapeutic dose, high therapeutic dose can often be used with most psychotropics and will be suggested throughout this book.
- A therapeutic trial implies the patient has received a middle to high dose of the drug for several weeks. Failing to use the full dose range and failing to use the drug for a sufficient time period often leads to treatment failure, partial response, or symptom relapse.
- If buspirone and an SSRI fail to fully treat the patient to GAD remission, then an SNRI is the next option in most situations.
- Again, these should be dosed and titrated similar to the SSRI approach noted above. The progression of aggressive monotherapy dosing and then a transition, if needed, from SSRI to SNRI is the standard of care for GAD, PTSD, and SAD.
- Failure of all of the above agents to remit a patient's GAD triggers a critical decision to combine drugs or switch to a monotherapy with greater risk and side effect burden. Section 2 of this chapter covers these more advanced approaches.

TIP: SAD Approved Medications

SSRIs:

Paroxetine (Paxil, Paxil CR)
Sertraline (Zoloft)

SNRIs:

Venlafaxine XR (Effexor XR)

TIP: SAD Prescribing

- The treatment guideline for SAD is similar to GAD except that buspirone is not an option due to lack of supportive evidence.
- Additionally, benzodiazepine (BZ) anxiolytics could be considered as second line options for GAD, SAD, and PD but carry the risk of addiction, respiratory suppression, psychomotor impairment, and increased risk for falls and serious injury.
- BZ do not carry risk of gastrointestinal upset, sexual dysfunction, weight gain, or insomnia or iatrogenic anxiety. They have a clear and unique profile compared to the SSRI and SNRI.

TIP: PD Approved Medications

SSRIs:

Paroxetine (Paxil, Paxil CR)
Sertraline (Zoloft)
Fluoxetine (Prozac)

SNRIs:

Venlafaxine XR (Effexor XR)

TIP: PD Prescribing

- The progression of SSRI to SNRI to possible BZ use is similar to that noted above for GAD and SAD.
- Failure of all of the above agents to remit a patient's PD triggers a critical decision whether to combine drugs or switch to a monotherapy associated with greater risk and side effect burden. These more advanced approaches are covered in Section 2.

TIP: PTSD Approved Medications

SSRIs:

Paroxetine (Paxil, Paxil CR)
Sertraline (Zoloft)

TIP: PTSD Prescribing

- PTSD approaches differ from the previous anxiety disorders in that only the SSRIs are approved. SNRIs are not approved and are poorly studied.
- BZ are generally contraindicated as up to 50% of PTSD patients are abusing controlled substances at the time of initial PTSD diagnosis. This makes BZ a riskier choice.
- Cognitive-behavioral therapy (CBT) is a good treatment for any anxiety disorder, but even more so for PTSD given the lack of approved medications.

TIP: OCD Approved Medications

SSRIs:

Fluoxetine (Prozac)
Fluvoxamine (Luvox, Luvox CR)
Paroxetine (Paxil, Paxil CR)
Sertraline (Zoloft)

TCAs:

Clomipramine (Anafranil)

TIP: OCD Prescribing

- Clinicians will often start with an SSRI and try all agents in succession instead of leaving the SSRI class after one or two treatment failures.
- OCD is commonly considered more difficult to treat, often requiring higher dosing for longer durations. It is not unusual for prescribers to use the highest doses and wait several weeks to a few months for effectiveness to gradually occur. A usual full titration trial of an SSRI for other anxiety disorders may take 10–12 weeks. For OCD, this may take 16 weeks or more.
- After a few weeks if there is full remission, the drug is continued for at least several months, but given the severity and tendency for OCD to recur, initial treatment may need to be continued for years.
- If the SSRIs fail to fully treat the OCD patient to remission, then the prescriber needs to make a decision whether to combine drugs or switch to a monotherapy that is associated with greater risk and side effect burden. Section 2 of this chapter covers these more advanced topics.
- Clomipramine, for example, is the tricyclic antidepressant (TCA) drug of choice after multiple SSRI failures.
- BZ are typically not effective for OCD and typically not used.

SECTION 2 Advanced Prescribing Practices

Introduction

In Section 1, the premise was to convince the reader that they must make an accurate diagnosis and pick an approved agent with well-defined dosing guidelines and expected clinical outcomes. This approach is largely one of pattern recognition: (1) identify the pattern of phenotypic symptoms, (2) choose from a finite list of available, proven effective drugs, (3) start dosing low and escalate through an approved dosing range, (4) assess for effectiveness, and (5) continue medication if effective or cross-titrate to a new drug if ineffective or not tolerated.

Section 2 is designed to provide a greater depth of neuroscience and pharmacodynamic knowledge to the reader. It is written for prescribers who are knowledgeable and competent in those skills outlined in Section 1. It is also written for those clinicians who treat patients who fail to respond to first level treatments. The section is generally intended for those patients found to be treatment resistant.

This section will address appropriate combinations and augmentations of medications which are usually reserved for those patients who have failed more easy and typical pharmacological approaches.

TIP: On-Label Prescribing

- Figuring out which medications are approved for specific DSM-5 disorders takes effort that is essentially memorization-based.
- On-label prescribing is always the frontline treatment approach.
- Off-label prescribing is valid and often necessary to get patients better as a second or third line approach.
- In the current era of medical prescribing it is easy to find "on-label" prescribing information.
    - Oftentimes this is seen on advertising commercials, embedded in written advertisements in journals, or seen on many medical websites. Essentially, prescribers are told what disease or diagnosis the drug is approved for and exactly how the regulators wish it to be dosed for that disorder.
    - Clinicians are told exactly how effective the drug will work in the patient at hand, assuming they have the single DSM disorder without comorbidity and only suffer a moderate degree of symptomatology.
    - In regulatory trials, mildly ill patients are not admitted as it is often felt that the risk of a new drug trial is too much for those who are only suffering to a mild degree.
    - On the contrary, those with the most significant symptom burden are often excluded as they are felt to lack capacity to agree to the risks

of the experimental drug trial, or they are felt to be unable to comply with the several trial visits and to be able to follow the protocol.
  - Finally, for on-label prescribing, clinicians are given a very clear set of side effects to monitor. These may range from common, daily side effects to end-organ damaging adverse effects that sometimes require laboratory monitoring.

TIP: Off-Label Prescribing

- It is more challenging, but vital, to become knowledgeable about off-label prescribing.
- Off-label prescribing is more difficult to become educated about as there are less clear resources available to describe and delineate best practices.
- It is imperative to document in your medical chart why you are choosing to go this route.
- Salespeople from pharmaceutical companies are not allowed to discuss these practices, and pharmaceutical advertising is not allowed to present non-approved, off-label approaches even if they have been proven effective and safe in the medical literature.
- In fact, many companies have been sued and/or fined in the past for off-label marketing and promoting.
- Interestingly, some recent court findings have agreed that sharing information about off-label prescribing is legal and warranted in improving patient care.
- Regardless, off-label information is frankly harder to obtain and validate.
- To become better informed, clinicians can read many journals or subscribe to a service that updates about new findings. Alternatively, reviewing articles or textbooks may serve to update the prescriber. Attending continuing medical education events (www.neiglobal.com, www.medscape.com, www.gmeded.com) or watching them online may be a more interactive alternative.

Table 2.6 Anxiety Disorder Lifetime Prevalences

Epidemiology	
ANXIETY DISORDER LIFETIME PREVALENCES	
Any Anxiety Disorder	28.8%
SAD	12.1%
PTSD	6.8%
GAD	5.7%
PTSD	4.7%
OCD	1.6%

Genetics

- All anxiety disorders exhibit high gene and environment interaction.
- PD is one of the most heritable of the anxiety disorders (up to 40%).
  - The most common genes associated with PD include COMT, *Adenosine 2A receptor*, *CCK*, CCK Receptor B, $5HT_{2A}$ receptor, Monoamine oxidase-A.
  - Interestingly, only some of these genes are related to the monoamines (serotonin, norepinephrine, dopamine) which are the target of many of our anti-anxiety treatment options.
- PTSD has a similar heritability but requires greater gene-environment interaction (a clear trauma).
  - One of the best studied genetic findings is that patients who develop PTSD have a short gene allele for the serotonin transporter (SERT) gene called *5-HTTLRP.* Transporter is another name for reuptake pump.
  - Theoretically, patients who carry this gene have defective proteins (reuptake pumps, enzymes, etc.) which predispose them to less resiliency in the face of stress and a greater likelihood of developing PTSD following a trauma.
  - Other genes (CRF-1, FKBP5) have also been implicated as risk factors for PTSD development.
- SAD appears to have a bit less heritability (20–40%) when compared to PD and PTSD.
  - Trauma and social experience seem to have little to do with gene by environment interactions in SAD.
  - Complicating the genetic studies of SAD is the clinical association that adults with SAD often suffer premorbid behavioral inhibition in childhood, low extroversion, and high neuroticism.
  - It is possible that SAD is a variant of avoidant personality disorder (AvPD) or mild autism spectrum disorder (ASD).
  - The most often studied and associated target genes are 5-HTTLPR and CRF-1. This commonality of serotonergic and HPA dysregulation is apparent with the above PD and PTSD discussions.
- GAD also appears to have less heritability according to experts in the field. Perhaps 30% of symptom development may be attributed to genetic loading. GAD also has the least amount of literature in this area for review.
- OCD may be more heritable, with some authors suggesting a 30–50% contribution of genetics.
  - SLC1A1 is the glutamate transporter gene which has recently been implicated in early onset OCD.
  - 5-HTTLPR has been implicated similar to other anxiety disorders noted above.
  - The serotonin receptor genes 5HT-1D and 5HT-2C as well.
  - COMT and DRD4 findings have also implicated abnormality in the CNS dopamine system.

TIP: Neuroanatomy Concepts

- The frontal cortex is the more evolved/advanced brain area thought to be the top-down control center of the brain that serves to control and contain our basic drives and impulses.
- The limbic system is the more primitive brain area responsible for basic drives and impulses. The anterior cingulates and insular cortex are the highest level of processing in this system. Their role is to integrate sensory, affective, and cognitive components of pain while processing information regarding the internal bodily state. The hippocampus manages the HPA stress response and the amygdala is a threat assessment center and serves to manage the fight or flight reaction in regard to environmental cues and stimuli.
- The *Dance Analogy* (borrowed from Philip T. Ninan, MD) involves the back and forth communication of these two systems. Ideally *the Dance* goes smoothly with both partners gracefully interacting.
- In the case of normal anxiety to normal situations, or high resiliency, both systems act in concert.
- For example, when anxiety develops the cortex analyzes the threat and with mild to moderate stressors it can interrupt fight or flight limbic signals to prevent inappropriate anxiety. Conversely, if the threat is bona-fide and dangerous then a fight or flight reaction proceeds.
- When DSM-5 anxiety disorder develops, *the Dance* is going horribly wrong, where one partner is too aggressive in their moves or too clumsy. With anxiety, if the amygdala is too aggressive or hyperactive, patients may burst into panic attacks at the innocuous grocery store, their school classroom, or at home on their couch. The amygdalae see threats everywhere, triggering panic. The cortical system may be too weak to override this and top-down, executive control is lost and allows the panic to continue again and again.

TIP: Functional Neuroanatomy Concepts

Cortical top down processing

These areas help to manage or prevent anxiety:

- **Dorsolateral Prefrontal Cortex (DLPFC)**—Provides executive functioning and complex planning.
- **Ventromedial Prefrontal Cortex (VMPFC)**—Provides higher level emotional experience processing.

- **Orbitofrontal Cortex (OFC)**—Provides impulse control, response prevention.

Limbic drive processing

These areas may promote anxiety:

- **Anterior Cingulate Cortex (ACC)**—Allows vigilance, concentration, and monitoring of internal states.
- **Insular Cortex (IC)**—Allows integration of sensory information.
- **Hippocampus (HC)**—Interacts with the hypothalamic-pituitary axis (HPA), regulates the stress response, and stores visceral and protective memory for fast reflexive responses to threats.
- **Amygdala (AM)**—Allows visceral, stimulus-driven fear, aggression, defensive behavior, and fight or flight.

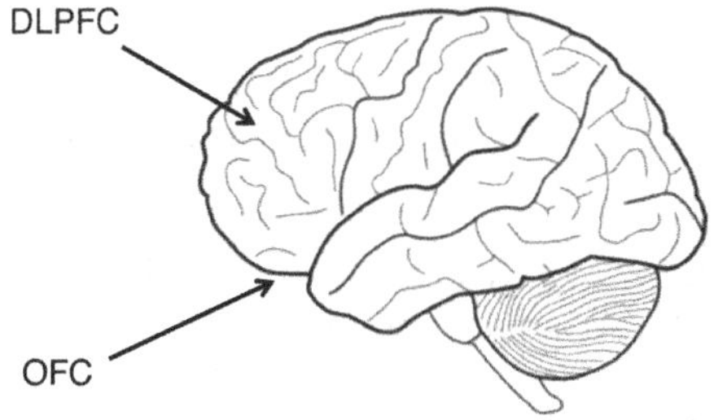

Figure 2.1a The Neuroanatomy of Anxiety

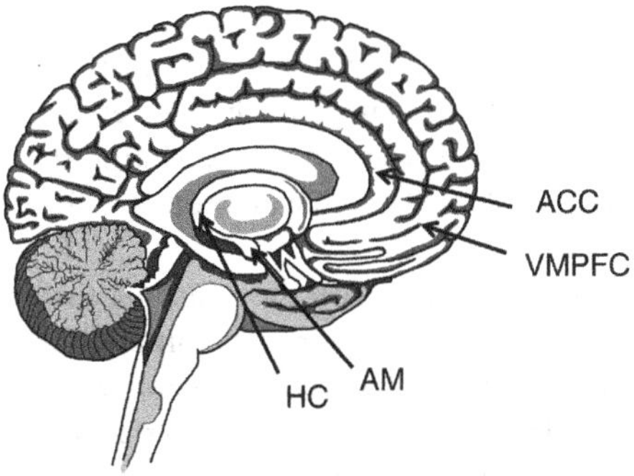

Figure 2.1b The Neuroanatomy of Anxiety

Table 2.7 Functional Neuroanatomy of Anxiety Disorder

PD	Increased activity in AM, HC, and ACC Lowered activity in DLPFC
SAD	Increased activity in AM Lowered activity in ACC and DLPFC
GAD	Increased activity in AM, ACC, and IC Increased activity in ventrolateral PFC
PTSD	Increased activity in the AM, ACC, and VMPFC
OCD	Increased activity in ACC, increased activity in OFC Lowered activity in caudate

Neuroscientific Background and Rationale for Medication Use

In treating anxiety disorder, there are ten families of medications that are often utilized. (**See Prescribing Table.**)

1) SSRIs (Selective Serotonin Reuptake Inhibitors)

MECHANISM OF ACTION

Fluoxetine (Prozac), sertraline (Zoloft), paroxetine (Paxil), citalopram (Celexa), escitalopram (Lexapro), fluvoxamine (Luvox)

- All SSRIs work by blocking serotonin reuptake pumps. This is called inhibition of the serotonin transporter (SERT). The net effect is an increase in serotonin (SR or sometimes abbreviated "5HT") availability in BOTH the frontal cortex and limbic system.
- Functionally, the SSRI increases SR activity, allowing increased neuronal firing with lessened hypervigilance and hyperarousal by ultimately calming the limbic system.
- Interestingly, the SSRI increases SR neuronal firing immediately, though these agents often take a few weeks to become effective.
- Increasing SR can create a more toxic or unusual environment for SR neurons in the brain. Each neuron likely registers this increase SR concentration as foreign and responds by activating transcription factors within said neurons. These factors will interact with neuronal DNA and create new proteins.
- Some of these proteins migrate to the neuronal surface and engulf the SR receptors. This is called downregulation and takes a few weeks to occur. This correlates to the length of time for DNA to RNA to protein synthesis (transcription and translation) to occur. It takes this length of time for a great enough volume of proteins to downregulate enough receptors to create a clinical anxiolytic effect.

- Sometimes brain or neuronal health protein genes are turned on, creating brain derived neurotrophic factor (BDNF) among others. These factors improve neuronal connectivity and allow different brain areas to communicate more effectively, thus lowering anxiety symptoms.
- This theory helps us appreciate *the Dance* between the frontal cortex and the limbic system. Improved growth factors and neuronal connectivity/integration may improve top down connectivity, allowing the cortex to limit limbic system overactivity.
- Antidepressants have been shown to downregulate SR receptors, increase BDNF, and restore atrophied brain tissue in those suffering from certain psychiatric conditions.

2) SNRIs (Serotonin-Norepinephrine Reuptake Inhibitors)

MECHANISM OF ACTION

Venlafaxine ER (Effexor XR), duloxetine (Cymbalta)

- All SNRIs work by blocking serotonin reuptake pumps just like SSRIs.
- Venlafaxine and duloxetine, even at low therapeutic doses, are as effective as the SSRI class in regard to serotonin reuptake inhibition (SRI) and treating anxiety. They essentially have the same ability as SSRIs.
- Norepinephrine reuptake inhibition (NRI) is also created by these agents. They have two mechanisms in place to treat anxiety disorder, SRI and NRI properties.
- There are three SNRIs that are approved for fibromyalgia (FM) or major depressive disorder (MDD) but not anxiety: milnacipran (Savella), levomilnacipran (Fetzima), and desvenlafaxine (Pristiq). These drugs are poorer at SRI but offer much greater NRI.
- For norepinephrine (NE), NRI is now more often called inhibition of the NE transporter (NET). The net effect of SERT and NET inhibition allows the SNRI anxiolytics to increase SR and NE availability in BOTH the frontal cortex and the limbic system.
- The frontal cortex governs higher levels of emotional processing, emotional thinking (VMPFC), anxiety response prevention (orbitofrontal cortex [OFC]), and executive functioning (dorsolateral prefrontal cortex [DLPFC]). Increased NE tone from NRI could theoretically improve cortical functioning and allow better top down control over the anxious and hyperactive limbic system, thus lowering anxiety symptoms.
- Similar to the SSRIs, SNRIs also increase SR activity in limbic structures and allow increased neuronal firing with lessened hypervigilance and hyperarousal by calming the limbic system.

- Metabolically speaking, NE can be converted to epinephrine. Both of these chemicals are thought to be arousing and to possibly make animals and humans more anxious and prone towards fight or flight reactions. If you think about a time when you were quite scared, you likely experienced dry mouth, palpitations, tremors, and hypervigilance. These symptoms are common to many of the anxiety disorders; it seems counter-intuitive to add NE to an anxious patient's brain.
- Adding any SSRI or SNRI too quickly may create iatrogenic anxiety and undermine initial treatment, which is why smart prescribers often will start SSRI or SNRI at very low doses. NRI properties are more likely to induce agitation, insomnia, and panic. Use of an SNRI can be very safe and very effective, but titration will need to be slow and monitored, and dose adjustments will be needed if anxiety is escalated at first.
- Sometimes SNRIs work better for anxiety at higher doses. As a rule, NRI activity increases for the two anxiety approved SNRIs (venlafaxine XR, duloxetine) at higher doses.
- Theoretically, a slow increase in NRI dosing will also slowly increase NE tone within the limbic system. Over time, this increased NE tone may be desensitizing, in that the limbic system has more NE *noise* and will perceive anxiety *signals* less often. This is analogous to calibrating a signal-to-noise ratio so that the brain may more accurately perceive real (truly fearful situations) versus anxious threats. If cortical function is strengthened for better control of limbic fearful activity and the limbic system is better calibrated to perceive real versus exaggerated threats, then anxiety may be better controlled through the dual reuptake blockade mechanism of the SNRI class of anxiolytics.

3) SPAs (Serotonin Partial Agonists)

MECHANISM OF ACTION

Buspirone (BuSpar)

- Buspirone is a unique anxiolytic that is neither an SSRI nor SNRI. It is only approved to treat GAD. Its ability to facilitate serotonergic systems, as with the SSRI and SNRI, lend to its ability to be a GAD monotherapy or to become one of the most commonly used augmentation strategies in those patients who are only partial responders to SSRI or SNRI monotherapy.
- Essentially, adding an SPA will further escalate the level of SR neurotransmission and theoretically lower anxiety further than monotherapy alone.

- Serotonin partial agonism (SPA), in the case of buspirone, occurs at the serotonin-1A (5HT-1A) autoreceptor found on the presynaptic ends of SR neurons. These autoreceptors (self-receptors) that slow the neuron down when bound by SR. This serves as an SR dampening system.
- As with DA (dopamine) discussed in chapter 1, the brain strives to have the correct amount of each transmitter, not too much and not too little. This homeostasis supports normal functioning. Similarly, if SR activity gets too high, side effects, mania, or serotonin syndrome might develop. If too low, depression may ensue.
- Activating 5HT-1a receptors is a routine response to normal upswings in SR activity in the brain. This is counter-intuitive to the concept that the SSRIs and SNRIs provide SRI activity which increases SR to combat anxiety symptoms. Slowing down SR activity is the opposite and should not treat anxiety at all.
- Buspirone initially *does* slow down neuronal SR firing rates but without clear deleterious effects, and only temporarily. SPA is a weak serotonin manipulation compared to the SRI property. After a few weeks of SPA, the 5HT-1a receptors bound to buspirone are tagged as abnormal and become engulfed and downregulated, thus eliminating them.
- As the SR slowing receptors disappear with the downregulation process, the SR neurons now can no longer slow/inhibit themselves and instead start to release even more serotonin. The net effect gives the SSRI or SNRI more SR to work with in the synapse, an additive amount of SR builds up in the CNS creating even greater SSRI and SNRI effects.
- 5HT-1a receptor partial agonism is the selective property of buspirone, but some other psychotropic agents possess this ability as well.
- Vilazodone (Viibryd) is an antidepressant with a weak SSRI and potent 5HT-1a pre- and post-synaptic partial agonist properties. It is approved for treating MDD, but looking at its SSRI and strong SPA profile it might also be considered as an off-label approach for those who only partially respond to an SSRI.
    - Vortioxetine (Trintellix) has similar 5HT-1a properties and is also an approved antidepressant.
    - Prescribers can choose to augment the SSRIs with buspirone or switch to vilazodone or vortioxetine as they appear to have SRI plus SPA together as a single pill.
    - Some of the second-generation antipsychotics (SGA) also possess this property and theoretically may be the more anxiolytic as such (ex. Quetiapine [Seroquel XR], aripiprazole [Abilify], brexpiprazole [Rexulti], cariprazine [Vraylar], lurasidone [Latuda]).

4) TCAs (Tricyclic Antidepressants)

MECHANISM OF ACTION

Amitriptyline (Elavil), clomipramine (Anafranil), imipramine (Tofranil)

- They share a similar mechanism with the SNRI.
- TCA, however, produce side effects that are more excessive.
- TCA can provide SRI and/or NRI properties to treat anxiety, but unfortunately also block or antagonize cholinergic muscarinic (ACHm), alpha-1 (A1), and histamine 1 (H1) receptors causing remarkable side effects when compared to SSRI, SNRI, and SPA classes of anxiolytics.

TIP: Receptor Blockade Side Effects

	Anticholinergic	**Antiadrenergic**	**Antihistaminergic**
Side Effects	Dry mouth, blurred vision, constipation, tachycardia, urinary retention	Fatigue, lightheadedness, hypotension syncope	Fatigue, somnolence, appetite and weight gain

TIP: Prescribing TCAs

- TCAs can be categorized and separated based upon the ability to provide either more or less NRI.
- In treating anxiety, it makes sense to use a TCA with greater serotonergic potential.
- Desipramine (Norpramin) and nortriptyline (Pamelor) are actually metabolites of imipramine and amitriptyline, respectively. Desipramine and nortriptyline are NRI predominant. Add protriptyline (Vivactil) as the third NE robust TCA and this makes a sub class within the TCA which are generally avoided in anxiety treatment.
- If a prescriber is looking to increase NE tone and activity in order to treat ADHD-like symptoms, improve frontal lobe functioning (change fatigue to alertness, inattention to vigilance, improve cortical control of limbic anxiety, etc.), then these may be the ideal TCAs to use.

- On the positive side, these NRI-based TCAs often have less anticholinergic, antihistaminergic, and anti-alpha adrenergic side effects.
- Imipramine, amitriptyline, clomipramine, and doxepin all start as potent SRI-based anxiolytic antidepressants and are more ideal for anxiety.
- Clomipramine is the only TCA actually approved for anxiety treatment (OCD).
- All of these agents are converted by the liver into metabolites that possess NRI properties: desipramine, nortriptyline, norclomipramine, nordoxepin.
- Many are sedating and can also provide relief for insomnia associated with the anxiety disorder.
- TCA use is limited as there is often a higher drop-out rate due to side effect burden as compared to SSRIs, SNRIs, and SPAs.
- TCAs must be given in limited doses to suicidal patients as they can induce ventricular arrhythmias and death.
- TCAs must be monitored with EKG and blood levels in most patients.
- TCAs require hepatic CYP4502D6 metabolic pathways to be cleared. The SSRIs paroxetine (Paxil) and fluoxetine (Prozac), being strong 2D6 inhibitors, may triple TCA levels and risk toxicity quickly. Citalopram (Celexa) is a moderate inhibitor and may double levels. The SSRIs with the least interaction include sertraline (Zoloft) and escitalopram (Lexpro), and the safest SNRIs are venlafaxine (effexor XR) and desvenlafaxine (Pristiq).

5) MAOIs (Monoamine Oxidase Inhibitors)

MECHANISM OF ACTION

Phenelzine (Nardil), isocarboxazid (Marplan), selegiline (EMSAM), tranylcypromine (Parnate)

- MAOIs are one of the original antidepressant treatments approved for use in major depressive disorder (MDD).
- MAOIs irreversibly inhibit rendering ineffective, monoamine oxidase A and B enzymes. These enzymes destroy serotonin, norepinephrine, and dopamine simultaneously, causing an increase in the levels of these monoamines in the central nervous system (CNS).
- MAOIs are used primarily for MDD, but MAOIs do have use in treating refractory social anxiety disorder (SAD) patients, perhaps as SAD has overlapping symptom similarity to atypical depressive states (rejection sensitivity). Sometimes MAOIs are used in the treatment of OCD as well.

TIP: Prescribing MAOIs

- See the depressive disorders chapter for greater details. MAOI agents have major *synergistic* interactions in combination with other agents that are effective at increasing serotonin in the CNS. Antidepressants with serotonin reuptake inhibition (SRI) and some theoretically with serotonin receptor modulation (i.e., 5HT-1a partial agonism) may create serotonin toxicity or syndrome. This adverse effect can be lethal as a result of hyperthermia and cardiovascular instability.
- MAOIs may have *additive* drug interactions when combined with other agents that facilitate increases in norepinephrine activity. This can cause gradual increases in blood pressure. Generally, these are not hypertensive crises, for example, adding an MAOI to an NRI (atomoxetine for ADHD, bupropion for MDD, pseudoephedrine for allergies, etc.).
- MAOI agents have a *synergistic* interaction when combined with foods that contain tyramine. In the GI tract, tyramine triggers a robust release of norepinephrine (NE) in the periphery, causing constriction of blood vessels leading to acute and extreme increases in blood pressure. This may lead to heart attack or stroke.
- Tyramine rich foods should be avoided if MAOIs are prescribed. The only exception is the use of the MAOI transdermal skin patch, selegiline (EMSAM). At the low, 6mg/day dose only, the MAOI diet needs not be adhered to.

6) BZ (Benzodiazepine Anxiolytics)

MECHANISM OF ACTION

Alprazolam (Xanax), clonazepam (Klonopin), lorazepam (Ativan)

- BZs are related to other sedatives (barbiturates, alcohol) which share similar properties: low doses may be disinhibiting, anxiety lowering, and therapeutic in several areas.
- At greater doses, psychomotor impairment, and respiratory and central nervous system suppression can occur.
- BZs are evidence-based for use in treating all anxiety disorders except for OCD and PTSD.
- BZs have specialized receptor sites on the GABA-A receptor. When a GABA neurotransmitter is bound to a GABA-A receptor (attached to a fast acting chloride channel), greater neuronal chloride influx occurs, hyperpolarizing (slows down) neurons so they are less likely to fire.

- If a BZ is bound at the same time to its site on the GABA-A receptor, even more chloride may enter the neuron as channels open more often and increase the hyperpolarization effect.
- This is called positive allosteric modulation (PAM), where a normal neuronal system's activity is amplified by the addition of a third entity (GABA + GABA-A receptor + BZ).
- Theoretically, if hyperpolarization occurs in the limbic system, then fight or flight (fear) responses can be dampened.

TIP: Prescribing BZs, Part 1

- BZ pharmacokinetics allow for clinical differences.
- First, there are "sedative-anxiolytics" and "sedative-hypnotics." The former lower anxiety and the latter induce sleep. This latter class is discussed in the insomnia chapter.
- BZs have different rates of absorption. The faster a BZ is absorbed through the GI system, the faster it can take effect. The difference could be alleviation of agitation, worry, or panic within 20 minutes versus 2 hours. The slower the absorption, the longer it takes to experience an abortive effect upon anxiety symptoms. (**See Prescribing Table.**)
- The faster the absorption, the faster the relief. The negative to this relates to the idea that faster absorption drugs can be associated with greater drug likeability and misuse. There is a greater risk of addiction.
- Generally, BZs are used on a daily basis and titrated to a dose that minimizes sedating side effects while providing for a remission of GAD, PD, or SAD symptoms.
- PRN (as needed) use may be advised when treating simple phobias or performance-based SAD if the panic is only experienced infrequently.
- For ongoing and impairing anxiety, BZs are dosed daily, using the same dose in order to achieve steady state blood plasma levels and ideally avoid experiencing any pathological anxiety at all. The concept is to treat the anxiety before it emerges and is clinically experienced rather than wait until the anxiety starts and treat after the fact with an as needed PRN dosing strategy.

TIP: Prescribing BZs, Part 2

- BZs may be divided based upon their half-life. (**See Prescribing Table.**)
- This pharmacokinetic term defines how fast a drug will be metabolized/inactivated within the patient. The number of hours it takes for a drug to lose half of its dose within the patient's blood stream is its half-life.

- Short half-life drugs can build up in the patient's system more quickly. After four to five half-life periods, the drug is said to be at a steady state and ideally optimally effective.
- At this time, side effects should be clearly identified. Dose-effectiveness can now be established as plasma levels are more steady and tend not to fluctuate as much within the patient's CNS.
- Unfortunately, short half-life drugs also leave the patient's system quickly, creating rebound effects (where greater amounts of anxiety are felt) or, frankly, BZ drug withdrawal may occur.
- Shorter half-life drugs often have to be taken a few times daily. This lowers compliance, possibly creating rebound or withdrawal effects between doses.
- Longer half-life drugs will take longer to accumulate, and effectiveness may sometimes be delayed. Side effects may emerge more gradually and well after treatment has started. If the patient develops side effects, it will take longer for these to abate as it takes the drug longer to be metabolized.
- Given the propensity for less rebound and withdrawal, the long half-life BZs could be less addicting.
- Generally, the fast absorption/short half-life drugs likely have a greater addiction potential.

TIP: Prescribing BZs, Part 3

- BZs can be divided into those that are oxidized by the liver versus those that are glucuronidized and excreted by the kidneys.
- The former requires patients to have good hepatic function and may be subject to genetic differences in the CYP450 pathways.
- Glucuronidized BZs are generally much safer on the liver and do not depend of CYP450 metabolic pathways. However, patients must have good renal function on these agents.
- Lorazepam (ativan), temazepam (Restoril), and oxazepam (Serax) are glucuronidized.

TIP: Prescribing BZs, Part 4

- Pharmacodynamically, some BZs have a greater affinity for BZ1 receptor subtypes, which are typically located in the hypothalamic sleep-wake switch (specifically in the ventrolateral preoptic area [VLPO]) and, when occupied, promotes sleep.
- Temazepam (Restoril) and flurazepam (Dalmane) are approved for insomnia (Sedative-Hypnotics) and have greater affinity for this sub-receptor.

7) AED (Anti-epileptic Drugs)

MECHANISM OF ACTION

Divalproex (Depakote), gabapentin (Neurontin), pregabalin (Lyrica)

- AEDs are not currently approved in the U.S. for the treatment of anxiety disorders; however, some approvals exist outside of the U.S.
- Some have a moderate evidence base to support their use in anxiety.
- AEDs that are used in psychiatry often share the common mechanism that they decrease neuronal firing in the CNS, theoretically in limbic areas.
- AEDs often close down neuronal sodium or calcium channels. Sometimes they lower glutamate activity by blocking glutamate NMDA receptors. Some agents may increase GABA neurotransmitter activity, but this is not accomplished via a GABA-A receptor BZ-like activity.
- For example: gabapentin and pregabalin block alpha-2-delta ligand calcium channels. This slows neuronal firing and may lower seizure activity. This mechanism in the periphery also lowers delta pain fiber firing to lower neuropathic pain. There are approvals for this type of prescribing for both gabapentin and pregabalin.
- The greatest evidence for use in anxiety among AEDs might be pregabalin for GAD. Alternatively, gabapentin has positive research for use in SAD and PD.
- Divalproex is an AED with an unclear mechanism of action. It is thought to increase GABA neuronal tone through multiple mechanisms, none of which is via GABA-A PAM. It is approved for treating absence seizures and for alleviating bipolar mania. In regard to anxiety, it may have the most supportive evidence for PTSD.

8) Alpha-2 Receptor Agonists and Alpha-1 Receptor Antagonists

MECHANISM OF ACTION

Clonidine (Catapres), guanfacine (Tenex), prazosin (Minipress)

- Alpha-2 agonists (clonidine and guanfacine) are better known for treating hypertension and were discussed in the ADHD chapter in detail.
- Their activity centrally lowers noradrenergic tone. Anxiety is hypothesized to begin with elevated NE activity via excessive neuronal firing. Theoretically, these agents are poised to directly lower NE firing and potentially improve anxiety symptoms.

- There are no approvals and limited evidence base in treating anxiety. Despite this, they are used frequently in psychopharmacological practice, sometimes as an alternative to using potentially addictive BZs.
- Alpha-1 antagonists are specifically used to treat nightmares associated with PTSD.
- Beta blockers (propranolol [Inderal], atenolol [Tenormin]) are antihypertensives with a reasonable evidence base for the treatment of SAD, performance anxiety types where palpitations and tremors may be best controlled.

9) Antihistamines

MECHANISM OF ACTION

Hydroxyzine (Vistaril, Atarax)

- This class of medication is better known for treating environmental allergies. Blocking or antagonism of the H1 histamine receptor will alleviate allergy symptoms peripherally. It also may create sedation and somnolence from activity in the CNS.
- Some of these drugs are formally approved for treating insomnia and are further discussed in that chapter. Similar to antihypertensives, the side effect of sedation may be utilized to treat anxiety where muscle tension, agitation, or insomnia exists as target anxiety symptoms.
- Stimulating H1 receptors in the hypothalamic tuberomammillary nuclei (TMN) essentially is a switch that convinces the brain it is daytime and that the patient should be alert. Blocking this receptor may remove alertness and arousal, thus causing fatigue and sedation. This may allow for a calming effect or even sleep onset.
- For anxiety, hydroxyzine is the only approved agent. Psychopharmacologists have become adept at using antihistamine properties in other classes of drugs which are well known to cause sedation (TCAs, first and second-generation antipsychotics [FGA/SGA], etc.). Light sedation is felt to be anxiolytic and calming, whereas heavy sedation may be a limiting side effect.
    - The SGAs quetiapine (Seroquel XR), olanzapine (Zyprexa), and asenapine (Saphris) are commonly used at low doses for this purpose.
    - The FGA chlorpromazine (Thorazine) and perphenazine (Trilafon) at low doses may be used as well.
    - The sedating antidepressants trazodone (Desyrel), nefazodone (Serzone), and mirtazapine (Remeron) may be helpful in this respect.

10) First- and Second-Generation Antipsychotics (FGA/SGA)

MECHANISM OF ACTION

Chlorpromazine (Thorazine), perphenazine (Trilafon), aripiprazole (Abilify), asenapine (Saphris), brexpiprazole (Rexulti), cariprazine (Vraylar), olanzapine (Zyprexa), quetiapine (Seroquel XR)

- This class of medication is discussed in greater detail in the schizophrenia chapter. Many of the antipsychotics are useful, and even approved for use, in other psychiatric disorders (MDD, bipolar disorder, autism). There are no approvals for their use in anxiety disorders but there is a small evidence base for this, and they are often used in an off-label manner to control anxiety and agitation symptoms, regardless of DSM-5 diagnosis.
- The greatest evidence exists for use of the SGA quetiapine (Seroquel XR) for GAD.
- The typical (first-generation) antipsychotics (FGA) were developed and clinically used to a great extent between 1950 and 1995. They chiefly antagonize the D2 receptor, which leads to a reduction in psychotic symptoms (delusions, hallucinations, and thought disorder). After 1995, the atypical (second-generation) antipsychotics (SGA) were developed and are the most utilized now.
- D2 blockage results in lower dopamine neuronal firing and can cause a calming effect.
- In addition to D2 receptor blockage, SGAs all antagonize the 5HT-2A serotonin receptor, which significantly lowers the risk for neuromuscular side effects (akathisia, Parkinsonism, dystonia, tardive dyskinesia, and neuroleptic malignant syndrome).
- Many of these agents antagonize the H1 receptor as well. This property can cause sedation and then somnolence at higher doses, but at lower doses may be anxiolytic and calming.
- *Low potency* FGAs (chlorpromazine and perphenazine) are more often used off-label for anxiety versus *higher potency* FGAs (haloperidol, thiothixene, fluphenazine) which have less H1 antagonism.
- SGA *-pines* have more of this activity as well (olanza*pine*, quetia*pine*, asena*pine*).
- Some SGAs contain properties akin to approved anxiolytic agents. For example, some (quetiapine, brexpiprazole, aripiprazole, cariprazine) contain 5HT-1a receptor partial agonism (SPA) similar to that employed by the approved GAD medication buspirone. Others have NRI (quetiapine) properties or weak SNRI (ziprasidone) properties.

Table 2.8 Prescribing Table for Anxiety Medications

Drugs listed in **BOLD** are approved agents for Adult ADHD. Dosing is based upon clinical application. Approved dosing guidelines should be further referenced by the prescriber.						
1. Antidepressants						
Brand	Generic	Indication (Bold for FDA Approved)	Drug Mechanism	Dosing Tips	Monitoring Tips	Medicolegal Tips
The Selective Serotonin Reuptake Inhibitors (SSRIs)						
Prozac	**Fluoxetine**	• **Obsessive-compulsive disorder (OCD)** • **Panic disorder (PD)** • Social anxiety disorder (SAD) • Post-traumatic stress disorder (PTSD) • Generalized anxiety disorder (GAD)	• Serotonin reuptake inhibitor	• Usual dose is 10–80mg/day • Increase 10–20mg every few weeks	• Common side effects include GI, headache, fatigue, anxiety, insomnia, weight gain, and sexual dysfunction • Serious side effects include (hypo)mania, increased suicidal ideation, easy bruising • Drug interactions as this is a major inhibitor of CYP4502D6	• In those age <25 there is increased risk of lethality, more frequent monitoring and safety planning is warranted
Zoloft	**Sertraline**	• **Panic disorder (PD)** • **Post-traumatic stress disorder (PTSD)** • **Social anxiety disorder (SAD)** • **Obsessive-compulsive disorder (OCD)** • Generalized anxiety disorder (GAD)	• Serotonin reuptake inhibitor	• Usual dose is 25–200mg/day • Increase 50mg every few weeks	• Same except higher possible rate of GI side effects • Drug interactions are minimal	• Same as above • Do not stop abruptly
Paxil **Paxil CR**	**Paroxetine**	• **Obsessive-compulsive disorder (OCD)** • **Panic disorder (PD)** • **Social anxiety disorder (SAD)** • **Post-traumatic stress disorder (PTSD)** • **Generalized anxiety disorder (GAD)**	• Serotonin reuptake inhibitor	• Usual dose is 10–50mg/day • Increase 10–20mg every few weeks	• Same except higher rates of mild anticholinergic effects and greater chance of serotonin withdrawal upon cessation • Drug interactions as this is a major inhibitor of CYP4502D6	• Same as above • Warning for birth defects

Luvox **Luvox CR**	**Fluvoxamine**	• **Obsessive-compulsive disorder (OCD)** • Social anxiety disorder (SAD) • Panic disorder (PD) • Post-traumatic stress disorder (PTSD) • Generalized anxiety disorder (GAD)	• Serotonin reuptake inhibitor	• Usual dose is 50–150mg twice daily or 100–300mg once daily for CR • Increase 100mg every few weeks	• Same as above except drug interaction as this agent is a major inhibitor of CYP1A2	• Same as above
Celexa	Citalopram	• Off-label for anxiety	• Serotonin reuptake inhibitor	• Usual dose is 10–40mg/day • Increase every few weeks • Do not exceed 40mg/day (or 20mg in elderly) due to cardiac QTc prolongation risks	• Same except for cardiac risks as this drugs increases QTc • Drug interaction is for moderate inhibition at CYP4502D6	• Same as above • If dosing at higher levels for better efficacy consider obtaining EKG and trough blood levels as a precaution
Lexapro	**Escitalopram**	• **Generalized anxiety disorder (GAD)** • Obsessive-compulsive disorder (OCD) • Social anxiety disorder (SAD) • Panic disorder (PD) • Post-traumatic stress disorder (PTSD)	• Serotonin reuptake inhibitor	• Usual dose is 5–20mg/day • Increase 5–10mg every few weeks	• Common side effects include GI, headache, fatigue, anxiety, insomnia, weight gain, and sexual dysfunction • Serious side effects include (hypo)mania, increased suicidal ideation, easy bruising	• Same as above but no cardiac warnings

(*Continued*)

Table 2.8 (Continued)

The Serotonin Norepinephrine Reuptake Inhibitors (SNRIs)						
Effexor Effexor XR	**Venlafaxine**	• **Generalized anxiety disorder (GAD)** • **Social anxiety disorder (SAD)** • **Panic disorder (PD)** • Obsessive-compulsive disorder (OCD) • Post-traumatic stress disorder (PTSD)	• Serotonin and norepinephrine reuptake inhibitor	• Usual dose is 37.5–225mg/day • Increase 37.5–75mg every few weeks • Maximal dose up to 375mg/day	• Common side effects same as SSRI but additional dry mouth, nausea, insomnia, anxiety may be experienced • Serious side effects same as SSRI but may include hypertension • Higher risk of serotonin withdrawal upon cessation	• Same as SSRI • Do not stop abruptly
Cymbalta	**Duloxetine**	• **Generalized anxiety disorder (GAD)** • Obsessive-compulsive disorder (OCD) • Social anxiety disorder (SAD) • Panic disorder (PD) • Post-traumatic stress disorder (PTSD) • Fibromyalgia (FM)	• Serotonin and norepinephrine reuptake inhibitor	• Usual dose is 30–120mg/day • Increase 30–60mg every few weeks	• Same as above but carries risk of liver damage in alcohol use disorder (AUD) patients	• Same as above
SSRI-PLUS Agents						
Viibryd	Vilazodone	• **Major depressive disorder** • Off-label for anxiety	• Weak serotonin reuptake inhibitor • Partial agonist action at serotonin 1A autoreceptor	• Usual dose is 10–40mg/day • Start at 10mg/day and increase to 10mg every week; 20–40mg/day is usual dose • Take with food	• Common side effects include GI, headache, fatigue, anxiety, insomnia dysfunction • Serious side effects include (hypo)mania, increased suicidal ideation, easy bruising	• In those age <25 there is increased risk of lethality, more frequent monitoring and safety planning is warranted • May have less weight gain and sexual dysfunction

Trintellix	Vortioxetine	• **Major depressive disorder** • Off-label for anxiety	• Serotonin reuptake inhibitor • Partial agonist action at serotonin 1A autoreceptor • Antagonist at serotonin 1b/d, 3, 7 receptors	• Usual dose is 5–20mg/day • Increase 10mg every few weeks • Usual dose is 10–20mg/day	• Same as above	• Same as above
Tricyclic Antidepressants (TCAs)						
Tofranil	Imipramine	• Off-label for all anxiety disorders	• Norepinephrine and serotonin reuptake inhibitor (predominantly serotonin reuptake inhibitor)	• Usual dose is 25–300mg/day • Start at 25mg/day at bedtime and increase by 25mg every 3–7 days	• Common side effects include sedation, weight gain, anticholinergic side effects, alpha adrenergic side effects (dizziness, orthostasis) • Serious side effects include QTc prolongation, activation of mania and suicidality • Monitor EKG prior to and periodically during use and obtain trough blood levels periodically	• Use in limited doses in those with suicidal symptoms • Use with caution in cardiac patients • Use with caution in suicidal patients • Avoid use with strong CYP4502D6 inhibitors such as fluoxetine/paroxetine/citalopram
Elavil	Amitriptyline	• Off-label for anxiety disorders	• Norepinephrine and serotonin reuptake inhibitor (predominantly serotonin reuptake inhibitor)	• Usual dose is 25–300mg/day • Start at 25mg/day at bedtime and increase by 25mg every 3–7 days	• Same as above	• Same as above

(*Continued*)

Table 2.8 (Continued)

Anafranil	Clomipramine	• **OCD** • Off-label for other anxiety disorders	• Norepinephrine and serotonin reuptake inhibitor (predominantly serotonin reuptake inhibitor)	• Usual dose is 25–250mg/day • Start at 25mg/day and increase by 25mg every 3–7 days	• Same as above	• Same as above
Sinequan	Doxepin	• Off-label for anxiety disorders	• Norepinephrine and serotonin reuptake inhibitor (predominantly serotonin reuptake inhibitor)	• Usual dose is 10–300mg/day • Start at 10–25mg/day and increase by 25mg every 3–7 days	• Same as above	• Same as above
Monoamine Oxidase Inhibitors (MAOIs)						
EMSAM	Selegiline	• Off-label for anxiety disorders	• Irreversibly inhibits MAO-A and MAO-B enzymes, increasing norepinephrine, serotonin, and dopamine	• Usual dose is 6–12mg/24 hrs for transdermal patch • Start at 6mg/24 hrs and increase by 6mg/24 hrs every few weeks	• Common side effects include application site reactions, insomnia, anxiety • Serious side effects include hypertensive crisis, serotonin syndrome, induction of mania and suicidality • Monitor for blood pressure changes	• Provide diet card and suggest patient use one pharmacy for all Rx and OTC medications • Document this and capacity to (1) follow diet and (2) patient ability to speak to pharmacist about every med utilized • This agent alone may create a false positive urine screen for methamphetamine

Marplan	Isocarboxazid	• Off-label for anxiety disorders	• Irreversibly inhibits MAO-A and MAO-B enzymes, increasing norepinephrine, serotonin, and dopamine	• Usual dose is 10–30mg twice a day • Increase by 10mg/day every 7 days	• Same as above but additionally may have greater weight gain and hypotension	• Same as above
Nardil	Phenelzine	• Off-label for anxiety disorders	• Irreversibly inhibits MAO-A and MAO-B enzymes, increasing norepinephrine, serotonin, and dopamine	• Usual dose is 15–30mg three times a day • Increase by 45mg every week	• Same as above	• Same as above
Parnate	Tranylcypromine	• Off-label for anxiety disorders	• Irreversibly inhibits MAO-A and MAO-B enzymes, increasing norepinephrine, serotonin, and dopamine	• Usual dose is 10mg–20mg three times a day • Increase by 10mg/day every week	• Same as above	• Same as above

(*Continued*)

Table 2.8 (Continued)

2. Serotonin partial agonist						
Brand	Generic	Indication (Bold for FDA Approved)	Drug Mechanism	Dosing Tips	Monitoring Tips	Medicolegal Tips
The Serotonin Partial Agonists (SPAs)						
BuSpar	**Buspirone**	• **Generalized anxiety disorder (GAD)**	• Partial agonist at presynaptic serotonin type 1A receptors	• Usual dose is 5–22.5mg twice a day • Increase 5mg twice daily every few weeks	• Common initial side effects include dizziness, headache, nervousness • Generally is felt to be least risky for sexual dysfunction or weight gain compared to SSRI, SNRI, TCA	

3. Benzodiazepines								
Brand	Generic	Indication (Bold for FDA Approved)	Average Dose Range for Anxiety	Equivalent Dose (to Lorazepam 1mg)	Onset of Action After Oral Dose	Half-life	Clinical Duration of Action	Medicolegal Tips
Benzodiazepines (BZs)								
Xanax **Xanax XR**	**Alprazolam** **Alprazolam XR**	• **Anxiety** • **Panic disorder**	0.5–4mg/day	0.5mg	(0.5 hrs) (1–2 hrs)	(11–16 hrs)	(3–4 hrs) (10 hrs)	• Consider alternatives for patients with addiction, fall, respiratory suppression, or cognitive risks • Monitor for abuse • Monitor for impairment in operating heavy machinery • Start low and use lowest effective dose
Librium	**Chlordiazepoxide**	• **Anxiety**	5–100mg/day	25mg	(2 hrs)	(>100 hrs)	(4–6 hrs)	• Same as above

Klonopin	**Clonazepam**	• **Panic disorder** • **Anxiety**	0.5–2mg/day	0.25mg	(1 hr)	(20–80 hrs)	(6–8 hrs)	• Same as above
Tranxene	**Clorazepate**	• **Anxiety**	15–60mg/day	7.5mg	(0.5–1 hr)	(>100 hrs)	(6–8 hrs)	• Same as above
Valium	**Diazepam**	• **Anxiety**	5–40mg/day	5–10mg	(0.5 hr)	(>100 hrs)	(4–6 hrs)	• Same as above
Ativan	**Lorazepam**	• **Anxiety**	1–4mg/day	1mg	(0.5–1 hr)	(10–20 hrs)	(4–6 hrs)	• Same as above
Serax	**Oxazepam**	• **Anxiety**	30–120mg/day	15mg	(2–4 hrs)	(5–14 hrs)	(6–8 hrs)	• Same as above

4. Anti-epileptics						
Brand	Generic	Indication (Bold for FDA Approved)	Drug Mechanism	Dosing Tips	Monitoring Tips	Medicolegal Tips
Calcium Channel Blockers						
Neurontin	Gabapentin	• Off-label for anxiety disorders	• Binds to alpha-2 delta subunit of voltage sensitive calcium channels	• Usual dose 100–1200mg three times daily • Increase by 300mg three times a day every few weeks	• Common side effects include sedation, dizziness, ataxia, tremor, headache, weight gain	• Avoid abrupt withdrawal due to seizure risk
Lyrica	Pregabalin	• Off-label for anxiety disorders	• Binds to alpha-2 delta subunit of voltage sensitive calcium channels	• Usual dose is 150–600mg/day in 2–3 divided doses • Titrate up to target dose from standard starting dose of 150mg in 2–3 divided doses.	• Same as above • Serious side effects include mild risk of addiction	• Same as above • Mild addictive properties, use same approach as for BZ anxiolytics

(*Continued*)

Table 2.8 (Continued)

GABA Enhancing Agents						
Depakote Depakote ER	Divalproex	• Off-label for anxiety disorders	• Increases CNS concentration of GABA via unknown mechanism	• Usual dose is 250mg–500mg three times a day • Increase by 250–500mg every few weeks for outpatient • For inpatient may load an 20mg/kg	• Common side effects include sedation, diarrhea, ataxia, tremor • Serious side effects include hepatotoxicity, pancreatitis, thrombocytopenia, polycystic ovarian syndrome, rashes, and activation of suicidality • Monitor for blood levels and obtain 50–125mg/day • Monitor liver, pancreas, and platelet function prior and during treatment	• Must monitor labs at baseline and then throughout use of this medication to avoid end-organ damage • Provide informed consent about these prior to treatment

5. The Alpha-2 Receptor Agonists and Alpha-1 Receptor Antagonists						
Brand	Generic	Indication (Bold for FDA Approved)	Drug Mechanism	Dosing Tips	Monitoring Tips	Medicolegal Tips
Alpha-2 Receptor Agonists						
Catapres/ Catapres-TTS/ Kapvay	Clonidine	• Off-label for anxiety disorders	• Stimulates central action of alpha-2A noradrenergic receptors, lowering peripheral noradrenergic tone	• Usual dose is 0.1mg–2.4mg/day given in twice daily dosing • Increase by 0.1mg every week	• Common side effects include dry mouth, dizziness, fatigue, lightheadedness • Serious side effects include hypotension, syncope, bradycardia, AV block, and abrupt withdrawal hypertensive crisis • Monitor vital signs	• Abrupt discontinuation may lead to rare hypertensive encephalopathy, stroke, and death • Taper over 2–4 days or longer to avoid rebound in blood pressure

Intuniv Tenex	Guanfacine	• Off-label for anxiety disorders	• Stimulates central action of alpha-2A noradrenergic receptors, lowering peripheral noradrenergic tone	• 1–3mg nightly • Increase 1mg every week	• Common side effects include dry mouth, dizziness, fatigue, lightheadedness • Serious side effects include hypotension, syncope, bradycardia, AV block, and abrupt withdrawal hypertensive crisis • Generally less side-vegetative effects compared to clonidine	• Same as above
Alpha-1 Receptor Antagonists						
Minipress	Prazosin	• Off-label for nightmares associated with PTSD	• Blocks alpha-1 receptors to reduce noradrenergic tone centrally	• Usual dose is 1–16mg/day • Start at 1mg at bedtime and increase dose until nightmares resolve	• Common side effects include dizziness, lightheadedness, fatigue • Serious side effects include hypotension, orthostasis, syncope	• Same as above

6. Antihistamines						
Brand	Generic	Indication (Bold for FDA Approved)	Drug Mechanism	Dosing Tips	Monitoring Tips	Medicolegal Tips
Antihistamines						
Atarax **Vistaril**	**Hydroxyzine**	• **Anxiety**	• Blocks histamine 1 receptors	• Usual dose is 10–100mg four times a day • Increase every few days in increments of 10–25mg	• Common side effects include dry mouth, sedation, and other anticholinergic effects • Serious side effects include dyspnea, seizures, cardiac conduction delay	• Warn of sedation and operating heavy machinery

(*Continued*)

Table 2.8 (Continued)

7. Antipsychotics						
Brand	Generic	Indication (Bold for FDA Approved)	Drug Mechanism	Dosing Tips	Monitoring Tips	Medicolegal Tips
Antihistamines						
Zyprexa Symbyax	Olanzapine, olanzapine/ fluoxetine	• Acute mania/mixed mania • Maintenance • Bipolar depression in combination with fluoxetine • Agitation/anxiety • Off-label for anxiety	• Blocks dopamine 2 receptors reducing psychosis and stabilizing mania; may provide calming effect • Blocks serotonin 2A receptors which may improve depression • Blocks H1 receptors which may provide sedation and anxiolysis	• Usual mania dose is 2.5–20mg/day • Increase by 5mg every few days	• Common initial side effects include dizziness, sedation, headache, GI side effects • Serious side effects include risk of diabetes, hyperlipidemia, hypertension, weight gain, transient and permanent neuromuscular side effects, hyperlipidemia, gynecomastia, agranulocytosis, increased risk of death in demented elderly, increased suicidality • Monitor at baseline and at least annually with CBC Diff, BMP, Lipid Panel; also conduct more routine weight and vital signs, AIMS tests or physical exam for EPS/TD neuromuscular symptoms	• Clearly explain life-threatening or serious side effects (e.g., TD/ EPS, metabolic side effects) • Provide treatments if side effects occur (e.g., weight loss agents, antiparkinson agents) • Considered one of the most metabolic syndrome inducing agents • Sedation risk is moderate • Risk of EPS is high

Seroquel (XR)	Quetiapine	• Acute mania • Maintenance • Bipolar depression • Off-label for agitation/anxiety	• Blocks dopamine 2 receptors reducing psychosis and stabilizing mania; may provide calming effect • Blocks serotonin 2A receptors which may improve depression • Blocks H1 receptors which may provide sedation and anxiolysis • Has potent NRI and 5HT-1a agonism as antidepressant properties which have been shown in other agents (SPA, SNRI) to lower anxiety	• Dosing is 25–400mg twice daily and for XR is 50–800mg/day • Depression dosing is 25–600 or 50–600, respectively, and both can be given once nightly	• Same as above	• Clearly explain life-threatening or serious side effects (e.g., TD/EPS, metabolic side effects) • Provide treatment if side effects occur (e.g., weight loss agents, antiparkinson agents) • Considered one of the most metabolic syndrome inducing agents • Risk of weight gain and metabolics is high • Risk of sedation is high • Risk of EPS/TD is lowest in SGA class
Abilify	Aripiprazole	• Acute mania/mixed mania • Maintenance • Off-label for agitation/anxiety	• Partially agonizes D2 and D3 receptors which may improve affect • Net effect may also block dopamine 2 receptors reducing psychosis, stabilizing mania, and allowing a calming effect • Blocks serotonin 2A receptors which may improve depression • Has 5HT-1a agonism similar to SPA anxiolytics (buspirone)	• Usual dose is 2–30mg/day • May increase 2–5mg every few days • Drug is a substrate for CYP2D6 and must be halved if 2D6 inhibitor concomitantly taken	• Same as above	• Clearly explain life-threatening or serious side effects (e.g., TD/EPS, metabolic side effects) • Provide treatment if side effects occur (e.g., weight loss agents, antiparkinson agents) • Risk of weight gain and metabolics is moderate • Risk of sedation is moderate • Risk of akathisia is high

(*Continued*)

Table 2.8 (Continued)

Rexulti	Brexpiprazole	• Schizophrenia • Major depression augmentation • Off-label for agitation/anxiety	• Partially agonizes D2 and D3 receptors which may improve affect • Net effect may also block dopamine 2 receptors reducing psychosis, stabilizing mania, and allowing a calming effect • Blocks serotonin 2A receptors which may improve depression • Has 5HT-1a agonism similar to SPA anxiolytics (buspirone)	• Usual dose is 0.25–4mg/day • May increase 0.5–1mg every few weeks • Drug is a substrate for CYP2D6 and must be halved if 2D6 inhibitor concomitantly taken	• Same as above	• Clearly explain life-threatening or serious side effects (e.g., TD/EPS, metabolic side effects) • Provide treatment if side effects occur (e.g., weight loss agents, antiparkinson agents) • Risk of weight gain and metabolics is moderate • Risk of sedation is moderate • Risk of akathisia is moderate
Vraylar	Cariprazine	• Acute mania/mixed mania • Maintenance • Off-label for agitation/anxiety	• Partially agonizes D2 and D3 receptors which may improve affect • Net effect may also block dopamine 2 receptors reducing psychosis, stabilizing mania, and allowing a calming effect • Blocks serotonin 2A receptors which may improve depression • Has 5HT-1a agonism similar to SPA anxiolytics (buspirone)	• Usual dose is 1.5–6mg/day • May increase 1.5mg every few weeks	• Same as above	• Clearly explain life-threatening or serious side effects (e.g., TD/EPS, metabolic side effects) • Provide treatment if side effects occur (e.g., weight loss agents, antiparkinson agents) • Risk of weight gain and metabolics is moderate • Risk of sedation is moderate • Risk of akathisia is high

Saphris	Asenapine	• Acute mania/mixed mania • Off-label for agitation/anxiety	• Blocks D2 receptors reducing psychosis, stabilizing mania, and allowing a calming effect • Blocks serotonin 2A receptors which may improve depression • Has 5HT-1a agonism similar to SPA anxiolytics (buspirone) • Blocks H1 receptors which may provide sedation and anxiolysis • Has similar antidepressant theoretical properties to mirtazapine (alpha-2 antagonism, 5HT-2c, 3 antagonism)	• Usual dose is 5–10mg twice daily • It is taken SL or will not be absorbed	• Same as above	• Clearly explain life-threatening or serious side effects (e.g., TD/EPS, metabolic side effects) • Provide treatment if side effects occur (e.g., weight loss agents, antiparkinson agents) • Risk of weight gain and metabolics is moderate • Risk of sedation is moderate

Final Advanced Prescribing Thoughts

Similar to the discussion for ADHD prescribing and management, comorbidity is key. Often, anxiety disorders can be so socially disruptive that distressed patients may develop MDD. Many anxious patients develop SUD to manage their symptoms, albeit maladaptively. Anxiety disorders are common in personality disorders due to poor defense mechanisms, coping strategies, and/or poor social support networks.

Despite the length of this chapter, which covers five separate disorders, there is some commonality. Using SSRIs and increasing serotonergic activity is a key initial strategy for any of the disorders. Use of full dose and monotherapy duration is good prescribing practice for all psychiatric disorders. If SSRI management fails over 3–4 months, then an escalation to an SNRI is a typical second step. GAD, PD, and SD all have SNRI approvals. PTSD and OCD have limited data for SNRIs, but they can be used here too. The use of TCAs was not discussed in great detail above, but many of TCAs (imipramine, amitriptyline, clomipramine) have robust SRI and NRI activity, and data supports their use in more resistant anxiety cases. Noradrenergic TCAs (desipramine, nortriptyline, protriptyline) are likely less effective. MAOIs may be used as well. SGAs have no approvals but many of these drugs improve sleep, lower agitation, and have serotonergic properties that can help anxiety symptoms. Quetiapine has the most extensive data for use in GAD, in particular. Other SGAs with greater 5HT-1A agonistic properties (aripiprazole, brexpiprazole, cariprazine) theoretically may help as well. Anti-epileptic drugs, especially gabapentin and pregabalin, have data and theoretical application in the management of anxiety. Pregabalin is approved in Europe for GAD treatment.

After SSRIs and SNRIs fail, the prescriber quickly runs out of approved options. This critical point has a key decision tree. One must choose to start a BZ with addiction risk or switch over to a non-addictive approach with agents that are not approved or have serious side effects. Anti-eplieptics can cause severe skin conditions and pancreas, liver, or bone marrow damage. SGAs may create permanent movement disorder and instigate metabolic disorder. Particularly for PD, GAD, and SAD, BZs likely have greater evidence to support their use here, but less so for PTSD and OCD. The prescriber must weigh the impact of addiction risk versus use of a less supported, off-label approach with different side effect risks.

Finally, rational polypharmacy should always occur in treatment resistant cases. Adding two medications from the same pharmacological family is rarely warranted. Adding together two SSRIs, two TCAs, two BZs, or two SGAs may not make sense versus simply maximizing the monotherapy. Redundantly manipulating the same brain mechanism of action that failed with the first monotherapy does not make clinical or statistical sense. Instead, drugs that are to be added together should have different mechanisms of anxiolytic action. Instead of adding two serotonergic SSRIs together, adding a GABAergic BZ to the SSRI makes rational pharmacodynamic sense. This polypharmacy allows two neurotransmitter systems to be manipulated complimentarily to lower anxiety. Adding buspirone (a SPA) to an SSRI makes more synergistic sense than adding two SSRIs together.

In the former, two different serotonin manipulations are added together, rather than a solely redundant double SRI mechanism. Unfortunately, there is very little data and more theoretical application when it comes to treating very resistant cases in this manner, where the goal is to add complementary medications of differing mechanisms of action. Throughout this book, polypharmacy approaches will be based upon known research trials, evidence base, or, at the minimum, this concept of rational polypharmacy.

Bibliography

Adamou, M., Puchalska, S., Plummer, W., & Hale, A. S. (2007) "Valproate in the treatment of PTSD: systematic review and meta analysis." *Current Medical Research and Opinion* 23(6), 1285-1291.

American Psychiatric Association. (2013) *Diagnostic and Statistical Manual of Mental Disorders: DSM-5.* (5th ed.). Washington, D.C.: American Psychiatric Association.

Bandelow B., et al. (2012). "Guidelines for the pharmacological treatment of anxiety disorders, obsessive-compulsive disorder and posttraumatic stress disorder in primary care." *International Journal of Psychiatry in Clinical Practice* 16, 77–84.

Bruce, S. E., Yonkers, K. A., Otto, M. W., Eisen, J. L., Weisberg, R. B., Pagano, M., & Keller, M. B. (2008) "Influence of psychiatric comorbidity on recovery and recurrence in generalized anxiety disorder, social phobia, and panic disorder: a 12-year prospective study." *Focus* 6(4), 539–548.

Caballo, V. E., Salazar, I. C., Arias, B., Irurtia, M. J., Calderero, M., & the CISO-A Research Team Spain. (2010) "Validation of the Social Anxiety Questionnaire for Adults (SAQ-A30) with Spanish university students: similarities and differences among degree subjects and regions." *Behavioral Psychology/Psicologia Conductual* 18, 5–34.

Caballo, V. E., Arias, B., Salazar, I. C., Irurtia, M. J., Hofmann, S.G., & the CISO-A Research Team. (2015) "Psychometric properties of an innovative self-report measure: the Social Anxiety Questionnaire for Adults." *Psychological Assessment* 27(3), 997–1012. http://dx.doi.org/10.1037/a0038828.

de Geus, E. J., van't Ent, D., Wolfensberger, S. P., Heutink, P., Hoogendijk, W. J., Boomsma, D. I., & Veltman, D. J. (2007) "Intrapair differences in hippocampal volume in monozygotic twins discordant for the risk for anxiety and depression." *Biological Psychiatry* 61(9), 1062–1071.

Foa, E. B., et al. (2002) "The Obsessive Compulsive Inventory: development and validation of a short version. *Psychological Assessment* 14, 485–496.

Kessler, R. C., Berglund, P., Demler, O., Jin, R., Merikangas, K. R., & Walters, E. E. (2005) "Lifetime prevalence and age-of-onset distributions of DSM-IV disorders in the National Comorbidity Survey Replication." *Archives of General Psychiatry* 62(6), 593–602.

Kingsbury, S. J., Yi, D., & Simpson, G. M. (2001) "Psychopharmacology: rational and irrational polypharmacy." *Psychiatric Services* 52(8), 1033–6.

Liebowitz, M. R., Gorman, J. M., Fyer, A. J., & Klein, D. F. (1985) "Social phobia: review of a neglected anxiety disorder." *Archives of General Psychiatry* 42(7), 729.

Marchesi C. (2008) "Pharmocologic management of panic disorder." *Neuropsychiatric Disease and Treatment* 4(1), 93–106.

Martin, E. I., Ressler, K. J., Binder, E., & Nemeroff, C. B. (2009) "The neurobiology of anxiety disorders: brain imaging, genetics, and psychoneuroendocrinology." *Psychiatric Clinics of North America* 32(3), 549–575.

Mavissakalian, M. R. (1996) "The relationship of plasma imipramine and N-desmethylimipramine to response in panic disorder." *Psychopharmacology Bulletin* 32(1), 143–7.

Pande, A. C., Pollack, M. H., Crockatt, J., Greiner, M., Chouinard, G., Lydiard, R. B., & Shiovitz, T. (2000) "Placebo-controlled study of gabapentin treatment of panic disorder." *Journal of Clinical Psychopharmacology* 20(4), 467–471.

Regier, D. A., Rae, D. S., Narrow, W. E., Kaelber, C. T., & Schatzberg, A. F. (1998) "Prevalence of anxiety disorders and their comorbidity with mood and addictive disorders." *The British Journal of Psychiatry* 34, 24–8.

Schwartz, T. L. (2011) "Vilazodone: a brief pharmacological and clinical review of the novel serotonin partial agonist and reuptake inhibitor." *Therapeutic Advances in Psychopharmacology* 1(3), 81–7.

Smoller, J. W., & Faraone, S. V. (2008) "Genetics of anxiety disorders: complexities and opportunities." *American Journal of Medical Genetics Part C: Seminars in Medical Genetics* 148(2), 85–88.

Spitzer, R. L., Kroenke, K., Williams, J. B. W., & Lowe, B. (2006) "A brief measure for assessing generalized anxiety disorder." *Archives of Internal Medicine* 166(10), 1092–1097.

Stahl, S. M. (1998) "Mechanism of action of serotonin selective reuptake inhibitors: serotonin receptors and pathways mediate therapeutic effects and side effects." *Journal of Affective Disorders* 51(3), 215–235.

Stahl, S. M. (2000) "The 7 habits of highly effective psychopharmacologists: overview." *The Journal of Clinical Psychiatry* 61(4), 1–478.

Stahl, S. M. (2003) "Selective actions on sleep or anxiety by exploiting GABA-A/benzodiazepine receptor subtypes." *The Journal of Clinical Psychiatry* 63(3), 1–478.

Stahl, S. M. (2013) *Stahl's Essential Psychopharmacology: Neuroscientific Basis and Practical Applications.* Cambridge, UK: Cambridge University Press.

CHAPTER 3

Bipolar Disorders: Bipolar 1, Bipolar 2, and Cyclothymic Disorder

SECTION 1 Basic Prescribing Practices

Essential Concepts

- Accurate diagnosis is essential for treatment of bipolar disorder.
- Sustained mania (7+ days) is definitively needed to confirm the diagnosis of bipolar disorder.
- Depressive episodes are common but are not absolutely needed for the diagnosis.
- Many patients will state they are "bipolar" because they have mood swings (lability). This is often due to personality disorder, anxiety, stress, or substance use instead.
- There are a few key diagnoses within this spectrum:
    - Bipolar 1 (B1D) patients have sustained (7+ days) of mania and usually major depressive episodes.
    - Bipolar 2 (B2D) patients have hypomania and usually major depressive episodes.
    - Cyclothymia (CT) patients have chronic (2+ years) hypomania spells and usually minor depressive episodes.
    - Some bipolar patients may be grandiose, paranoid, and psychotic (delusions, hallucinations, etc.).
    - Some bipolar patients may have mixed features where 3+ mania symptoms intrude upon a depression episode or 3+ depressive symptoms intrude into a mania episode.
- Comorbid bipolar disorder (BD) and substance use disorder (SUD) are common.
- Borderline personality disorder (BPD) and ADHD are not variants of BD.
- Mania generally requires pharmacotherapy.
- Depressive episodes may respond to psychotherapy and/or pharmacotherapy.

Phenomenology, Diagnosis, Clinical Interviewing

For any new practitioner in any field, the goal is to be able to make an accurate diagnosis. All of psychiatric prescribing at this beginning level is based on regulatory findings, approvals, and indications that are psychiatric disorder specific. Psychotropics will only deliver the outcomes promised if the patient at hand actually has been accurately identified as having BD. Mania is the hallmark of BD, which is definitively needed to confirm the diagnosis. Depressive episodes are more common than manic or hypomanic spells but are not absolutely needed for the diagnosis. BD patients more often present in outpatient venues as depressed compared to being manic. Unipolar depressive symptoms are similar to those of bipolar depression, and telling them apart is extremely difficulty even for experts. Up to 10% of BD patients never experience depressive episodes and only have manic events. Furthermore, distractibility (poor concentration), hyperactivity, insomnia, and increased self-esteem are also symptoms that are not unique to BD. These symptoms can be prevalent in major depressive disorder (MDD), post-traumatic stress disorder (PTSD), generalized anxiety disorder (GAD), and narcissistic personality disorder (NPD). This can make diagnosis difficult, especially when the patient presents in a depressed state identical to MDD. Typically, the average BD patient spends more time predominantly depressed rather than in a manic state.

Commonly, BD in adults is confounded by other psychiatric disorders such as anxiety, substance misuse, or depression. Similar to previous chapters, this chapter will teach diagnosis and treatment of BD initially as a simplified, single-disorder state, then progress toward more advanced treatment of comorbid psychiatric states. This chapter assumes that the reader is adept and comfortable with descriptive DSM-5 interviewing and diagnostic assessment. Furthermore, in the absence of DSM-5 mastery, patient administered rating scales should become more the standard of care.

TIP: Bipolar Disorder Screening Questions

Screening for (hypo)mania

- Have there been times lasting at least several days when you feel high, on top of the world, euphoric, or overly happy?
- What about a period lasting several days where you needed little sleep but were full of energy and never tired, despite not sleeping?

DSM-5 Diagnosis

People with B1D and B2D typically show patterns of sustained mood elevation (excessive happiness, expansiveness, euphoria, etc.) and mood depressions (sadness, loss of enjoyment, etc.). Major depressive episodes (MDE) will be thoroughly discussed in the major depressive disorder (MDD) chapter, but in brief are considered to occur when at least two weeks of pervasive low mood, low self-worth, low interest, low energy, poor concentration, alterations in appetite, psychomotor functioning change, and suicidal thinking occur. Prior to defining DSM-5 bipolar disorder, hypomanic and manic episodes must be precisely defined. (**See below.**)

Manic Episodes Include:

A. A distinct period of abnormally and persistently elevated, expansive, or irritable mood, occurring daily and lasting at least one week (or any duration if hospitalization is necessary or psychosis occurs).

B. During the period of mood disturbance *and* increased energy/activity, three (or more) of the following symptoms are present and a change from normal behavior (four if the mood is only irritable):
- inflated self-esteem or grandiosity
- decreased need for sleep
- more talkative than usual or pressure to keep talking
- flight of ideas or subjective experience that thoughts are racing
- distractibility
- increase in goal-directed activity or psychomotor agitation
- excessive involvement in pleasurable activities that have a high potential for painful consequences

TIP: Commonly Used Mnemonics for DSM-5 Manic Episode Criteria

- **DTRHIGH** = **D**istractibility, **T**alkativeness, **R**acing thoughts, **H**yperactivity, **I**mpulsivity, **G**randiosity, and **H**yposomnia
- **DIGFAST** = **D**istractibility, **I**rresponsibility, **G**randiosity, **F**light of ideas, **A**ctivity increase, **S**leep decrease, **T**alkativeness

TIP: Interviewing a Bipolar Patient

- Ask about *sustained* mood elevation to distinguish mania from *transient* mood swings that are normal reactions to life events.
- Patients with BD may be in psychotic denial or may purposefully deceive practitioners because they like the "natural high" associated with (hypo) mania. Patients often answer negatively about previous mania events. It is key to attempt to gain permission to talk to family members, colleagues, or friends about mood patterns as such.

- Rapid, shallow, or even extreme mood swings (lability) are often due to histrionic, borderline, or antisocial personalities or substance misuse.
- Patients who present depressed may have a greater chance of bipolarity if they have:
  - Prepubertal onset of symptoms
  - Brief duration of depressed episodes
  - High frequency of depressed episodes
  - Seasonal pattern
  - Postpartum symptom onset
  - Multiple antidepressant failures
  - Nonresponse to antidepressant treatment
  - Rapid response to antidepressant treatment
  - Erratic response to antidepressant treatment
  - Dysphoric response to antidepressant treatment with agitation and insomnia
  - Family history of bipolar disorder
  - History of unstable interpersonal relationships
  - Frequent vocational problems
  - Frequent legal problems
  - Alcohol and drug use

Finally, patients in mania are felt to be in a state of psychotic denial. As with other psychotic illnesses (schizophrenia) there is a frank loss of memory for present or past manic events. Unfortunately, patients do not remember their past manic transgressions. In less severe manic events (hypomania), some patients do remember events, and these less severe episodes are looked upon as positive. These patients feel really good. They are mood elevated, happy, energetic, with increased self-esteem. They do not need sleep and are overly productive. These hypomanic episodes are felt to be less impairing (may actually benefit the patient) but are a clear change in their usual functioning, and people in their environment take notice. Mild mannered patients appear to change to a hyperthymic temperament and become goal driven and more the life of the party in their actions. They feel like they are on extra caffeine or even cocaine, but without actually having used those substances. Hypomania is a natural high with fewer consequences than a full-blown manic event. Unfortunately, some patients will deceive their prescribers and state they are not hypomanic, have not suffered such events, as they purposefully want these experiences and do not want them removed by medication management. Therefore, despite excellent interviewing and/or rating scale use, a sizeable minority of BD patients will forget manic episodes or will deny the existence of hypomania, making a retrospective diagnosis difficult if they present in a euthymic or depressed state. Given this, a secondary interview with a significant other or family member, or obtaining past psychiatric records, robustly increases the accuracy of diagnosis.

Hypomanic Episodes

A hypomania episode must last for most of the day each day for at least four days (but may last longer). The patient must experience a clear change in personality and function that is readily apparent to others in their environment. Unlike mania, a patient in a hypomanic spell generally has less impact or psychosocial consequence due to hypomanic activity. In addition to mood elevation, three or more of the following symptoms must be present:

- Inflated self-esteem or grandiosity
- Decreased need for sleep
- More talkative
- Experience of thoughts/ideas racing
- Distractibility
- Increase in goal-directed activity or psychomotor agitation
- Excessive involvement in pleasurable activities with a high potential of painful consequences
- Experiences unequivocal change in function that is uncharacteristic and noticeable by others

Rating Scales

There are very few mania rating scales. Generally, if a patient arrives in a manic state, everyone in the office is aware of the rapid speech, grandiosity, and extreme mood elevation. Office staff or clinicians may actually feel the patient is high or intoxicated on cocaine or a stimulant. One possible scale that may be considered is the Altman Self-Rating Mania Scale (ASRM).

Altman Self-Rating Mania Scale (ASRM)

- This scale is used to determine the amount and severity of current mania symptoms present.
- A positive score of six or more is suggestive of hypomania or mania being present. Scores may be followed sequentially over time to track treatment outcomes.
- It is simple to use, takes approximately 1–2 minutes for the patient to complete and several seconds to score. The article containing the scale can be purchased for a small amount at http://www.biologicalpsychiatryjournal.com/article/S0006-3223(96)00548-3/abstract. The author may also be reached for permission to use. Several web site resources offer downloads.

Table 3.1 The Altman Self-Rating Mania Scale

Appendix: Altman Self-Rating Scale for Mania (ASRM)		
Name______________Date________Score________		
Instructions		
1.	On this questionnaire, there are groups of five statements; read each group carefully.	
2.	Choose the one statement in each group that best describes the way you have been feeling for the past week.	
3.	Circle the number next to the statement you picked.	
4.	Please note: The word "occasionally" used here means once or twice, "often" means several times or more, "frequently" means most of the time.	
1)	0	I do not feel happier or more cheerful than usual.
	1	I occasionally feel happier or more cheerful than usual.
	2	I often feel happier or more cheerful than usual.
	3	I feel happier or more cheerful than usual most of the time.
	4	I feel happier or more cheerful than usual all of the time.
2)	0	I do not feel more self-confident than usual.
	1	I occasionally feel more self-confident than usual.
	2	I often feel more self-confident than usual.
	3	I feel more self-confident than usual most of the time.
	4	I feel extremely self-confident all of the time.
3)	0	I do not need less sleep than usual.
	1	I occasionally need less sleep than usual.
	2	I often need less sleep than usual.
	3	I frequently need less sleep than usual.
	4	I can go all day and night without any sleep and still do not feel tired.
4)	0	I do not talk more than usual.
	1	I occasionally talk more than usual.
	2	I often talk more than usual.
	3	I frequently talk more than usual.
	4	I talk constantly and cannot be interrupted.
5)	0	I have not been more active (either socially, sexually, at work, home, or school) than usual.
	1	I have occasionally been more active than usual.
	2	I have often been more active than usual.
	3	I have frequently been more active than usual.
	4	I am constantly active or on the go all the time.

The Mood Disorders Questionnaire (MDQ)

- The Mood Disorders Questionnaire (MDQ) is an alternative that asks historical questions which help detect previous mania episodes. This scale may be more useful if the patient presents in a depressive state, and especially if it is difficult to distinguish between an ongoing unipolar or bipolar depressive episode.

- If a patient scores seven or more in Item 1, answers YES to Item 2, and answers MODERATE or higher in Item 3, then a historical diagnosis of bipolar 1 or 2 is likely valid.
- To obtain this scale, please refer to Hirschfeld, R. M., Williams, J. B., Spitzer, R. L., Calabrese, J. R., Flynn, L., Keck, Jr., P. E., & Zajecka, J. (2000) "Development and validation of a screening instrument for bipolar spectrum disorder: the Mood Disorder Questionnaire." *American Journal of Psychiatry*, 157(11), 1873–1875 to contact the author directly.

Table 3.2 The Mood Disorders Questionnaire

Instructions: Please answer each question to the best of your ability.		
	YES	NO
1. Has there ever been a period of time where you were not your usual self and. . .		
. . . you felt so good or so hyper that other people thought you were not your normal self, or you were so hyper that you got into trouble?	☐	☐
. . . you were so irritable that you shouted at people or started fights or arguments?	☐	☐
. . . you felt much more self-confident than usual?	☐	☐
. . . you got much less sleep that usual and found you didn't really miss it?	☐	☐
. . . you were much more talkative or spoke much faster than usual?	☐	☐
. . . thoughts raced through your head or you couldn't slow your mind down?	☐	☐
. . . you were so easily distracted by things around you that you had trouble concentrating or staying on track?	☐	☐
. . . you had much more energy than usual?	☐	☐
. . . you were much more active or did many more things than usual?	☐	☐
. . . you were much more social or outgoing than usual; for example, you telephoned friends in the middle of the night?	☐	☐
. . . you were much more interested in sex than usual?	☐	☐
. . . you did things that were unusual for you or that other people might have thought were excessive, foolish, or risky?	☐	☐
. . . spending money got you or your family into trouble?	☐	☐
2. If you checked YES to more than one of the above, have several of these things ever happened during the same period of time?	☐	☐
3. How much of a problem did any of these cause you—like being unable to work; having family, money or legal troubles; getting into arguments or fights? *Please circle one response only* No Problem Minor Problem Moderate Problem Serious Problem		
4. Have any of your blood relatives (i.e., children, siblings, parents, grandparents, aunts, uncles) had manic-depressive illness or bipolar disorder?	☐	☐
5. Has a health professional ever told you that you have manic-depressive illness or bipolar disorder?	☐	☐

Treatment Guidelines

TIP: Essential Concepts

- Know the FDA indications for specific phases of bipolar disorder.
- It is best to use a medication that can safely treat both the highs and lows of BD, ideally in a single agent.
- Mood stabilizing, anti-epileptic drugs (AEDs) and second-generation antipsychotics (SGA) are monotherapy treatments of choice for mania and depressive spells.
- Antidepressant monotherapy treatments are not advised, and their use in combination with a stabilizing agent is controversial.
- Strongly consider obtaining past psychiatric treatment records or interview collateral resources.

TIP: Guidelines

- The CANMAT guideline is fairly modern and straightforward.
- Clinicians must take a history and make an accurate diagnosis based upon lifetime mood events and associated impairments.
- DSM-5 criteria and, ideally, rating scales should be used.
- Comorbidities should be ruled out.
- Pharmacotherapy should be started after reasonable informed consent.
    - Lithium and some SGAs can stop mania and also treat depression. They are considered first line treatments.
    - AEDs (anti-epileptic drugs) such as carbamazepine (Tegretol/ Equetro) and divalproex (Depakote) are more effective in treating mania versus depression.
    - Lamotrigine, divalproex, and some SGAs are effective in decreasing the amount of cycles a patient will experience and are considered maintenance drugs.
- Both mania and depressive episodes must be treated aggressively, and it is most important to avoid multiple mania episodes, as BD tends to become more resistant to treatment and more disabling as the number of mania events increase.
- Comorbidities should be treated with appropriate pharmacotherapy and/or psychotherapy.
- Bipolar disease management counseling, sleep-wake hygiene, Cognitive-Behavioral Therapy (CBT), or Family Therapy (FT) may be added as augmentation strategies, particularly in the euthymic or depressed phases of BD.

- BD is a psychiatric disorder where medication management often shows greater effect sizes in clinical trials than psychotherapy where mania is concerned.
- For bipolar depression, psychotherapy can be very effective. Medication can be used for mild, moderate, or severe BD in adults.

TIP: Approved Anti-Mania Agents

- Lithium
- Anti-epileptic Drugs (AED)
  - Divalproex (Depakote)
  - Carbamazepine (Equetro)
  - Lamotrigine (Lamictal)
    - Approved to maintain stability, not alleviate depression or mania
- Second-Generation Antipsychotics (SGA)
  - Risperidone(Risperdal)
  - Olanzapine (Zyprexa)
  - Quetiapine XR (Seroquel XR)
  - Ziprasidone (Geodon)
  - Aripiprazole (Abilify)
  - Asenapine (Saphris)
  - Cariprazine (Vraylar)

Second line treatments for mania are the remaining SGAs, other anti-epileptics, benzodiazepine sedative-hypnotics, and electroconvulsive therapy (ECT).

TIP: Approved Bipolar Antidepressants

- Olanzapine-Fluoxetine Combination (Symbyax)
- Quetiapine (Seroquel XR)
- Lurasidone (Latuda)

The above are all SGAs. Second line treatments for bipolar depression include some of the remaining SGAs, lithium, MDD/unipolar antidepressants, and electroconvulsive therapy (ECT). If an antidepressant is to be used, an SSRI or NDRI is warranted. Other antidepressants carry much higher risks of inducing mania, mixed features, or rapid cycling. Antidepressants are only used if another mood stabilizer is already present, especially in B1D.

Table 3.3 Prescribing Table for Bipolar Mania

Drugs listed in BOLD are approved agents. Dosing is based upon clinical application. Approved dosing guidelines should be further referenced by the prescriber.

Drug Mechanism	Dosing and Monitoring	Side Effects
Lithium—*Stabilizes neuronal membranes likely via calcium modulation.*	• 300mg twice a day is a suggested starting dose with a range to 2400mg/day • It is more important to dose for a safe blood level rather than a total mg/day dose • Lithium levels should be drawn at trough and kept within 0.08 and 1.2. This can be done 4–5 days after a dose increase • After mood stability, sometimes a lower range of 0.6–0.8 can be used • Requires bloodwork to monitor renal, thyroid, parathyroid, and bone marrow toxicity • Conduct baseline and follow-up monitoring of Cre, TSH, calcium, and WBC • QTc prolongation may occur and EKGs may be warranted. Baseline, post titration, and then annually are suggested and may be paired with blood work above • Avoidance of dehydration, diuretics, and NSAID anti-inflammatories is warranted	• Initial side effects may include GI upset, thirst, increased urination, intent tremor, skin changes/psoriasis, weight gain • Toxicity manifests by progression of polyuria, polydipsia, and tremor to confusion, stupor, and coma • Interestingly, lithium is approved to lower suicidality in B1D patients • End-organ damage includes cardiac, renal, thyroid, parathyroid, or bone marrow dysfunction. Informed consent and routine monitoring are necessary • Cardiac defects are possible if dosed in pregnant women
Divalproex (Depakote)—*Improves GABA tone, may inhibit sodium neuronal channels.*	• 250mg twice a day is a suggested starting dose with a range up to 50mg/kg/day • Levels should be kept between 50–125. Levels may be checked 4–5 days after dose increases and follow-up blood work can be obtained after final titration and then annually • Requires bloodwork to monitor hepatic, pancreatic, and bone marrow toxicity • Conduct baseline and follow-up monitoring of AST, ALT, amylase, lipase, platelets • Blood ammonia levels may rise	• Initial side effects include GI upset and fatigue • Some experience hair loss, tremor, or ataxia • Like other anti-epileptics, it has a greater chance of severe skin rashes • Toxicity often presents with the progression from sedation, confusion, stupor, coma but generally is not lethal as is lithium toxicity • End-organ damage includes hepatic, pancreatic, and bone marrow dysfunction. Polycystic ovarian syndrome has been noted in younger female patients. Informed consent and routine monitoring are necessary • Neural tube defects are possible if dosed in pregnant women

Drug Mechanism	Dosing and Monitoring	Side Effects
Carbamazepine (Equetro/ Tegretol)—*Inhibits neuronal sodium channels.*	• 200mg twice a day is a suggested starting dose with a range to 1600mg/day • Levels should be between 8–12. Dosing carbamazepine too low will be ineffective and dosing too high may yield toxicity • It may lower red blood cell (RBC) counts and cause aplastic anemia, which should be monitored with blood work at baseline, after titration and annually • It is a CYP3A4 enzyme inducer and will lower blood levels of many other concomitant drugs	• Initially, patients most often complain of drowsiness, dizziness, or unsteadiness • Others may develop tremor or ataxia • May have a greater chance of serious skin rashes • Toxicity often presents as the progression from sedation, to confusion, stupor, coma • End-organ damage includes bone marrow dysfunction • Informed consent and routine monitoring are necessary • Neural tube defects are possible if dosed in pregnant women
Lamotrigine (Lamictal)—*Inhibits neuronal sodium channels and may inhibit glutamate release.*	• It is not approved for treating acute mania like the above medications. It is approved to be started in a euthymic state and added to other mood stabilizing treatments to decrease recurrence of mania or depression • It takes several weeks to slowly titrate to avoid serious skin rashes such as Stevens-Johnson Syndrome (SJS) or Toxic Epidermal Necrolysis (TEN) • Strict dosing involves taking 25mg/day for 2 weeks, then 50mg/day for 2 weeks, 100mg/day for 2 weeks, then advancing to a standing dose of 200mg/day	• Initially, patients may experience drowsiness, dizziness, or unsteadiness • Others may develop tremor or ataxia • End-organ damage includes severe skin rashes • Any rash of any kind requires cessation • Any break in therapy of >5 days requires re-titration • There are no blood level or EKG monitoring requirements • Clinicians should always ask about rashes and skin changes

(*Continued*)

Table 3.3 (Continued)

Drug Mechanism	Dosing and Monitoring	Side Effects
Second-Generation Antipsychotics (SGAs)—*Block dopamine-2 (D2) receptors lowering DA neuronal activity.*	• Several, but not all, SGAs are approved to treat mania: ◦ Risperidone: 1–6mg/day ◦ Olanzapine: 5–20mg/day ◦ QuetiapineXR150: 800mg/day ◦ Ziprasidone: 40–80mg twice daily ◦ Aripiprazole: 5–30mg/day ◦ Asenapine: 5–10mg twice daily (sublingual) ◦ Cariprazine: 1.5–6mg/day • SGAs are associated with risks for increasing metabolic syndrome (elevated blood sugars, lipids, blood pressure, and weight). The first three agents listed above carry the greatest risk • Vitals should be monitored • Suggest baseline and follow-up monitoring of fasting blood glucose, lipids, and WBC (subtle risk of agranulocytosis) • EKG may be considered as ziprasidone can elevate QTc approximately 20 msec • SGAs all may create drug induced Parkinsonism, dystonia, akathisia (restlessness), or hyperthermia neuroleptic malignant syndrome. Permanent movement disorder (tardive dyskinesia TD) may occur over time as well. Monitoring frequently for new onset of these side effects is warranted and sometimes mandated (ex. AIMS testing for TD)	• The SGA class is quite varied regarding side effects • Typically, any SGA ending in a *-done, -ole, -zine* may carry more akathisia and extrapyramidal side effects • Those ending in *-pine* may be more sedating and weight gain prone • Patients often report some level of fatigue, headaches, and stomach upset

Practical Application

TIP: Mania Prescribing

- Treatment of mania = choose any of the above except lamotrigine
- Presence of psychosis = choose a SGA
- Treatment of severe mania = choose a SGA or divalproex as high initial loading dose strategies have been studied and are better tolerated than that of lithium or carbamazepine
- Lamotrigine is not an acute treatment but may be added to any of the above treatments to ideally delay or prevent future mania relapses

Patients in mania deserve solid monotherapy trials of successive agents. Dosing must be therapeutic, achieving adequate blood levels, or using full FDA dose range when levels are not defined. Guidelines support polypharmacy where two of the above agents are combined to stop resistant mania. Of course, patients who are grandiose and delusional will need an SGA. Non-psychotic patients may be started on any agent. If drugs are to be combined, two combined SGAs do not make sense as they all work by blocking dopamine-2 (D2) receptors, making this mechanism of drug action redundant. It would make clinical sense to add lithium or an anti-epileptic based anti-manic to the first SGA so there are complementary mechanisms of action instead of overlapping ones. This method has been termed rational polypharmacy by psychopharmacology expert Stephen Stahl.

Finally, an anti-manic may be chosen based on side effect profile. Obese patients or those with metabolic disease should not take risperidone, olanzapine, or quetiapine unless it is unavoidable. The more weight friendly option of carbamazepine (Equetro), divalproex (Depakote), or lithium may be considered, but the clinician should be aware that all of these agents are more or less weight gain prone. Those with pre-existing movement disorder may avoid SGAs. Those with renal or thyroid problems should not take lithium. Those with liver disease should not take divalproex (Depakote). Those with skin conditions should not take lithium, divalproex (Depakote), lamotrigine (Lamictal), or carbamazepine (Equetro).

Bipolar Depression Pharmacotherapy

Second-Generation Antipsychotics (SGA)

These drugs are fully discussed in the schizophrenia chapter. Many were initially approved for treating psychosis associated with schizophrenia. Secondarily, these drugs have also been found to halt mania as discussed above. Thirdly, many SGAs possess pharmacodynamic properties with antidepressant potential. Currently, there are 11 approved SGAs, of which only a few are approved to treat bipolar depression. The benefit here is that SGAs often possess the ability to stop or prevent mania and may also be able to treat depressive episodes. Unlike the use of unipolar SSRIs or SNRIs, these bipolar depressive agents have some built-in safety to help avoid escalating the depressed BD patient into a new mania episode via D2 receptor blockade. For warnings, side effects, and monitoring issues regarding SGAs, see the **Prescribing Table** above concerning mania pharmacotherapy or see the schizophrenia chapter.

TIP: Bipolar Depression Prescribing

- Olanzapine-Fluoxetine Combination (Symbyax) 6/25mg–12/50mg/day
- Quetiapine (Seroquel XR) 150–600mg/day
- Lurasidone (Latuda) 20–120mg/day
- Typically, lower doses of the SGA possess its antidepressant properties, while medium to high doses stop and prevent mania or psychosis. It is important to dose the SGA being used as an antidepressant in BD to the approved middle dose range in order to gain the anti-manic protection needed.

TIP: Bipolar Prescribing Off-Label Antidepressants

- Aggressive treatment is warranted for bipolar depression to prevent escalating the patient into mania, creation of mixed features, or rapid cycling.
- Data regarding antidepressant use in BD is controversial. If a formal unipolar antidepressant is used, it must be combined simultaneously with an anti-manic regimen already in place. Failure to use a mood stabilizer first is called unopposed antidepressant use, as there is no safety mechanism to prevent mania escalation as a side effect.
- If an antidepressant is used, consider removing it once depression remits, leaving just the mood stabilizing anti-manic agent in place as a monotherapy.
- Tricyclic antidepressants (TCAs) are the most likely class to worsen bipolar mood swings, and selective serotonin reuptake inhibitors (SSRIs) and norepinephrine-dopamine reuptake inhibitors (NDRIs) (bupropion [Wellbutrin XL]) possibly being the least likely.
- The most convincing evidence for the treatment of bipolar depression rests with SGAs.
- Lithium is not approved for bipolar depression but does have a reasonable evidence base for it to be used in bipolar depressed phases.
- Lamotrigine (Lamictal) is not approved for any acute bipolar state (depression/mania). It is approved for maintenance only and has some limited data for the treatment of depressive states.

TIP: Lamotrigine (Lamictal) as Maintenance Therapy

- It is typically added once another mood stabilizer has provided for a stable euthymic state or if the patient has gone into euthymia on their own.
- Needs to be titrated very slowly to avoid risk of serious rashes, making an acute antidepressant response unlikely.
- The goal is to lower the long-term frequency of mania and depression events. If lamotrigine does not decrease cycling over time, it should be stopped.
- Clinicians often like this agent as it may have the lowest risk of weight gain and cognitive dulling. It does not induce metabolic disorder, tardive dyskinesia, extrapyramidal symptoms, thyroid, parathyroid, or renal disease.
- Lithium, divalproex (Depakote), and some SGAs are also approved to be added in polypharmacy as maintenance drugs and may lower the frequency of future mania or depressive episodes as well.

TIP: Prescribing for Bipolar 2 (B2D) Disordered Patients

- It is better to treat all bipolar patients conservatively as if the patient is a bipolar 1 disorder (B1D) patient to prevent progression from a milder spectrum illness into a full clinical B1D diagnosis
- Additionally, some clinicians do prefer to use safer MDD antidepressants in those with milder (B2D) disorder. Again, there is risk of escalating the patient into full mania. Sometimes antidepressants create greater mood instability such as:
    - Rapid cycling—>4 mania or depressive episodes per year
    - Mixed features—3+ mania symptoms intruding upon a depressive episode

SECTION 2 Advanced Prescribing Practices

Introduction

In Section 1, the premise is to convince the reader that they must make an accurate diagnosis and pick an approved agent with well-defined dosing guidelines and expected clinical outcomes. This approach is largely one of pattern recognition: (1) identify the pattern of phenotypic symptoms, (2) choose from a finite list of available, proven effective drugs, (3) start dosing low and escalate through an approved dosing range, (4) assess for effectiveness, and (5) continue medication if effective or cross-titrate to a new drug if ineffective or not tolerated. This methodical and mathematical approach can improve the standard of care and, ideally, patient outcomes when treated by the novice psychopharmacologist.

Section 2 is designed to provide a greater depth of neuroscience and pharmacodynamic knowledge to the reader and is written for prescribers who are knowledgeable and competent in those skills outlined in Section 1. The section is generally intended for those patients who are felt to be treatment resistant and comorbid with other disorders.

Epidemiology

- Bipolar disorder (BD) is thought to have a clinical onset in the second or third decade of life and is hallmarked by the onset of a hypomanic or manic episode.
- In retrospect, many patients often experience a depressive or anxiety disorder starting in their teens.
- Sometimes these early depressive disorders will have a few (hypo)mania symptoms buried within suggesting a depressive disorder with mixed features.
- BD is generally considered to be a disorder where a relapsing and recurring illness course is expected.
- Approximately 1% of the U.S. population suffers from classic bipolar 1 disorder (B1D) and higher for type 2 bipolar disorder (B2D).

Genetics

- B1D is one of the most heritable psychiatric disorders (60–85%).
- There is no single gene that causes BD.
- Strongest evidence supports possible genetic vulnerabilities in certain genes (ex. DAOA(G72), BDNF, ANK3, and CACNA1C) when compared to non-bipolar patients.
- Many of these genes convey risks by way of altering dopamine metabolism, interneuronal growth and connectivity, and neuronal membrane excitability.
- Serotonin and norepinephrine neurotransmission risk genes have been identified as well.

TIP: Genetic Risk and Symptom Development

- Many genes code for many central nervous system (CNS) proteins that, when each mutated, creates a subtle risk for the development of certain BD symptoms, i.e., grandiosity versus dangerous impulsivity.
- As genetic risks build, more brain neurocircuitry malfunction occurs and more phenotypic, externally noticeable symptoms may develop.
- Theoretically, a patient inherits genes from both parents, called *a genotype*. If a gene is mutated, it often yields an abnormal protein.
- These proteins might be enzymes, receptors, ion channels, etc. If enough of these function improperly in the brain, it may cause hyperfunctioning or hypofunctioning within or between certain brain areas that may be able to be detected with neuroimaging (ex. fMRI or PET scans), called *an endophenotype*.
- This alteration in brain neurocircuitry function may lead to specific psychiatric symptoms that can be detected by interviewing (ex. distractibility, talkativeness, goal directed hyperactivity, elevated mood).
- These outward symptoms that the DSM-5 is based upon are considered the patient's *phenotype*.

Neuroanatomy

- Early in the course of BD there are findings of abnormal fronto-cortical, striatal (caudate, putamen, nucleus accumbens, olfactory tubercle), and amygdala activity.
- After repeated and chronic cycling, other functional neuroanatomic abnormalities may be seen. Generally speaking, there appears to be frontal lobe volume loss (left side > right side) and a hypofunctioning of advanced prefrontal cortical structures.
- The subgenual prefrontal cortex is associated with higher mood functioning, and this is observed to be smaller in bipolar patients when compared to controls.
- Further, there is often a volume increase and hyperactivity in the deeper, limbic system structures (amygdala, anterior striatum, thalamus).

Neuroscientific Background and Rationale for Medication Use

In treating bipolar mania, there are three families of medications that are often utilized to treat mania and three families for treating depression. (**See Prescribing Table.**)

TIP: Bipolar Prescribing

- For mania consider:
  - Lithium
  - Anti-epileptic Drugs (AEDs)
    - Carbamazepine (Equetro)
    - Divalproex (Depakote)
    - Lamotrigine (Lamictal) (for maintenance only)
  - Second-Generation Antipsychotics (SGAs)
    - Risperidone (Risperdal), olanzapine (Zyprexa), quetiapine (Seroquel XR), ziprasidone (Geodon), aripiprazole (Abilify), asenapine (Saphris), cariprazine (Vraylar)
- For depression consider:
  - Second-Generation Antipsychotics (SGAs)
    - Olanzapine/fluoxetine combination (Symbyax), quetiapine (Seroquel XR), lurasidone (Latuda)
  - Lithium
  - Antidepressants are off-label
    - SSRI (fluoxetine [Prozac], sertraline [Zoloft], paroxetine [Paxil], escitalopram [Celexa/Lexapro])
    - NDRI (bupropion [Wellbutrin XL])

1) Lithium

MECHANISM OF ACTION

Lithium

- Largely unknown, but used to treat both manic and depressed states in BD.
- Thought to stabilize neuronal membranes (calcium inositol pathway) thus reducing hyperactive firing rates perhaps in the limbic system thus lowering mania.
- May downregulate the serotonin-1a receptor (5HT-1a) with a downstream effect of elevating CNS serotonin (5HT) for mood elevation and depression treatment.
- Has ability to improve neuronal health, growth factors, and connectivity between brain areas associated with affective dysfunction.
- Interestingly, lithium also has specific regulatory language that it may lower suicidality in B1D patients.

2) Mood Stabilizers (AEDs)

MECHANISM OF ACTION

Divalproex (Depakote), carbamazepine (Equetro), lamotrigine (Lamictal)

- Typically, AEDs may lower mania but are often minimally effective for the treatment of bipolar depressed states.
- Carbamazepine is one of the initially studied agents and is thought to lower neuronal firing by blocking sodium channels. In the cortex this may lower tonic-clonic seizure activity. This activity in the limbic system may possibly lower mania.
- Lamotrigine also has the ability to block sodium channels. It is also purported to dampen glutamate activity as another way to lower abnormally elevated neuronal firing. It may antagonize 5HT-3 receptors which could passively increase cortical monoamines further downstream. This drug is not approved for manic or depressive states but for maintenance, decreasing cycling in either direction.
- Divalproex may increase the synthesis of GABA. Increases in GABA neurotransmission may also have a dampening effect on mania-induced hyperactive limbic structures. It may also lower glutamate neuronal firing by inhibiting NMDA receptors.
- Some AEDs do not treat mania and did fail in regulatory trials (ex. lamotrigine [Lamictal], topiramate [Topamax], gabapentin [Neurontin]).
- Clonazepam (Klonopin) is a benzodiazepine (BZ) and is both an AED and an anxiolytic. It has limited data as a monotherapy but some positive trials as an augmentation approach for more refractory mania.

3) Second-Generation Antipsychotics (SGA)

MECHANISM OF ACTION

Risperidone (Risperdal), olanzapine (Zyprexa), quetiapine (Seroquel XR), ziprasidone (Geodon), aripiprazole (Abilify), asenapine (Saphris), cariprazine (Vraylar)

- Regarding mania, all of these agents block the D2 receptor and, in the limbic system, this should restore a lower, more normal activity, thus alleviating mania. All SGAs have this effect, but the above drugs have approval and indication for mania.

- All first-generation antipsychotics (FGAs) (ex. haloperidol [Haldol], fluphenazine [Prolixin]) also effectively antagonize D2 and may stop mania.

Olanzapine/fluoxetine Combination (Symbyax), quetiapine (Seroquel XR), lurasidone (Latuda)

- Antidepressant effects are more complicated and varied across the SGAs.
- All of these block 5HT-2a serotonin receptors, which is a purported mechanism of antidepressant action for the approved unipolar antidepressants trazodone (Desyrel), nefazodone (Serzone), and mirtazapine (Remeron). Activity here may improve both serotonergic and noradrenergic functioning to lower depressive symptomatology.
- Quetiapine and lurasidone seem to have more activity in partially agonizing the 5HT-1a receptor. This activity may initially lower serotonin activity but ultimately causes downregulation of this autoreceptor and then a resultant robust increase in serotonin neuronal firing. This activity is employed by the antidepressants vilazodone (Viibryd) and vortioxetine (Trintellix) and the anxiolytic buspirone (BuSpar).
- Lurasidone may be unique in its robust activity to block the 5HT-7 receptor. This activity is felt to improve cognitive symptoms and circadian symptoms of depression.
- Finally, quetiapine may be unique in that it has potent norepinephrine reuptake pump blocking activity/inhibition (NRI). This is an antidepressant mechanism utilized by the NDRI bupropion (Wellbutrin XL) and serotonin-norepinephrine reuptake inhibitors (SNRI), including venlafaxine (Effexor XR) and duloxetine (Cymbalta) and many of the TCAs.
- From an off-label perspective, it is unclear if other SGAs possess antidepressant properties that may be useful in BD.
  - Risperidone (Risperdal) has a positive trial in unipolar depression.
  - Ziprasidone (Geodon) has a small positive trial in BD depression.
  - Aripiprazole (Abilify) and brexpiprazole (Rexulti) have approvals for major depressive disorder (MDD) as an augmentation strategy.
  - Asenapine (Saphris) is under investigation for BD depression and has many similarities to the unipolar antidepressant mirtazapine (Remeron).

Table 3.4 Prescribing Table for Bipolar Disorder

Drugs listed in BOLD are approved agents. Approved dosing guidelines should be further referenced by the prescriber.						
1. Lithium						
Brand	Generic	Indication (Bold for FDA Approved)	Drug Mechanism	Dosing Tips	Monitoring Tips	Medicolegal Tips
Lithium						
Eskalith **Lithobid** **Lithostat**	**Lithium carbonate**	• **Mania** • **Maintenance** • **Bipolar depression**	• **May stabilize neuronal membranes, reducing limbic firing rates** • **Downregulates serotonin-5HT-1a receptors** • **May promote monoamine synthesis and availability in CNS** • **Improves neuronal health, growth factors, and connectivity**	• **Acute mania: usual dose is 600–1800mg/day in divided doses initially** • **Maintenance: usual dose may be lowered and converted to once daily** • **Increase dose 300mg every 4–5 days**	• **Common initial side effects include increased thirst and urination, tremor, GI side effects** • **Other notable side effects include acne, psoriasis, weight gain** • **Serious side effects include lithium toxicity, thyroid and kidney dysfunction, lymphocytosis, arrhythmia** • **Monitor blood levels 4–5 days after dose increases (steady state), then annually** • **Therapeutic trough plasma levels should be 0.8–1.2mEq/l for acute mania and 0.6–1.2mEq/l for maintenance** • **Monitor EKG, CBC, TSH, CRE, calcium at baseline, after titration and then annually**	• **Clearly explain life-threatening toxicity, drug interactions, and side effects** • **Should be discontinued before pregnancies (risk category D) due to evidence of increased risk of birth defects and cardiac anomalies (Ebstein's anomaly)** • **Drug interactions include the use of concomitant NSAIDS or diuretics that may increase lithium levels.** • **Can be lethal in suicidal overdose**

(*Continued*)

Table 3.4 (Continued)

2. Anti-epileptic Drugs (AEDs)

Brand	Generic	Indication (Bold for FDA Approved)	Drug Mechanism	Dosing Tips	Monitoring Tips	Medicolegal Tips
Sodium Channel Blockers						
Equetro **Tegretol**	**Carbamazepine**	• **Acute mania/ mixed features** • Maintenance	• Blocks voltage sensitive sodium channels and dampens excessive neuronal firing	• Usual dose is 200–800 mg twice daily • Increase 200mg every few days	• Common initial side effects include sedation, GI side effects, ataxia, tremor, dysarthria • Serious side effects include serious rashes, aplastic anemia, agranulocytosis, SIADH. Monitor at baseline, after titration and then annually for CBC and differential. Trough blood levels should be between 8–12mg/dl	• Clearly explain life-threatening or serious side effects (e.g., rash, blood dyscrasia, 3A4 interactions) • Should be discontinued before pregnancies (risk category D) due to evidence of increased risk of birth defects (neural tube defects) • CYP3A4 hepatic inducer will lower plasma levels of many other drugs
Trileptal	Oxcarbazepine	• Acute mania/ mixed features • Maintenance	• Blocks voltage sensitive sodium channels and dampens excessive neuronal firing	• Usual dose is 150–1200mg twice daily • Increase 150mg twice daily every few days	• Common initial side effects include sedation, GI side effects, ataxia, tremor, dysarthria • Serious side effects include serious rashes, aplastic anemia, agranulocytosis, SIADH • Monitoring for blood dyscrasias may not be warranted	• Clearly explain life-threatening or serious side effects (e.g., rash, blood dyscrasia) • Should be discontinued before pregnancies (risk category D) due to evidence of increased risk of birth defects (neural tube defects)

Lamictal **Lamictal XR**	**Lamotrigine**	• **Maintenance** • Bipolar depression • Bipolar mania	• Blocks voltage sensitive sodium channels and dampens excessive neuronal firing • May dampen glutamatergic activity	• Usual dose is 25–200mg/day as monotherapy • Start at 25mg/day for two weeks, increase to 50mg/day for 2 weeks, increase to 100mg/day for 2 weeks and then to 200mg/day at week 6. Must follow exactly • Any 5 day period of missed doses must retitrate	• Common side effects include headache, sedation, GI side effects, tremor, ataxia, weight gain • Serious side effects include serious rash, increased suicidality • Monitor for rashes. Must be discontinued for any rash	• Clearly explain life-threatening or serious side effects (e.g., rash) • Should be discontinued before pregnancies (risk category C) • Dosing must be changed if used in conjunction with divalproex and carbamazepine
GABA Enhancing Agents						
Depakote **Depakote ER**	**Divalproex**	• **Acute mania and mixed episodes** • **Maintenance**	• Increases CNS GABA tone	• Usual dose is 250mg–500mg 3 times a day • Increase by 250–500mg every few weeks for outpatient • For inpatient, may load at 20mg/kg	• Common side effects include sedation, diarrhea, ataxia, tremor • Serious side effects include hepatotoxicity, pancreatitis, thrombocytopenia, polycystic ovarian syndrome, rashes, and activation of suicidality • Monitor for blood levels and obtain 50–125mg/dl • Monitor liver, pancreas, and platelet function prior and during treatment	• Must monitor labs at baseline and then throughout use of this medication to avoid end-organ damage • Provide informed consent about these prior to treatment

(*Continued*)

Table 3.4 (Continued)

Klonopin	Clonazepam	• Adjunct for acute mania	• Binds to benzodiazepine receptors on GABA-receptors and enhances chloride channel activity and neuronal hyperpolarization	• Usual dosing is 0.25–4mg/day • Increase 0.25–0.5mg every few days	• Common side effects include sedation, psychomotor impairment, cognitive slowing • Serious side effects include respiratory suppression, addiction • Monitor pill counts, controlled drug databases, consider urine drug screens	• Clearly explain life-threatening or serious side effects (e.g., respiratory suppression and addiction) • Should be discontinued before pregnancies (risk category D) • Should not be used in patients with addictive histories

3. Second-Generation Antipsychotics (SGAs)

Brand	Generic	Indication (Bold for FDA Approved)	Drug Mechanism	Dosing Tips	Monitoring Tips	Medicolegal Tips
Second-Generation Antipsychotics						
Risperdal	**Risperidone**	• **Acute mania/mixed mania** • **Maintenance** • Bipolar depression	• Blocks dopamine 2 receptors reducing psychosis and stabilizing mania • Blocks serotonin 2A receptors which may improve depression	• Usual dose is 0.25–6mg/day • Maximum daily dose is 16mg/day • For more severe mania load at 2–3mg/day and increase 1mg every few days	• Common initial side effects include dizziness, sedation, headache, GI side effects • Serious side effects include risk of diabetes, hyperlipidemia, hypertension, weight gain, transient and permanent neuromuscular side effects, hyperlipidemia, gynecomastia, agranulocytosis, increased risk of death in demented elderly, increased suicidality • Monitor at baseline and at least annually with CBC Diff, BMP, Lipid Panel. Also conduct more routine weight and vital signs, AIMS tests or physical exam for EPS/TD neuromuscular symptoms	• Clearly explain life-threatening or serious side effects (e.g., TD/EPS, metabolic side effects) • Provide treatments if side effects occur (e.g., weight loss agents, antiparkinson agents) • Risk of weight gain and metabolics is high • Risk of EPS is high

Zyprexa Symbyax	**Olanzapine, olanzapine/ fluoxetine**	• **Acute mania/ mixed mania** • **Maintenance** • **Bipolar depression in combination with fluoxetine** • **Agitation**	• Blocks dopamine 2 receptors reducing psychosis and stabilizing mania • Blocks serotonin 2A receptors which may improve depression	• Usual mania dose is 2.5–20mg/day • Increase by 5mg every few days • For more severe mania may load 10–15mg/day • Usual depression dose (olanzapine mg/ fluoxetine mg) is 3/25–12/50, increasing by 3/25 every few weeks • For combative agitation, 10mg IM q 2–4 hrs with max 30mg/day with warning NOT TO MIX WITH SEDATIVES	• Same as above	• Clearly explain life-threatening or serious side effects (e.g., TD/ EPS, metabolic side effects) • Provide treatments if side effects occur (e.g., weight loss agents, antiparkinson agents) • Considered one of the most metabolic syndrome inducing agents • Sedation risk is moderate • Risk of EPS is high

(*Continued*)

Table 3.4 (Continued)

Seroquel (XR)	**Quetiapine**	• **Acute mania** • **Maintenance** • **Bipolar depression**	• Blocks dopamine 2 receptors reducing psychosis and stabilizing mania • Blocks serotonin 2A receptors which may improve depression • Has potent NRI and 5HT-1a agonism as antidepressant properties (metabolite norquetiapine)	• Dosing is 25–400mg twice daily and for XR is 50–800mg/day • May load for severe mania within 4 days to 400mg or XR may load at 300mg • Depression dosing is 25–600mg or 50–600mg, respectively, and both can be given once nightly	• Same as above but increased risk of cataracts • Monitoring is same and consider optometry for cataract warning	• Clearly explain life-threatening or serious side effects (e.g., TD/EPS, metabolic side effects) • Provide treatment if side effects occur (e.g., weight loss agents, antiparkinson agents) • Considered one of the most metabolic syndrome inducing agents • Risk of weight gain and metabolics is high • Risk of sedation is high • Risk of EPS/TD is lowest in SGA class

Geodon	**Ziprasidone**	• **Acute mania/ mixed mania** • **Maintenance** • Bipolar depression • Agitation	• Blocks dopamine 2 receptors reducing psychosis and stabilizing mania • Blocks serotonin 2A receptors which may improve depression • Has mild SNRI and 5HT-1a agonism as antidepressant properties	• Must be taken with food • Usual dose is 20–80mg twice daily • May increase 20–40mg every few days for mania, every few weeks for depression • For severe mania, may escalate to 80mg twice daily on day 2 • For agitation in schizophrenia it may be used intramuscular 10mg q 2 hr with 40mg/day max	• Common initial side effects include dizziness, sedation, headache, GI side effects, akathisia • Serious side effects include risk of diabetes, hyperlipidemia, hypertension, weight gain, transient and permanent neuromuscular side effects, hyperlipidemia, gynecomastia, agranulocytosis, increased risk of death in demented elderly, increased suicidality, cardiac QTc prolongation • Monitor at baseline and at least annually with CBC Diff, BMP, Lipid Panel. Also conduct more routine weight and vital signs, AIMS tests or physical exam for EPS/ TD neuromuscular symptoms, and consider baseline EKG and after titration for those at cardiac risk	• Clearly explain life-threatening or serious side effects (e.g., TD/ EPS, metabolic side effects) • Provide treatment if side effects occur (e.g., weight loss agents, antiparkinson agents) • Considered one of the least metabolic syndrome inducing agents • Sedation risk is moderate • Akathisia rates are moderate

(*Continued*)

Table 3.4 (Continued)

Abilify	**Aripiprazole**	• **Acute mania/ mixed mania** • **Maintenance** • **Agitation**	• Partially agonizes D2 and D3 receptors which may improve affect • Net effect may also block dopamine 2 receptors reducing psychosis and stabilizing mania • Blocks serotonin 2A receptors which may improve depression • Has 5HT-1a agonism as antidepressant properties	• Usual dose is 2–30mg/day • May increase 2–5mg every few days • For severe mania may load at 15mg/day and increase to 30mg on day 2 or 3 • Start 10–15mg/day. Maximum daily dose is 30mg/day • Intramuscular for agitation is 9.75–15mg q 2hr, max 30mg/day • Drug is a substrate for CYP2D6 and must be halved if 2D6 inhibitor concomitantly taken	• Same as above but EKG monitoring is not needed	• Clearly explain life-threatening or serious side effects (e.g., TD/EPS, metabolic side effects) • Provide treatment if side effects occur (e.g., weight loss agents, antiparkinson agents) • Risk of weight gain and metabolics is moderate • Risk of sedation is moderate • Risk of akathisia is high

Rexulti	Brexpiprazole	• Schizophrenia • Major depression augmentation • Agitation/ anxiety	• Partially agonizes D2 and D3 receptors which may improve affect • Net effect may also block dopamine 2 receptors reducing psychosis, stabilizing mania and allowing a calming effect • Blocks serotonin 2A receptors which may improve depression • Has 5HT-1a agonism similar to SPA anxiolytics (buspirone)	• Usual dose is 0.25–4mg/day • May increase 0.5–1mg every few weeks • Drug is a substrate for CYP2D6 and must be halved if 2D6 inhibitor concomitantly taken	• Same as above though akathisia rates are much lower	• Clearly explain life-threatening or serious side effects (e.g., TD/ EPS, metabolic side effects) • Provide treatment if side effects occur (e.g., weight loss agents, antiparkinson agents) • Risk of weight gain and metabolics is moderate • Risk of sedation is moderate • Risk of akathisia is moderate

(*Continued*)

Table 3.4 (Continued)

Vraylar	**Cariprazine**	• **Acute mania/ mixed mania** • **Maintenance** • **Agitation/ anxiety**	• Partially agonizes D2 and D3 receptors which may improve affect • Net effect may also block dopamine 2 receptors reducing psychosis, stabilizing mania, and allowing a calming effect • Blocks serotonin 2A receptors which may improve depression • Has 5HT-1a agonism similar to SPA anxiolytics (buspirone)	• Usual dose is 1.5–6mg/day • May increase 1.5mg every few weeks	• Same as above	• Clearly explain life-threatening or serious side effects (e.g., TD/ EPS, metabolic side effects) • Provide treatment if side effects occur (e.g., weight loss agents, antiparkinson agents) • Risk of weight gain and metabolics is moderate • Risk of sedation is moderate • Risk of akathisia is high

Saphris	**Asenapine**	• **Acute mania/ mixed mania** • Depression	• Blocks dopamine 2 receptors reducing psychosis and stabilizing mania • Blocks serotonin 2A receptors which may improve depression • Has similar antidepressant theoretical properties to mirtazapine (alpha-2 antagonism, 5HT-2c,3 antagonism)	• Usual dose is 5–10 mg twice daily • May load dose at 10mg twice daily for severe mania • It is taken sublingually (SL) or will not be absorbed	• Common initial side effects include taste bud dysfunction, dizziness, sedation, headache, GI side effects • Serious side effects include risk of diabetes, hyperlipidemia, hypertension, weight gain, transient and permanent neuromuscular side effects, hyperlipidemia, gynecomastia, agranulocytosis, increased risk of death in demented elderly, increased suicidality • Monitor at baseline and at least annually with CBC Diff, BMP, Lipid Panel. Also conduct more routine weight and vital signs, AIMS tests or physical exam for EPS/TD neuromuscular symptoms	• Clearly explain life-threatening or serious side effects (e.g., TD/ EPS, metabolic side effects) • Provide treatment if side effects occur (e.g., weight loss agents, antiparkinson agents) • Risk of weight gain and metabolics is mild to moderate • Risk of sedation is moderate

(Continued)

Table 3.4 (Continued)

Invega	Paliperidone	• Acute mania/ mixed mania • Maintenance	• Blocks dopamine 2 receptors reducing psychosis and stabilizing mania • Blocks serotonin 2A receptors which may improve depression	• Dosing is 3–12mg/day • May increase 3mg every few days	• Same as above	• Clearly explain life-threatening or serious side effects (e.g., TD/ EPS, metabolic side effects) • Provide treatments if side effects occur (e.g., weight loss agents, antiparkinson agents) • Risk of weight gain and metabolics is moderate • Risk of EPS is high

Fanapt	Iloperidone	• Acute mania/ mixed mania • Bipolar maintenance	• Blocks dopamine 2 receptors reducing psychosis and stabilizing mania • Blocks serotonin 2A receptors which may improve depression	• Usual dose is 12–24mg/day in 2 divided doses • Due to high hypotension risk, start at 2mg in 2 divided doses on day 1 and increase to 4mg on day 2, 8mg on day 3, 12mg on day 4, 16mg on day 5, 20mg on day 6, and 24mg on day 7, all on divided doses. Maximum daily dose is 32mg/ day	• Same as above and consider EKG monitoring for QTc prolongation and after titration for those at cardiac risk	• Clearly explain life-threatening or serious side effects (e.g., TD/ EPS, metabolic side effects) • Provide treatment if side effects occur (e.g., weight loss agents, antiparkinson agents) • Risk of weight gain and metabolics is moderate • Risk of sedation is moderate • Risk of orthostasis may be highest in class • Akathisia rates are low

(*Continued*)

Table 3.4 (Continued)

Latuda	**Lurasidone**	• **Bipolar depression** • **Mixed features** • Mania	• Blocks dopamine 2 receptors reducing psychosis and stabilizing affective symptoms • Blocks serotonin 2A receptors which promotes dopamine release that improves cognitive and affective symptoms without marked EPS • Blocks serotonin-7 receptors which may improve cognition and circadian rhythm • Partially agonizes serotonin-1a receptors to treat depression	• Usual dose is 20–120mg/day for bipolar depression • Must be taken with food to absorb • May increase 20–40mg every few weeks	• Same as above but does not include EKG monitoring	• Clearly explain life-threatening or serious side effects (e.g., TD/EPS, metabolic side effects) • Provide treatment if side effects occur (e.g., weight loss agents, antiparkinson agents) • Risk of weight gain and metabolics is minimal • Risk of sedation is low

Practical Applications

Good Polypharmacy to Be Used to Gain Remission in Resistant Patients

DO

- Start low dose to minimize side effects.
- May use a loading dose/high dose at initiation strategy for severe mania or psychotic mania for most AED and SGA mania treatments.
- Escalate dosing within full range for optimal effectiveness. Again, escalate more slowly for better tolerability in outpatients and faster for greater symptom control in inpatients.
- Monitor for weight gain, skin changes, abnormal movements, and end-organ damage.
- Add drugs from different anti-manic classes for treatment-resistant cases or improved maintenance.
    - Lithium + AED or SGA
    - AED + SGA
    - Lithium + AED + SGA
- Escalate to higher doses with caution and maximize within normal blood levels.
- Check blood levels of any drug to confirm compliance.

DON'T

- Add two SGAs together for mania.
- Add two sodium channel blocking AEDs together for mania.
- Add an unopposed antidepressant without proper prior mood stabilizer titration.

Good Polypharmacy to Be Used to Gain Remission in Comorbid Patients

Bipolar + ADHD

- **Use of NDRI:** bupropion (Wellbutrin XL)
- **Use of NRI:** atomoxetine (Strattera)
- **Use second-generation antipsychotic (SGA) augmentation:** aripiprazole (Abilify), brexpiprazole (Rexulti), cariprazine (Vraylar) (has partial dopamine receptor 2/3 agonism), quetiapine (Seroquel XR) (has potent NRI)
- **Use of stimulant medication** (ex. amphetamine [Adderall XR], methylphenidate [Concerta]). There is risk of mania escalation but this is felt to be lower than that antidepressant use.

Bipolar + Anxiety Disorder

- **Use of SSRI:** fluoxetine (Prozac), sertraline (Zoloft), paroxetine (Paxil), citalopram (Celexa), escitalopram (Lexapro) only after mood stabilization.
- **Use of BZ:** alprazolam (Xanax XR), clonazepam (Klonopin). These have no risk of worsening mania in BD and may be considered more front line unless addiction is also a comorbid condition.
- **Use alpha-2 agonists:** guanfacine (Tenex), clonidine (Catapres).
- **Use of antihistamine (H1 receptor antagonist):** hydroxyzine (Vistaril/ Atarax).
- **Avoid use of SNRIs, TCAs, MAOIs due to potential higher risk of mania escalation**

Bipolar + Schizophrenia (Schizoaffective) Disorder

- Use second-generation antipsychotic (SGA) monotherapy.
- If remaining affective symptoms, may utilize strategies listed throughout this chapter to better control residual mania or depression.

Bipolar + Borderline Personality

- Use second-generation antipsychotic (SGA) monotherapy or anti-epileptic drug (AED) monotherapy.
- If remaining affective symptoms, may utilize strategies listed throughout this chapter to better control residual mania or depression.
- SSRIs may be helpful but likely have lowest effect sizes.

TIP: Bipolar Depression Prescribing

- Use of approved SGAs as monotherapy is the gold standard, frontline approach.
- Use of SSRI or NDRI augmentation to Lithium, SGAs, or AEDs may be considered.
    - Consider removing antidepressant several weeks after depression remits.
    - Monitor for induction of rapid cycling or mixed features.
    - Use low doses, titrate slowly.
- N-acetyl cysteine (NAC) may be considered at 1000mg twice daily as a complementary alternative medication (CAM) augmentation as well.
- Pramipexole (Mirapex) up to 5mg/day may help more resistant depressions.
- Modafinil (Provigil) and armodafinil (Nuvigil) have a reasonable evidence base for use.
- Most AEDs will not treat depression. Lamotrigine has controversial data and may take many weeks to see an effect.

Final Advanced Prescribing Thoughts

Comorbidity is key. If a patient has three or four psychiatric conditions, you may not need three or four medications if you plan wisely and spend time understanding the transmitter and receptor profiles that are unique to each psychotropic. Alternatively, you could use a polypharmacy approach whereby each diagnostic entity gets its own medication.

It should also be clear to the reader that there is often more than one guideline-based answer to each clinical question or scenario. There are often one or two wrong ways to treat a patient pharmacologically, but within each case at certain critical points a clinician can choose wisely among several reasonable protocols.

For example, one can err on the side of aggressive, sequential monotherapeutic approaches, especially if the prescriber can keep track of FDA approvals and indications, the availability and knowledge of stringent drug trials, and possibly by knowing the pharmacodynamic nuances of the monotherapy at hand. Alternatively, one can add drugs together in rational polypharmacy. Use of drugs that are FDA approved for each specific condition makes intuitive sense. Off-label and theoretical prescribing is also warranted in more resistant and refractory cases.

Misdiagnosis of addiction, anxiety, and personality disorder as being BD is common. Missed diagnosis of mixed features is common. BD commonly has psychiatric comorbidity. Accurate diagnoses and aggressive psychopharmacology as noted above is paramount. Depressed BD states are more common, clinically harder to treat, and are more risky for worsening of symptoms. Prescribers should try to treat depression in BD while keeping close observation for the onset of mixed features or (hypo)manic activation.

Bibliography

Altman, E. G., Hedeker, D., Peterson, J. L., & Davis, J. M. (1997) "The Altman self-rating mania scale." *Biological Psychiatry* 42(10), 948–955.

American Psychiatric Association. (2013) *Diagnostic and Statistical Manual of Mental Disorders: DSM-5*. Washington, D.C.: American Psychiatric Association.

Compton, M. T. & Nemeroff, C. B. (2000) "The treatment of bipolar depression." *Journal of Clinical Psychiatry* 61(9), 57–67.

Craddock, N., O'Donovan, M. C., & Owen, M. J. (2005) "The genetics of schizophrenia and bipolar disorder: dissecting psychosis." *Journal of Medical Genetics* 42(3), 193–204.

Ferreira, M. A., O'Donovan, M. C., Meng, Y. A., Jones, I. R., Ruderfer, D. M., Jones, L., & Farmer, A. (2008) "Collaborative genome-wide association analysis supports a role for ANK3 and CACNA1C in bipolar disorder." *Nature Genetics* 40(9), 1056–1058.

Geddes, J. R., Calabrese, J. R., & Goodwin, G. M. (2009) "Lamotrigine for treatment of bipolar depression: independent meta-analysis and meta-regression of individual patient data from five randomised trials." *The British Journal of Psychiatry* 194(1), 4–9.

Gijsman, H. J., Geddes, J. R., Rendell, J. M., Nolen, W. A., & Goodwin, G. M. (2014) "Antidepressants for bipolar depression: a systematic review of randomized, controlled trials." *American Journal of Psychiatry* 161(9), 1537–1547.

Grant, B. F., Stinson, F. S., Hasin, D. S., Dawson, D. A., Chou, S. P., Ruan, W., & Huang, B. (2005) "Prevalence, correlates, and comorbidity of bipolar I disorder and axis I and II disorders: results from the National Epidemiologic Survey on Alcohol and Related Conditions." *Journal of Clinical Psychiatry* 66(10), 1205–1215.

Hirschfeld, R. M., Williams, J. B., Spitzer, R. L., Calabrese, J. R., Flynn, L., Keck Jr., P. E., & Zajecka, J. (2000) "Development and validation of a screening instrument for bipolar spectrum disorder: The Mood Disorder Questionnaire." *American Journal of Psychiatry* 157(11), 1873–1875.

Keck, Jr., P. E., & McElroy, S. L. (2002) "Clinical pharmacodynamics and pharmacokinetics of antimanic and mood-stabilizing medications." *Journal of Clinical Psychiatry* 63(4), 3–11.

Manning, J. S. (2010) "Tools to improve differential diagnosis of bipolar disorder in primary care." *Primary Care Companion to the Journal of Clinical Psychiatry* 12(1), 17.

Merikangas, K. R., Akiskal, H. S., Angst, J., Greenberg, P. E., Hirschfeld, R. M., Petukhova, M., & Kessler, R. C. (2007) "Lifetime and 12-month prevalence of bipolar spectrum disorder in the National Comorbidity Survey replication." *Archives of General Psychiatry* 64(5), 543–552.

Psychiatric Times. (2014) "Tipsheet: Bipolar Depression Versus Unipolar Depression." www.psychiatrictimes.com/bipolar-disorder/tipsheet-bipolar-depression-versus-unipolar-depression#sthash.kkVluz1y.dpuf.

Smoller, J. W., & Finn, C. T. (2003) "Family, twin, and adoption studies of bipolar disorder." *American Journal of Medical Genetics Part C: Seminars in Medical Genetics* 123(1), 48–58.

Stahl, S. M. (2003) "Deconstructing psychiatric disorders, part 1: Genotypes, symptom phenotypes, and endophenotypes." *Journal of Clinical Psychiatry* 64(9), 982–983.

Stahl, S. M. (2003) "Deconstructing psychiatric disorders, part 2: An emerging, neurobiologically based therapeutic strategy for the modern psychopharmacologist." *Journal of Clinical Psychiatry* 64(10), 1145–1152.

Stahl, S. M. (2012) "Antipsychotic polypharmacy: never say never, but never say always." *Acta Psychiatrica Scandinavica* 125(5), 349–351.

Strakowski, S. M., Delbello, M. P., & Adler, C. M. (2005). "The functional neuroanatomy of bipolar disorder: a review of neuroimaging findings." *Molecular Psychiatry* 10(1), 105–116.

Yatham, L. N., Kennedy, S. H., Schaffer, A., Parikh, S. V., Beaulieu, S., O'Donovan, C., & Kapczinski, F. (2009) "Canadian Network for Mood and Anxiety Treatments (CANMAT) and International Society for Bipolar Disorders (ISBD) collaborative update of CANMAT guidelines for the management of patients with bipolar disorder: update 2009." *Bipolar Disorders* 11(3), 225–255.

CHAPTER 4

Borderline Personality Disorder

SECTION 1 Basic Prescribing Practices

Essential Concepts

- There are no approvals or regulatory studies that guide us toward choosing a psychotropic to treat borderline personality disorder (BPD).
- Psychotherapy is often considered the treatment of choice and clinicians should aim to avoid overmedicating BPD patients.
- Self-injurious behaviors (SIB) tend to alert the clinician toward the diagnosis of BPD. These may be confused with suicide attempts (SA).
- BPD often presents with comorbid psychopathology, especially PTSD (56%), PD (48%), GAD, and substance use disorders (SUD) (64%).
- Clinicians often easily detect these other psychiatric disorders but either miss or make a very delayed diagnosis of BPD, unless the BPD severity is high with very apparent SIB activity.
- BPD has more abrupt, labile mood swings that can easily be confused with the sustained manic and depressive episodes of bipolar disorder (BD).
- Pharmacotherapy is aimed at lowering mood lability, aggression, SIB, depression, impulsivity, or quasi-psychotic/dissociative symptoms.
- Finally, it should be noted that BPD patients will have a 40% greater likelihood of carrying at least three other psychiatric diagnoses at the time of evaluation. When meeting a patient who appears to have much psychiatric comorbidity, the index of suspicion for an ultimate BPD diagnosis should be elevated.

Phenomenology, Diagnosis, Clinical Interviewing

BPD patients often present to busy emergency rooms, primary practice offices, or psychopharmacological practices. They appear distressed and may be seen as difficult to office staff, medical assistants, and clinicians. These patients have chronic maladaptive coping skills and interpersonal difficulty causing them to clearly meet DSM-5 criteria for a depressive or anxiety disorder, and they are often started on SSRIs. These diagnoses are felt to be the "tip of the iceberg," and symptoms are usually triggered by interpersonal or environmental crises. (See figure below for the base of the iceberg.) If the clinician is pressed for time and does not investigate a social history or illicit a longitudinal history comparing the timeline of depressive spells versus interpersonal stressors, then the diagnosis of BPD will likely be missed unless there is a finding of excessive SIB (cutting) that is detected on a physical exam. If attention is not given to the social history, including investigating relationships with parents, peers, or employers, then the BPD diagnosis is likely to be missed. These patients generally have problems relating to others in all spheres of their lives, and their interactions and relationships tend not to be smooth, supportive, flexible, or even-keeled. BPD patients are plagued by feelings of threatened abandonment and tend to react to stress with extreme, excessive emotions. They tend to idealize and devalue individuals quickly and project their issues, feelings, and concerns onto others. These patients are often known by hospital and office staff as being difficult, demanding, manipulative, etc. Like every psychiatric disorder, this condition may range from mild to severe. Students who train in inpatient settings often see the most severe cases and assume all BPD patients are difficult, time-consuming, and impossible to manage. Like other psychiatric disorders, early detection and illiciting of milder symptoms may actually provide for better long-term outcomes as psychotherapy becomes a greater priority than psychopharmacological management.

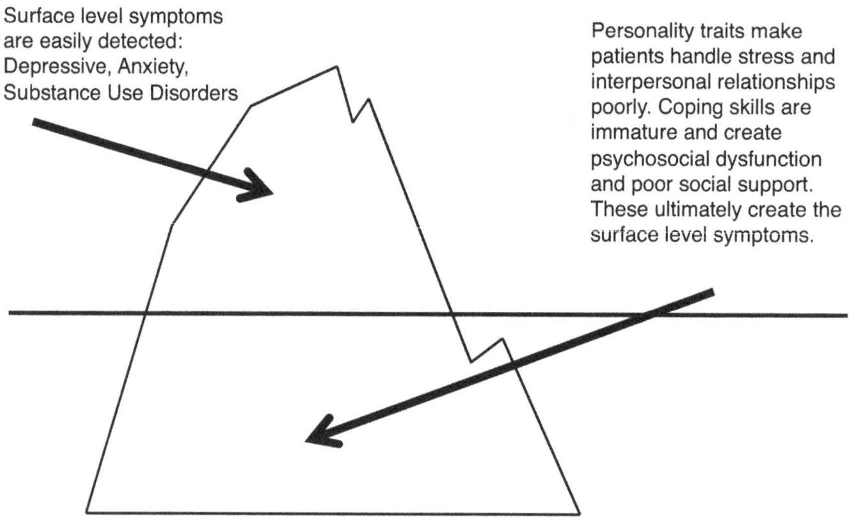
Surface level symptoms
are easily detected:
Depressive, Anxiety,
Substance Use Disorders
Personality traits make
patients handle stress and
interpersonal relationships
poorly. Coping skills are
immature and create
psychosocial dysfunction
and poor social support.
These ultimately create the
surface level symptoms.

Figure 4.1 The Iceberg Analogy for Personality Disorder

TIP: Borderline Personality Disorder (BPD) Screening Questions

Screening for affective instability

- Do you often have days when your mood changes a great deal—days when you shift back and forth from feeling like your usual self to feeling angry or depressed or anxious?

Screening for pattern of unstable relationships

- Do your relationships with friends and lovers tend to be intense and stormy with lots of ups and downs?

Screening for recurrent self-injurious behaviors

- Have you ever been so upset or tense that you deliberately hurt yourself by cutting, burning, or hitting yourself?

Screening for chronic feelings of emptiness

- Do you feel empty and depressed much of the time?

DSM-5 Diagnosis

People with BPD typically will have patterns of remarkable instability in their interpersonal relations and emotional states, often exhibiting patterns of impulsivity. As with other personality disorders, these behaviors should be pervasive across time and across a variety of social contexts and situations. The severity and chronicity of symptoms must cause psychosocial distress to reach the level of a true disorder.

DSM-5 Diagnosis of Borderline Personality Disorder

A pervasive pattern of instability of interpersonal relationships, self-image, and affects, and marked impulsivity beginning by early adulthood and present in a variety of contexts as indicated by five (or more) of the following:

1. Frantic efforts to avoid real or imagined abandonment.
2. A pattern of unstable and intense interpersonal relationships characterized by alternating between extremes of idealization and devaluation.
3. Identity disturbance: markedly and persistently unstable self-image or sense of self.
4. Impulsivity in at least two areas that are potentially self-damaging (e.g., spending, sex, substance abuse, reckless driving, binge eating).

5. Recurrent suicidal behavior, gestures, threats, or self-mutilating behavior.
6. Affective instability due to a marked reactivity of mood (e.g., intense episodic dysphoria, irritability, or anxiety usually lasting a few hours and only rarely more than a few days).
7. Chronic feelings of emptiness.
8. Inappropriate, intense anger or difficulty controlling anger.
9. Transient, stress-related paranoid ideation or severe dissociative symptoms.

TIP: Commonly Used Mnemonics for DSM-5 BPD Criteria

AM SUICIDE

A: Abandonment
M: Mood instability (marked reactivity of mood)
S: Suicidal (or self-mutilating) behavior
U: Unstable and intense relationships
I: Impulsivity
C: Control of anger
I: Identity disturbance
D: Dissociative (or paranoid) symptoms that are transient and stress-related
E: Emptiness (chronic feelings of)

TIP: Diagnosis

- Unlike bipolar disorder (BD), patients with borderline personality disorder (BPD) never truly have discrete "episodes" as they live with BPD symptoms longitudinally and daily.
- BPD patients will often idealize and then devalue other people. They sway between all-or-none, or black-and-white thinking. People or situations may be 100% excellent at one point and then 100% awful the next.
- Sometimes, abrupt affective changes or identity disturbances are misconstrued for dissociative identity disorder (DID) (multiple personality). Unlike DID, the BPD patient is fully aware of themselves and their emotional state. BPD patients do not adopt a new persona or alter personality.
- Sustained mania spells are never present.
- Sustained depressions, "empty feelings," or other negativities may be prevalent.
- It may take several sessions to link together the differing clinical presentations to appreciate the breadth of BPD DSM-5 symptoms.

Rating Scales

The Upstate Borderline Questionnaire (UBQ)

- There are very few BPD rating scales available. Most of those are difficult to obtain and may not be public domain. The Upstate Borderline Questionnaire (UBQ) is a newer scale that has been validated and is comparable to those in the private domain.
- This scale takes approximately 1–2 minutes for the patient to complete and several seconds to score. The scale may be obtained via author permission at www.upstate.edu/ddp.
- A positive score of five or more is suggestive of BPD being present. Scores may be followed sequentially over time to track treatment outcomes.

Table 4.1 The Upstate Borderline Questionnaire

UBQ—DSM-5 VERSION

INSTRUCTIONS
Circle "YES" or "NO" if the question completely or mostly applies to you. If you do not understand a question, leave it blank.

In the PAST YEAR:

1. Have you often become so preoccupied with fears of abandonment or separation from important people in your life that it's been hard to think about or do anything else?
   NO YES
2. Have you often found with people you are getting to know that they seem at first like the most special and understanding person you have ever met, but then later they do something to disappoint you?
   NO YES
3. Have you often wondered who you really are as a person, or noticed that you seem like a different person around different people?
   NO YES
4. Have you often done the following activities? (Circle all that apply.)
   1. Spent a lot of money on things that you later regretted?
      NO YES
   2. Driven a vehicle well over the speed limit?
      NO YES
   3. Had five or more drinks containing alcohol or used drugs to get high?
      NO YES
   4. Binged on food?
      NO YES
   5. Had sex with someone you hardly knew?
      NO YES

(*Continued*)

Table 4.1 (Continued)

5. On at least two occasions, have you tried to hurt yourself or kill yourself (e.g., choking, cutting, burning, overdose, etc.) or threatened to do so?
   NO YES
6. Have you often had mood swings or noticed that your mood can suddenly shift from happy or angry to depressed and then back again?
   NO YES
7. Have you usually felt empty inside?
   NO YES
8. Have you often had anger outbursts during which you say things or do things that you later regret?
   NO YES
9. At times when you have been stressed, did you ever develop any of the following reactions? (Circle all that apply.)
   - Become very suspicious of people around you?
     NO YES
   - Feel detached from what is going on around you, as if it isn't real?
     NO YES
   - Feel disconnected from your body or as if you are floating above it?
     NO YES

Treatment Guidelines

TIP: APA GUIDELINES

- The BPD APA guideline suggests that the negative affective states (depression, dysphoria, anger, etc.) of BPD should be treated with SSRI antidepressant, as they are the simplest and least risky psychopharmacologic intervention. This approach may be applied to anxious states as well.
- For impulsive BPD symptoms, if the SSRI fails then addition of an antipsychotic (at the time of this guideline, the atypical antipsychotics were new and not often utilized) or mood stabilizing anti-epileptic drug (AED) could be combined.
- For cognitive, paranoid, or dissociative symptoms, an antipsychotic should be added.
- This relatively simple guideline suggests starting with the safest class of medication and then adding further, more aggressive medications as needed.
- Clinically, routine psychodynamic psychotherapy or dialectical behavior therapy (DBT) is the most warranted treatment.
- This reflects the stance that there are no FDA approvals for BPD, and that the evidence base is moderate at best.

- It also reflects the psychiatric and psychologic bias that personality disorder requires psychotherapy. Clearly psychotherapy is effective, is evidence based, and is also in the treatment guidelines. With these biases in mind, it would make sense to use the least dangerous medication and strive, ideally, for monotherapy, thus minimizing the need for medication and stressing the importance of weekly psychotherapy.
- The 2010 NICE guidelines are more modern and extensively review many of the medications that will be discussed later in this chapter.
- Most recently, Gunderson's textbook (2014) succinctly describes an easy way to pick appropriate medications for those with BPD symptoms that incorporates the available literature well. This is outlined below.

TIP: Prescribing Practices

For mild overall symptoms

- If a patient has mild BPD symptoms and appears to not want, or will not ask for, medications, then no medications are warranted and psychotherapy is the best treatment option.
- If the patient asks for a pharmacological treatment, then SSRIs are a low-risk option despite the evidence base being the weakest for antidepressants as a pharmacologic approach.

For moderate to severe symptoms

- If depression/anxiety is predominant, then defaulting to an SSRI (ex. fluoxetine [Prozac], sertraline [Zoloft], etc.) is practical.
- If cognitive/perceptual symptoms such as transient psychosis, paranoia, hallucinations, dissociation, and derealization are present, then an atypical antipsychotic (SGA) is warranted (ex. ziprasidone [Geodon], aripiprazole [Abilify], etc.).
- If impulsive/anger-driven symptoms are most apparent, then use of a mood stabilizing epilepsy medication (AED) is a reasonable frontline intervention (ex. divalproex [Depakote]). Alternatively, an SGA may be used.
- Of note, the overall evidence base and effect-size analysis would suggest use of these niches for the above medication classes. Generally, the mood stabilizing epilepsy medications seem to have the most impact across all BPD symptoms when weighed collectively.

TIP: BPD Prescribing

- Comorbidities should be treated with appropriate pharmacotherapy and/or psychotherapy as indicated.
- Crises can be treated with psychotherapy or medication, though clinicians should lean toward support instead of immediately and reflexively medicating.
- Generally, BPD patients have a greater addiction risk, so benzodiazepine (BZ) anxiolytics and hypnotics are avoided.
  - Hydroxyzine (Vistaril/Atarax) is an anxiolytic antihistamine which may be utilized.
  - Many SGAs can have a calming, sedating, or anxiolytic effect due to their dopamine, histamine, and/or noradrenergic blocking potential.
    - These may be used as needed to target specific symptoms that flare up with interpersonal distress.
  - The goal is to ultimately have the patient self-monitor and detect the events that characteristically trigger BPD symptoms and to avoid or mitigate these situations psychosocially instead of treating mood swings with a PRN medication.

Practical Application

Essential Concepts: Antidepressants

- If a patient presents with BPD, the suggested starting point is often to use an antidepressant given the lower side effect risk.
- Use solid monotherapy approaches where doses are started low and escalated through the full dosing range as if the patient were suffering solely from an anxiety or depressive disorder. These strategies are found in both the anxiety and depressive disorders chapters.
- If a full SSRI trial fails to be effective then perhaps another serotonergic antidepressant can be tried next using an approach similar to the anxiety or depressive disorders.
  - Consider using *SSRI-Plus* medications (vortioxetine [Trintellix], vilazodone [Viibryd]) if greater serotonergic activity is desired.
  - Consider a sedating antidepressant (trazodone [Desyrel], nefazodone [Serzone], mirtazapine [Remeron]) if insomnia or agitation are severe.
- If one of these fails and the patient continues with impairing BPD, the next step is to taper off the antidepressant and choose the next class of medications.
- The antidepressants have the least effectiveness among the types of medications used to treat BPD.

- BPD patients tend to collect many medications in their regimen and end up on several marginal medications (irrational polypharmacy).
- Attempts should be made to remove any drug that does not have a definitive moderate to excellent effect.

Essential Concepts: Antipsychotics

- If the patient has predominant psychotic-like symptoms, perceptual problems, or uses distortion or dissociation defenses, then an SGA may be the best choice.
- The SGA may also help with anger, aggression, and impulsivity.
- Some SGAs have greater antidepressant effects and, theoretically, may be considered more advantageous. These include olanzapine (Zyprexa), quetiapine (Seroquel XR), aripiprazole (Abilify), brexpiprazole (Rexulti), lurasidone (Latuda), and risperidone (Risperdal).
- Clinicians again may try two to three medications in this class in successive, aggressive monotherapy trials. Lower doses likely treat depression, but higher doses may be needed to treat other BPD symptoms.
- Notice that these SGAs also have three main families: the *-dones*, the *-pines*, and the *-pips/rips*. If a patient fails to respond to one pharmacological class of SGA, then a cross titration to a different family makes intuitive sense. Combining two SGAs together is neither rational nor warranted.

Essential Concepts: Mood Stabilizing Anti-epileptics

- If a patient has more predominant mood lability and impulsivity, then use of an epilepsy-based mood stabilizer makes sense per the available evidence base.
- These agents may also lower aggression to some degree.
- These agents may not help depression or anxiety.
- Divalproex (Depakote), carbamazepine (Equetro), or lamotrigine (Lamictal) (sodium channel blockers) may be dosed and utilized as discussed in the previous BD chapter.
- Theoretically, calcium channel blocking agents (gabapentin [Neurontin], pregabalin [Lyrica]) may alleviate anxiety and insomnia better than aggression, impulsivity, or lability.
- Sequential use of these as monotherapies may be warranted though adding a calcium channel blocker to a sodium channel blocker may work for more treatment-resistant cases.
- These agents generally can be added to any antidepressant or SGA for the most severe BPD symptoms.

Table 4.2 Prescribing Table for Borderline Personality

Brand	Generic	Indication (Bold for FDA Approved)	Drug Mechanism	Dosing Tips	Monitoring Tips	Medicolegal Tips
Drugs listed in BOLD are approved agents. In this chapter, none are in BOLD! Dosing is based upon clinical application. Approved dosing guidelines should be further referenced by the prescriber.						
Antidepressants						
The Selective Serotonin Reuptake Inhibitors (SSRIs)						
Prozac	Fluoxetine	• **Obsessive-compulsive disorder (OCD)** • **Panic disorder (PD)** • Depression/anxiety associated with BPD	• Serotonin reuptake inhibitor	• Usual dose is 10–80mg/day • Increase 10–20mg every few weeks	• Common side effects include GI, headache, fatigue, anxiety, insomnia, weight gain, and sexual dysfunction • Serious side effects include (hypo)mania, increased suicidal ideation, easy bruising • Drug interactions as this is a major inhibitor of CYP4502D6	• In those age <25 there is increased risk of lethality, more frequent monitoring, and safety planning is warranted
Zoloft	Sertraline	• **Panic disorder (PD)** • **Post-traumatic stress disorder (PTSD)** • **Social anxiety disorder (SAD)** • **Obsessive-compulsive disorder (OCD)** • Depression/anxiety associated with BPD	• Serotonin reuptake inhibitor	• Usual dose is 25–200 mg/day • Increase 50mg every few weeks	• Same as above except higher possible rate of GI side effects • Drug interactions are minimal	• Same as above • Do not stop abruptly

Paxil Paxil CR	Paroxetine	• **Obsessive-compulsive disorder (OCD)** • **Panic disorder (PD)** • **Social anxiety disorder (SAD)** • **Post-traumatic stress disorder (PTSD)** • **Generalized anxiety disorder (GAD)** • Depression/anxiety associated with BPD	• Serotonin reuptake inhibitor	• Usual dose is 10–50 mg/day • Increase 10–20mg every few weeks	• Same as above except higher rates of mild anticholinergic effects and greater chance of serotonin withdrawal upon cessation • Drug interactions as this is a major inhibitor of CYP4502D6	• Same as above
Celexa	Citalopram	• Major depressive disorder (MDD) • Depression/anxiety associated with BPD	• Serotonin reuptake inhibitor	• Usual dose is 10–40 mg/day • Increase every few weeks • Do not exceed 40mg/day (or 20mg in elderly) due to cardiac QTc prolongation risks	• Same as above except for cardiac risks as this drug increases QTc • Drug interaction is for moderate inhibition at CYP4502D6	• Same as above • If dosing at higher levels for better efficacy, consider obtaining EKG and trough blood levels as a precaution
Lexapro	Escitalopram	• **Generalized anxiety disorder (GAD)** • Depression/anxiety associated with BPD	• Serotonin reuptake inhibitor	• Usual dose is 5–20 mg/day • Increase 5–10mg every few weeks	• Common side effects include GI, headache, fatigue, anxiety, insomnia, weight gain, and sexual dysfunction • Serious side effects include (hypo)mania, increased suicidal ideation, easy bruising	• Same as above but no cardiac warnings

(*Continued*)

Table 4.2 (Continued)

SSRI-Plus						
Viibryd	Vilazodone	• Major depressive disorder • Depression/anxiety associated with BPD	• Weak serotonin reuptake inhibitor • Partial agonist action at serotonin 1A autoreceptor	• Usual dose is 10–40 mg/day • Start at 10mg/day and increase by 10mg every week. 20–40mg/day is usual dose • Take with food	• Common side effects include GI, headache, fatigue, anxiety, insomnia. • Serious side effects include (hypo)mania, increased suicidal ideation, easy bruising	• In those age <25 there is increased risk of lethality, more frequent monitoring and safety planning is warranted • May have less weight gain and sexual dysfunction
Trintellix	Vortioxetine	• Major depressive disorder • Depression associated with BPD	• Serotonin reuptake inhibitor • Partial agonist action at serotonin 1A autoreceptor • Antagonist at serotonin 1b/d, 3, 7 receptors	• Usual dose is 5–20 mg/day • Increase 10mg every few weeks • Usual dose is 10–20mg/day	• Same as above	• Same as above
Sedating Antidepressants						
Desyrel	Trazodone	• Major depressive disorder • Insomnia • Depression/anxiety associated with BPD	• Blocks serotonin 2A receptors • Weak serotonin reuptake inhibitor • Alpha-1 norepinephrine receptor antagonist • H-1 histamine receptor antagonist	• Usual dose is 50–600 mg/day • May be dosed at night for insomnia 50–300mg • For depression is generally dosed 50–300mg twice daily	• Common side effects include dizziness, sedation, hypotension • Serious side effects include priapism, induction of (hypo) mania, and suicidal ideation	• In those age <25 there is increased risk of lethality, more frequent monitoring, and safety planning is warranted • Warn of psychomotor impairment

Serzone	Nefazodone	• Major depressive disorder • Insomnia • Depression/anxiety associated with BPD	• Blocks serotonin 2A receptors • Weak erotonin reuptake inhibitor	• Usual dose is 50–300 mg/day	• Same as above • Monitor liver functions as rare cases of hepatitis occur. Obtain AST and ALT at baseline, after titration, and annually	• Same as above • Clearly explain life-threatening or serious side effects (e.g., hepatotoxicity)
Remeron	Mirtazapine	• Major depressive disorder • Insomnia • Depression/anxiety associated with BPD	• Blocks alpha 2 adrenergic presynaptic receptor and increases norepinephrine and serotonin in the cortex via serotonin2c, 3 receptor blockade • Blocks H1 histamine receptors	• Usual dose is 7.5–45 mg/day at nighttime	• Common side effects include dizziness, sedation, hypotension, weight gain • Serious side effects include excessive weight gain and metabolic syndrome, induction of (hypo) mania, and suicidal ideation • Monitor at baseline and at least annually with CBC Diff, BMP, Lipid Panel. Also conduct more routine weight and vital sign assessment	• Clearly explain life-threatening or serious side effects (e.g., weight gain, metabolic side effects)

(*Continued*)

Table 4.2 (Continued)

SNRI						
Effexor Effexor XR	Venlafaxine	• Generalized anxiety disorder (GAD) • Social anxiety disorder (SAD) • Panic disorder (PD) • Obsessive-compulsive disorder (OCD) • Post-traumatic stress disorder (PTSD) • Depression/anxiety associated with BPD	• Serotonin and norepinephrine reuptake inhibitor • SRI > NRI	• Usual dose is 37.5–225 mg/day • Increase 37.5–75mg every few weeks • Maximal dose up to 375mg/day	• Common side effects same as SSRI but additional dry mouth, nausea, insomnia, anxiety may be experienced • Serious side effects same as SSRI but may include hypertension • Higher risk of serotonin withdrawal upon cessation	• Same as SSRI • Do not stop abruptly
Pristiq	Desvenlafaxine	• Major depressive disorder • Depression/anxiety associated with BPD	• Serotonin and norepinephrine reuptake inhibitor • NRI roughly equal to SRI	• Usual dose is 50–400mg/day • Increase 50mg every few weeks	• Same as above	• Same as above

Cymbalta	Duloxetine	• Generalized anxiety disorder (GAD) • Obsessive-compulsive disorder (OCD) • Social anxiety disorder (SAD) • Panic disorder (PD) • Post-traumatic stress disorder (PTSD) • **Fibromyalgia (FM)** • **Major depressive disorder** • Depression/anxiety associated with BPD	• Serotonin and norepinephrine reuptake inhibitor • NRI roughly equal to SRI	• Usual dose is 30–120mg/day • Increase 30mg every few weeks	• Same as above but carries risk of liver damage in alcohol use disorder (AUD) patients	• Same as above
Fetzima	Levomilnacipran	• Major depressive disorder • Depression associated with BPD	• Serotonin and norepinephrine reuptake inhibitor • NRI > SRI	• Usual dose is 20–120mg/day once daily • Start at 20mg once daily for 2 days and increase to 40mg once daily and increase by 40mg/day every 2 or more days to therapeutic effect	• Same as above except no liver abnormalities noted	• Same as above

(Continued)

Table 4.2 (Continued)

2. Mood Stabilizing Anti-epileptics

Brand	Generic	Indication (Bold for FDA Approved)	Drug Mechanism	Dosing Tips	Monitoring Tips	Medicolegal Tips
Calcium Channel Blockers						
Neurontin	Gabapentin	• Off-label for BPD anxiety and lability	• Binds to alpha 2 delta subunit of voltage sensitive calcium channels	• Usual dose 100–1200mg three times daily • Increase by 300mg three times a day every few weeks	• Common side effects include sedation, dizziness, ataxia, tremor, headache	• Avoid abrupt withdrawal due to seizure risk
Lyrica	Pregabalin	• Off-label for BPD anxiety and lability	• Binds to alpha 2 delta subunit of voltage sensitive calcium channels	• Usual dose is 150–600mg/day in 2–3 divided doses • Titrate up to target dose from standard starting dose of 150mg in 2–3 divided doses	• Same as above • Serious side effects include mild risk of addiction	• Same as above • Mild addictive properties, use same approach as for BZ anxiolytics
Sodium Channel Blockers						
Lamictal Lamictal XR	Lamotrigine	• Bipolar maintenance • Bipolar depression • Bipolar mania • Off-label for BPD lability/impulsivity	• Blocks voltage sensitive sodium channels and dampens excessive neuronal firing • May dampen glutamatergic activity	• Usual dose is 25–200mg/day as monotherapy • Start at 25mg/day for two weeks, increase to 50mg/day for 2 weeks, increase to 100mg/day for 2 weeks, and then to 200mg/day at week 6. Must follow exactly to avoid serious rashes • Any 5-day period of missed doses must re-titrate	• Common side effects include headache, sedation, GI side effects, tremor, ataxia, weight gain • Serious side effects include serious rash, increased suicidality • Monitor for rashes. Must be discontinued for any rash	• Clearly explain life-threatening or serious side effects (e.g., rash) • Should be discontinued before pregnancies (risk category C)

Equetro Tegretol	Carbamazepine	• Acute mania/ mixed features • Maintenance	• Blocks voltage sensitive sodium channels and dampens excessive neuronal firing	• Usual dose is 200–800 mg twice daily • Increase 200mg every few days	• Common initial side effects include sedation, GI side effects, ataxia, tremor, dysarthria • Serious side effects include serious rashes, aplastic anemia, agranulocytosis, SIADH • Monitor at baseline, after titration and then annually for CBC and differential. Trough blood levels should be between 8-12mg/dl	• Clearly explain life-threatening or serious side effects (e.g., rash, blood dyscrasia, 3A4 interactions) • Should be discontinued before pregnancies (risk category D) due to evidence of increased risk of birth defects (neural tube defects) • CYP3A4 hepatic inducer will lower plasma levels of many other drugs
Trileptal	Oxcarbazepine	• Acute mania/ mixed features • Maintenance	• Blocks voltage sensitive sodium channels and dampens excessive neuronal firing	• Usual dose is 150–1200mg twice daily • Increase 150mg twice daily every few days	• Common initial side effects include sedation, GI side effects, ataxia, tremor, dysarthria • Serious side effects include serious rashes, aplastic anemia, agranulocytosis, SIADH • Monitoring for blood dyscrasias may not be warranted	• Clearly explain life-threatening or serious side effects (e.g., rash, blood dyscrasia) • Should be discontinued before pregnancies (risk category D) due to evidence of increased risk of birth defects (neural tube defects)

(*Continued*)

Table 4.2 (Continued)

Topamax	Topiramate	• Off-label for affective instability and impulsivity associated with BPD	• Blocks voltage sensitive sodium channels and dampens excessive neuronal firing	• Usual dose is 25–200mg twice daily • Start at 25–50mg/day and increase every week by 50mg/day. Give in 2 divided doses	• Common initial side effects include sedation, dizziness, GI side effects, weight loss, psychomotor retardation, cognitive dulling • Serious side effects include metabolic acidosis, kidney stone formation, secondary angle closure glaucoma, activation of suicidality, and excessive weight loss, oligohydrosis • Monitor blood at baseline and annually with basic metabolic panel for renal function and acidosis. Check weights routinely	• Clearly explain life-threatening or serious side effects (e.g., metabolic acidosis, weight loss, oligohydrosis, glaucoma)

GABA Enhancing Agents						
Depakote Depakote ER	Divalproex	• Bipolar mania • Bipolar maintenance • Bipolar depression • Bipolar mania • Off-label for BPD lability/impulsivity	• Increases CNS concentration of GABA via unknown mechanism	• Usual dose is 250mg–500mg twice daily • Increase by 250–500mg every few weeks for outpatients • For inpatient may load an 20mg/kg	• Common side effects include sedation, diarrhea, ataxia, tremor • Serious side effects include hepatotoxicity, pancreatitis, thrombocytopenia, polycystic ovarian syndrome, rashes, and activation of suicidality • Monitor for blood levels and obtain 50–125mg/dl • Monitor liver, pancreas, and platelet function prior and during treatment	• Must monitor labs at baseline and then throughout use of this medication to avoid end-organ damage • Provide informed consent about these prior to treatment

(*Continued*)

Table 4.2 (Continued)

3. Second-Generation Antipsychotics

Brand	Generic	Indication (Bold for FDA Approved)	Drug Mechanism	Dosing Tips	Monitoring Tips	Medicolegal Tips
Second-Generation Antipsychotics						
Risperdal	Risperidone	• Schizophrenia • Acute mania/ mixed mania • Maintenance • Bipolar and unipolar depression • Off-label for BPD psychosis, lability, impulsivity	• Blocks dopamine 2 receptors reducing psychosis and stabilizing mania • Blocks serotonin 2A receptors which may improve depression	• Usual dose is 0.25–6mg/day • Maximum daily dose is 16mg/day • For more severe mania load at 2–3mg/day and increase 1mg every few days	• Common initial side effects include dizziness, sedation, headache, GI side effects • Serious side effects include risk of diabetes, hyperlipidemia, hypertension, weight gain, transient and permanent neuromuscular side effects, hyperlipidemia, gynecomastia, agranulocytosis, increased risk of death in demented elderly, increased suicidality • Monitor at baseline and at least annually with CBC Diff, BMP, Lipid Panel. Also conduct more routine weight and vital signs, AIMS tests or physical exam for EPS/TD neuromuscular symptoms	• Clearly explain life-threatening or serious side effects (e.g., TD/ EPS, metabolic side effects) • Provide treatments if side effects occur (e.g., weight loss agents, antiparkinson agents) • Risk of weight gain and metabolics is high • Risk of EPS is high

Zyprexa Symbyax	Olanzapine, olanzapine/fluoxetine	• Schizophrenia • Acute mania/mixed mania • Maintenance • Bipolar depression in combination with fluoxetine • Agitation • Off-label for BPD psychosis, lability, impulsivity	• Blocks dopamine 2 receptors reducing psychosis and stabilizing mania • Blocks serotonin 2A receptors which may improve depression	• Usual mania dose is 2.5–20mg/day • Increase by 5mg every few days • For more severe mania may load 10–15mg/day • Usual depression dose (olanzapine/fluoxetine) is 3/25–12/50, increasing by 3/25 every few weeks • For combative agitation, 10mg IM q 2–4 hrs with max 30mg/day with warning NOT TO MIX WITH SEDATIVES	• Same as above	• Clearly explain life-threatening or serious side effects (e.g., TD/EPS, metabolic side effects) • Provide treatments if side effects occur (e.g., weight loss agents, antiparkinson agents) • Considered one of the most metabolic syndrome inducing agents • Sedation risk is moderate • Risk of EPS is high
Seroquel (XR)	Quetiapine	• Schizophrenia • Acute mania • Maintenance • Bipolar and unipolar depression • Off-label for BPD psychosis, lability, impulsivity	• Blocks dopamine 2 receptors reducing psychosis and stabilizing mania • Blocks serotonin 2A receptors which may improve depression • Has potent NRI and 5HT-1a agonism as antidepressant properties (metabolite norquetiapine)	• Dosing is 25–400mg twice daily and for XR is 50–800mg/day • May load for severe mania within 4 days to 400mg or XR may load at 300mg • Depression dosing is 25–600 or 50–600, respectively, and both can be given once nightly	• Same as above but increased risk of cataracts • Monitoring is same and consider optometry for cataract warning	• Clearly explain life-threatening or serious side effects (e.g., TD/EPS, metabolic side effects) • Provide treatment if side effects occur (e.g., weight loss agents, antiparkinson agents) • Considered one of the most metabolic syndrome inducing agents • Risk of weight gain and metabolics is high • Risk of sedation is high • Risk of EPS/TD is lowest in SGA class

(*Continued*)

Table 4.2 (Continued)

Geodon	Ziprasidone	• Schizophrenia • Acute mania/ mixed mania • Maintenance • Bipolar depression • Agitation • Off-label for BPD psychosis, lability, impulsivity	• Blocks dopamine 2 receptors reducing psychosis and stabilizing mania • Blocks serotonin 2A receptors which may improve depression • Has mild SNRI and 5HT-1a agonism as antidepressant properties	• Must be taken with food • Usual dose is 20–80mg twice daily • May increase 20–40mg every few days for mania, every few weeks for depression • For severe mania may escalate to 80mg twice daily on day 2 • For agitation in schizophrenia it may be used IM 10mg q 2 hr with 40mg/day max	• Common initial side effects include dizziness, sedation, headache, GI side effects, akathisia • Serious side effects include risk of diabetes, hyperlipidemia, hypertension, weight gain, transient and permanent neuromuscular side effects, hyperlipidemia, gynecomastia, agranulocytosis, increased risk of death in demented elderly, increased suicidality, cardiac QTc prolongation • Monitor at baseline and at least annually with CBC Diff, BMP, Lipid Panel. Also conduct more routine weight and vital signs, AIMS tests or physical exam for EPS/TD neuromuscular symptoms, and consider baseline EKG and after titration for those at cardiac risk	• Clearly explain life-threatening or serious side effects (e.g., TD/ EPS, metabolic side effects) • Provide treatment if side effects occur (e.g., weight loss agents, antiparkinson agents) • Considered one of the least metabolic syndrome inducing agents • Sedation risk is moderate • Akathisia rates are moderate

Abilify	Aripiprazole	• Schizophrenia • Acute mania/mixed mania • Maintenance • Unipolar depression • Agitation • Off-label for BPD psychosis, lability, impulsivity	• Partially agonizes D2 and D3 receptors which may improve affect • Net effect may also block dopamine 2 receptors reducing psychosis and stabilizing mania • Blocks serotonin 2A receptors which may improve depression • Has 5HT-1a agonism as antidepressant properties	• Usual dose is 2–30mg/day • May increase 2–5mg every few days • For severe mania may load at 15mg/day and increase to 30mg on day 2 or 3 • Start 10–15mg/day. Maximum daily dose is 30mg/day • Intramuscular for agitation is 9.75–15mg q 2 hr, max 30mg/day • Drug is a substrate for CYP2D6 and must be halved if 2D6 inhibitor concomitantly taken	• Same but EKG monitoring is not needed	• Clearly explain life-threatening or serious side effects (e.g., TD/EPS, metabolic side effects) • Provide treatment if side effects occur (e.g., weight loss agents, antiparkinson agents) • Risk of weight gain and metabolics is moderate • Risk of sedation is moderate • Risk of akathisia is high
Rexulti	Brexpiprazole	• Schizophrenia • Major depression augmentation • Off-label for BPD psychosis, lability, impulsivity	• Partially agonizes D2 and D3 receptors which may improve affect • Net effect may also block dopamine 2 receptors reducing psychosis, stabilizing mania and allowing a calming effect • Blocks serotonin 2A receptors which may improve depression • Has 5HT-1a agonism similar to SPA anxiolytics (buspirone)	• Usual dose is 0.25–4mg/day • May increase 0.5–1mg every few weeks • Drug is a substrate for CYP2D6 and must be halved if 2D6 inhibitor concomitantly taken	• Same though akathisia rates are much lower	• Clearly explain life-threatening or serious side effects (e.g., TD/EPS, metabolic side effects) • Provide treatment if side effects occur (e.g., weight loss agents, antiparkinson agents) • Risk of weight gain and metabolics is moderate • Risk of sedation is moderate • Risk of akathisia is moderate

(*Continued*)

Table 4.2 (Continued)

Vraylar	Cariprazine	• Schizophrenia • Acute mania/ mixed mania • Off-label for BPD psychosis, lability, impulsivity	• Partially agonizes D2 and D3 receptors which may improve affect • Net effect may also block dopamine 2 receptors reducing psychosis, stabilizing mania and allowing a calming effect • Blocks serotonin 2A receptors which may improve depression • Has 5HT-1a agonism similar to SPA anxiolytics (buspirone)	• Usual dose is 1.5–6mg/ day • May increase 1.5mg every few weeks	• Same as above	• Clearly explain life-threatening or serious side effects (e.g., TD/ EPS, metabolic side effects) • Provide treatment if side effects occur (e.g., weight loss agents, antiparkinson agents) • Risk of weight gain and metabolics is moderate • Risk of sedation is moderate • Risk of akathisia is high

Saphris	Asenapine	• Schizophrenia • Acute mania/ mixed features • Off-label for BPD psychosis, lability, impulsivity	• Blocks dopamine 2 receptors reducing psychosis and stabilizing mania • Blocks serotonin 2A receptors which may improve depression • Has similar antidepressant theoretical properties to mirtazapine (alpha-2 antagonism, 5HT-2c,3 antagonism)	• Usual dose is 5–10 mg twice daily • May load dose at 10mg twice daily for severe mania • It is taken SL or will not be absorbed	• Common initial side effects include taste bud dysfunction, dizziness, sedation, headache, GI side effects • Serious side effects include risk of diabetes, hyperlipidemia, hypertension, weight gain, transient and permanent neuromuscular side effects, hyperlipidemia, gynecomastia, agranulocytosis, increased risk of death in demented elderly, increased suicidality • Monitor at baseline and at least annually with CBC Diff, BMP, Lipid Panel. Also conduct more routine weight and vital signs, AIMS tests or physical exam for EPS/TD neuromuscular symptoms	• Clearly explain life-threatening or serious side effects (e.g., TD/ EPS, metabolic side effects) • Provide treatment if side effects occur (e.g., weight loss agents, antiparkinson agents) • Risk of weight gain and metabolics is mild to moderate • Risk of sedation is moderate

(*Continued*)

Table 4.2 (Continued)

Invega	Paliperidone	• Schizophrenia • Off-label for BPD psychosis, lability, impulsivity	• Blocks dopamine 2 receptors reducing psychosis and stabilizing mania • Blocks serotonin 2A receptors which may improve depression	• Dosing is 3–12mg/day • May increase 3mg every few days	• Same as above	• Clearly explain life-threatening or serious side effects (e.g., TD/EPS, metabolic side effects) • Provide treatments if side effects occur (e.g., weight loss agents, antiparkinson agents) • Risk of weight gain and metabolics is moderate • Risk of EPS is high
Fanapt	Iloperidone	• Schizophrenia • Off-label for BPD psychosis, lability, impulsivity	• Blocks dopamine 2 receptors reducing psychosis and stabilizing mania • Blocks serotonin 2A receptors which may improve depression	• Usual dose is 12–24mg/day in 2 divided doses • Due to high hypotension risk, start at 2mg in 2 divided doses on day 1 and increase to 4mg on day 2, 8mg on day 3, 12 mg on day 4, 16mg on day 5, 20mg on day 6, and 24mg on day 7, all on divided doses. Maximum daily dose is 32mg/day	• Same as above and consider EKG monitoring for QTc prolongation and after titration for those at cardiac risk	• Clearly explain life-threatening or serious side effects (e.g., TD/EPS, metabolic side effects) • Provide treatment if side effects occur (e.g., weight loss agents, antiparkinson agents) • Risk of weight gain and metabolics is moderate • Risk of sedation is moderate • Risk of orthostasis may be highest in class • Akathisia rates are low

Latuda	Lurasidone	• Schizophrenia • Bipolar depression • Off-label for BPD psychosis, lability, impulsivity	• Blocks dopamine 2 receptors reducing psychosis and stabilizing affective symptoms • Blocks serotonin 2A receptors which promotes dopamine release that improves cognitive and affective symptoms without marked EPS • Blocks serotonin-7 receptors which may improve cognition and circadian rhythm • Partially agonizes serotonin-1a receptors to treat depression	• Usual dose is 20–120mg/day for bipolar depression • Must be taken with food to absorb • May increase 20–40mg every few weeks	• Same as above but does not include EKG monitoring	• Clearly explain life-threatening or serious side effects (e.g., TD/EPS, metabolic side effects) • Provide treatment if side effects occur (e.g., weight loss agents, antiparkinson agents) • Risk of weight gain and metabolics is minimal • Risk of sedation is low

(*Continued*)

Table 4.2 (Continued)

4. The Alpha-2 Receptor Agonists and Alpha-1 Receptor Antagonists

Brand	Generic	Indication (Bold for FDA Approved)	Drug Mechanism	Dosing Tips	Monitoring Tips	Medicolegal Tips
Alpha-2 Receptor Agonists						
Catapres / Catapres-TTS/Kapvay	Clonidine	• Off-label for anxiety	• Stimulates central action of alpha 2A noradrenergic receptors, lowering peripheral noradrenergic tone	• Usual dose is 0.1mg–2.4mg/day, given in twice daily dosing • Increase by 0.1mg every week	• Common side effects include dry mouth, dizziness, fatigue, lightheadedness • Serious side effects include hypotension, syncope, bradycardia, AV block, and abrupt withdrawal hypertensive crisis • Monitor vital signs	• Abrupt discontinuation may lead to rare hypertensive encephalopathy, stroke, and death • Taper over 2–4 days or longer to avoid rebound in blood pressure
Intuniv Tenex	Guanfacine	• Off-label for anxiety	• Stimulates central action of alpha 2A noradrenergic receptors, lowering peripheral noradrenergic tone	• 1–3mg nightly • Increase 1mg every week	• Same as above • Generally less vegetative effects compared to clonidine	• Same as above

Alpha-1 Receptor Antagonists						
Minipress	Prazosin	• Off-label for nightmares associated with PTSD	• Blocks alpha 1 receptors to reduce noradrenergic tone centrally	• Usual dose is 1–16mg/day • Start at 1mg at bedtime and increase dose until nightmares resolve	• Common side effects include dizziness, lightheadedness, fatigue • Serious side effects include hypotension, orthostasis, syncope	• Same as above

5. Antihistamines

Brand	Generic	Indication (Bold for FDA Approved)	Drug Mechanism	Dosing Tips	Monitoring Tips	Medicolegal Tips
Antihistamines						
Atarax Vistaril	Hydroxyzine	• Anxiety	• Blocks histamine 1 receptors	• Usual dose is 10–100mg four times a day • Increase every few days in increments of 10–25mg	• Common side effects include dry mouth, sedation, and other anticholinergic effects • Serious side effects include dyspnea, seizures, cardiac conduction delay	• Warn of sedation and operating heavy machinery

SECTION 2 Advanced Prescribing Practice

Introduction

In Section 1, the premise is to convince the reader that they must make an accurate diagnosis and pick an approved agent with well-defined dosing guidelines and expected clinical outcomes. This approach is largely one of pattern recognition: (1) identify the pattern of phenotypic symptoms, (2) choose from a finite list of available, proven effective drugs, (3) start dosing low and escalate through an approved dosing range, (4) assess for effectiveness, and (5) continue medication if effective or cross-titrate to a new drug if ineffective or not tolerated. This is a methodical and mathematical approach that can improve the standard of care and, ideally, patient outcomes when treated by the novice psychopharmacologist.

Section 2 is designed to provide a greater depth of neuroscience and pharmacodynamic knowledge to the reader and is written for prescribers who are knowledgeable and competent in those skills outlined in Section 1. The section is generally intended for those patients who are felt to be treatment resistant and comorbid with other disorders.

Epidemiology

- BPD lifetime prevalence is as high as 6%.
- It is one of the most commonly presenting personality disorders in clinical practice.
- BPD is associated with one of the highest medical utilization rates given the frequent need for hospitalizations and team-based approaches.
- There are high rates of comorbidity with mood disorders, anxiety disorders, substance use, and other personality disorders.

Genetics

- Heritability of BPD based upon more recent twin studies has been found to be approximately 40%.
- There is high amount of gene-environment interaction where a history of trauma or neglect may increase the risk for BPD.
- The serotonergic system is often implicated as being abnormal but risk-gene findings have been inconsistent (serotonin transporter, tryptophan hydroxylase 1, and serotonin-1b).
- Most positive findings suggest abnormalities for monoamine oxidase-A (MAOA) and catechol-O-methyltransferase (COMT) genes implicating the monoamines in general.
- The dopamine transporter (DAT1) and several dopamine receptor genes (DRD2, DRD4) have been implicated as being abnormal.

Neuroanatomy

- Neuroimaging suggests a loss of top down cortical control over emotional monitoring and expression.
- Abnormal limbic-cortical neurocircuitry involving abnormal activity within and between the limbic bilateral amygdala, hippocampus and the anterior cingulate (ACC), orbitofrontal (OFC), and dorsolateral prefrontal cortices (DLPFC) has been found.
- The OFC and DLPFC are felt to be weakened and underactive.
- The amygdala appears to lose volume but gain abnormal hyperactivity.
- ACC may be over active.
- This suggests a neuroanatomic tendency toward emotionality and impulsivity while increased scanning of the environment for potential threats occurs.

TIP: Environment and Gene Interaction

- This is sometimes called Stress-Diathesis, which equates to social stress and risk genes interacting to create symptoms or disorders.
- Epigenetics is an emerging field of science that studies heritable changes caused by the activation and deactivation of genes. Here, environment stress may cause certain genes to turn on or off.
- DNA possesses structures called histones. Sometimes during environmental stress, they become methylated, essentially turning genes off. If enough gene deactivation occurs, psychiatric symptoms may develop. In this case, gene mutations are not needed as the gene itself no longer functions.
- Patients may not require true mutations that yield abnormal proteins (enzymes, receptors, ion channels, etc.) if they no longer have an active gene making these structures.
- If enough genes are turned off and cause improperly functioning circuits in the brain, it may cause hyperfunctioning or hypofunctioning within or between certain brain areas that may be able to be detected with neuroimaging: *an endophenotype*.
- This alteration in brain neurocircuitry function may lead to specific psychiatric symptoms that can be detected by interviewing (distractibility, talkativeness, goal directed hyperactivity, elevated mood).
- Regarding BPD (which has a high association with trauma), social trauma may increase stress and possibly cortisol. Cortisol itself may cause atrophy of certain brain structures (hippocampi) but theoretically may start the process of epigenetics discussed above.
- These outward symptoms that the DSM-5 is based upon are considered the patient's *phenotype*. The ultimate cause of this may be gene mutuations or the fact that genes have been inappropriately turned off or on.

Neuroscientific Background and Rationale for Medication Use

In treating BPD, there are five main classes frequently utilized. (**See Prescribing Table**):

TIP: BPD Prescribing

- For depression/anxiety symptoms consider:
  - SSRI (fluoxetine [Prozac], sertraline [Zoloft], paroxetine [Paxil], escitalopram [Celexa/Lexapro])
  - SNRI (venlafaxine [Effexor XR], desvenlafaxine [Pristiq], duloxetine [Cymbalta], levomilnacipran [Fetzima])
  - SSRI-Plus (vilazodone [Viibryd], vortioxetine [Trintellix])
  - Sedating antidepressants (trazodone [Desyrel], nefazodone [Serzone], mirtazapine [Remeron])
  - Alpha-2 agonists (clonidine [Catapres], guanfacine [Tenex]) theoretically may lower hyperarousal.
  - H1 antagonists (hydroxyzine [Vistaril/Atarax]) may lower anxiety and agitation.
- For impulsivity and mood lability consider:
  - Anti-epileptic drugs (AEDS)/mood stabilizers (divalproex [Depakote], carbamazepine [Equetro/Tegretol], gabapentin [Neurontin], pregabalin [Lyrica])
  - The latter two agents may have a niche for improved anxiety control.
- For anger, psychosis, mood lability consider:
  - Second-generation antipsychotics (SGAs)—risperidone, paliperidone, olanzapine, quetiapine, ziprasidone, aripiprazole, asenapine, iloperidone, lurasidone, brexpiprazole, cariprazine.
  - Risperidone (Risperdal), olanzapine (Zyprexa), quetiapine (Seroquel XR), ziprasidone (Geodon), aripiprazole (Abilify), brexpiprazole (Rexulti), and lurasidone (Latuda) all have antidepressant properties and may have a niche for better control of these symptoms.
  - Quetiapine (Seroquel XR) has the most evidence for treating anxiety symptoms in general.

1) Antidepressants

MECHANISM OF ACTION

SSRI, SNRI, SSRI-Plus, Sedating Antidepressants

- The reader is referred to the depression chapter for further details.
- The mechanism of anxiety and/or depressive symptom reduction is likely due to the increase of serotonin (5HT) and/or norepinephrine (NE) in the synapse, ultimately.

- All of the above medications inhibit these associated transporters (reuptake inhibition).
- The SSRI-Plus agents also agonize 5HT-1a receptors and may antagonize 5HT-1d, 3, 7 (vortioxetine).
- The sedating antidepressants antagonize 5HT-2a similar to the SGA and may antagonize 5HT-3 (mirtazapine).

2) Mood Stabilizers (Anti-epileptic Drugs—AED)

MECHANISM OF ACTION

Divalproex (Depakote), carbamazepine (Tegretol), lamotrigine (Lamictal), gabapentin (Neurontin), pregabalin (Lyrica)

- The reader is referred to the bipolar chapter for further details.
- Most AEDs block neuronal sodium channels (carbamazepine, lamotrigine) and may best control impulsivity and mood lability.
- Some block calcium channels (gabapentin and pregabalin) and may control anxiety-based mood lability.
- Divalproex is a bit different. It may increase the synthesis of GABA. Increases in GABA neurotransmission may also have a dampening effect on BPD induced hyperactive limbic structures. It may also lower glutamate neuronal firing by inhibiting NMDA receptors.

3) Second-Generation Antipsychotics

MECHANISM OF ACTION

Risperidone (Risperdal), paliperidone (Invega), olanzapine (Zyprexa), quetiapine (Seroquel XR), ziprasidone (Geodon), aripiprazole (Abilify), asenapine (Saphris), iloperidone (Fanapt), lurasidone (Latuda), brexpiprazole (Rexulti), cariprazine (Vraylar)

- The reader is referred to the bipolar and the schizophrenia chapters for further detail.
- This class of medication may be utilized to treat psychosis and mood lability in BPD.
- All of these agents block limbic D-2 receptors, which should restore a lower, more normal activity, thus alleviating mood swings, hostility, aggression, and psychosis. All SGAs, therefore, may help treat these core symptoms of BPD.
- Antidepressant effects are more complicated and varied across SGAs. For antidepressant effects aripiprazole, brexpiprazole, lurasidone, quetiapine,

and olanzapine (when combined with fluoxetine) are approved for various other forms of depressive episodes. All of these block 5HT-2a serotonin receptors, which is a purported mechanism of antidepressant action for the approved unipolar antidepressants trazodone, nefazodone, and mirtazapine. Activity here may improve both serotonergic and noradrenergic functioning to lower depressive symptomatology.

- Quetiapine and lurasidone seem to have more activity in partially agonizing the 5HT-1a receptor. This activity may initially lower serotonin activity but ultimately causes downregulation of this autoreceptor with a resultant increase in serotonin neuronal firing. This activity is employed by the antidepressant vilazodone and vortioxetine.
- Lurasidone may be unique in its robust activity to block the 5HT-7 receptor. This activity is felt to improve cognitive symptoms and circadian symptoms of depression.
- Quetiapine may be unique in that it has potent norepinephrine reuptake pump blocking activity. This is an antidepressant mechanism utilized by NDRI, (bupropion), serotonin-norepinephrine reuptake inhibitors (SNRI), and many of TCAs.
- Finally, aripiprazole, brexpiprazole, and cariprazine may have the ability to stimulate dopamine activity at the D2 and D3 receptor. This could improve drive, motivation, and concentration from an antidepressant perspective.

4. Antihistamines

MECHANISM OF ACTION

Hydroxyzine (Atarax/Vistaril)

- Blocking (antagonism) of the H1 histamine receptor may create sedation and somnolence.
- This may treat insomnia or agitation associated with BDP.
- Further discussion of this agent is found in the anxiety chapter.

5. Alpha-2 Receptor Agonists

MECHANISM OF ACTION

Clonidine (Catapres), guanfacine (Tenex), prazosin (Minipress)

- Further discussion of these agents are found in the ADHD and the anxiety chapters.
- Drug activity here centrally lowers noradrenergic tone. Anxiety is hypothesized to begin with elevated NE activity and neuronal firing. Theoretically, these agents can directly lower NE firing and potentially improve anxiety symptoms.

Practical Applications

Good Polypharmacy to Be Used to Gain Remission in Resistant Patients

DO

- Start low dose to minimize side effects.
- Escalate dosing within full range for optimal effectiveness.
- Monitor for weight gain, blood pressure, skin changes, abnormal movements, and end-organ damage depending on medication chosen.
- In BPD it is prudent to refer for psychotherapy as a key treatment and strive for more aggressive monotherapies in general. Validated therapies include dialectical behavioral therapy (DBT) and dynamic deconstructive psychotherapy (DDP).
- Polypharmacy may be required for more complex and severe cases. The five classes of medications often can be combined with each other for rational polypharmacy to address key symptoms. It generally is not wise to combine medications from within a class of agents unless:
  - Add anti-epileptics together if they have different mechanisms of action (ex. add calcium channel blockers to sodium channel blockers).
  - Add non-SSRI/SNRI antidepressants together (ex. mirtazapine/trazodone/nefazodone to an SSRI or SNRI).
- Cautiously escalate to higher doses using caution with blood level monitoring for resistant cases.
- As all BPD prescribing is off-label, clearly define a target symptom you wish to control (lability, impulsivity, anger, psychosis, etc.) and measure it in some manner prior to prescribing. Re-check after titration and continue the medication only if there is a clinically meaningful response (>30% definitive improvement).

DON'T

- Add an SSRI to an SSRI or an SSRI to an SNRI.
- Add two SGAs together.
- Add two sodium channel blocking anti-epileptics together.
- Let BPD patients collect and stay on a series of medications without definitive proof each medication is clearly effective!

Good Polypharmacy to Be Used in Comorbid Patients

BPD + ADHD

- **Use of NDRI:** bupropion (Wellbutrin XL)
- **Use of NRI:** atomoxetine (Strattera)

- **Use second-generation antipsychotic (SGA) augmentation:** aripiprazole (Abilify), brexpiprazole (Rexulti), and cariprazine (Vraylar) have partial dopamine receptor 2/3 agonism; quetiapine XR has potent NRI.
- **Use of stimulant medications** are usually avoided in BPD patients as there is risk of mood lability and likely an increased risk of substance misuse.
- **Use alpha-2 agonists:** guanfacine, clonidine.

BPD+ Anxiety Disorder

- **Use of SSRIs:** fluoxetine, sertraline, paroxetine, citalopram, escitalopram.
- **Use of SSRI-Plus:** vilazodone, vortioxetine.
- **Use of BZs** are generally avoided due to addiction risk and misuse.
- **Use alpha-2 agonists:** guanfacine, clonidine.
- **Use of antihistamine (H1 receptor antagonist):** hydroxyzine.

BPD + Schizophrenia (Schizoaffective) Disorder

- **Use second-generation antipsychotic (SGA) monotherapy.**
- If remaining affective symptoms, may utilize strategies listed throughout this chapter or the BD chapter to better control residual mania or depression.

BPD + Bipolar Disorder

- **Use of epilepsy-based mood stabilizer monotherapy (AEDs).**
- **Use second-generation antipsychotic (SGA) monotherapy.**
- **Possible use of lithium.**
- If remaining affective symptoms, may utilize strategies listed throughout this chapter to better control residual mania or depression.

BPD + Major Depressive Disorder

- Use of SSRI or SSRI-Plus.
- Use of sedating antidepressants.
- TCAs and MAOIs may be too risky to use due to threat of self-harm overdoses, and greater medication non-compliance due to self-medication.

Final Advanced Prescribing Thoughts

Patients with BPD can be very difficult yet very rewarding to treat. In training, clinicians often see the most severe and hospitalized BPD patients, but in the outpatient setting there is wide ranging severity. This disorder has hallmarks of anxiety, depression, psychosis, impulsivity, and very primitive defense mechanisms. Non-compliance rates and medical utilization of psychiatric services are high. Utilizing an approach of aggressive monotherapy and minimal polypharmacy can appear to be a lofty goal, but many of the medications suggested have wide ranging abilities to treat these symptom clusters and must be attempted. It should also be clear to the reader that there is often more than one guideline-based answer to each clinical question. There are often one or two wrong ways to treat a patient pharmacologically, but each case contains critical points where a clinician can choose wisely among several better protocols. More emphasis on compliance and use of psychotherapy should be a key goal. In conclusion, suffering from a personality disorder often affords less acute and sustained effectiveness from psychopharmacologic management alone. Patients with BPD likely should be enrolled in a bona fide, outcomes-based weekly psychotherapy regimen, such as dialectical behavior therapy (DBT) or dynamic deconstructive psychotherapy (DDP), to obtain the best outcomes.

Bibliography

Amad, A., Ramoz, N., Thomas, P., Jardri, R., & Gorwood, P. (2014) "Genetics of borderline personality disorder: systematic review and proposal of an integrative model." *Neuroscience & Biobehavioral Reviews* 40, 6–19.

American Psychiatric Association. (2001) *Practice Guideline for the Treatment of Patients with Borderline Personality Disorder*. Worcester, MA: American Psychiatric Pub.

American Psychiatric Association. (2013) *Diagnostic and Statistical Manual of Mental Disorders: DSM-5*. Washington, D.C.: American Psychiatric Association.

Distel, M. A., Trull, T. J., Derom, C. A., Thiery, E. W., Grimmer, M. A., Martin, N. G., & Boomsma, D. I. (2008) "Heritability of borderline personality disorder features is similar across three countries." *Psychological Medicine* 38(9), 1219–1229.

Grant, B. F., Chou, S. P., Goldstein, R. B., Huang, B., Stinson, F. S., Saha, T. D., & Ruan, W. J. (2008) "Prevalence, correlates, disability, and comorbidity of DSM-IV borderline personality disorder: results from the Wave 2 National Epidemiologic Survey on Alcohol and Related Conditions." *The Journal of Clinical Psychiatry* 69(4), 533.

Gregory, R. J., DeLucia-Deranja, E., & Mogle, J. A. (2010) "Dynamic deconstructive psychotherapy versus optimized community care for borderline personality disorder co-occurring with alcohol use disorders: a 30-month follow-up." *The Journal of Nervous and Mental Disease* 198(4), 292–298.

National Collaborating Centre for Mental Health (UK). (2009) *Borderline Personality Disorder: Treatment and Management*. Leicester, UK: British Psychological Society.

Strakowski, S. M., Delbello, M. P., & Adler, C. M. (2005) "The functional neuroanatomy of bipolar disorder: a review of neuroimaging findings." *Molecular Psychiatry* 10(1), 105–116.

Verheul, R., van den Bosch, L. M., Koeter, M. W., De Ridder, M. A., Stijnen, T., & van den Brink, W. (2003) "Dialectical behaviour therapy for women with borderline personality disorder." *The British Journal of Psychiatry* 182(2), 135–140.

Zanarini, M. C., Frankenburg, F. R., Dubo, E. D., Sickel, A. E., Trikha, A., Levin, A., & Reynolds, V. (2014) "Axis I comorbidity of borderline personality disorder." *American Journal of Psychiatry* 155(12), 1733–1739.

CHAPTER 5

Depressive Disorders: Major Depressive Disorder, Persistent Depressive Disorder, Premenstrual Dysphoric Disorder, and Seasonal Depressive Disorder

SECTION 1 Basic Prescribing Practices

Essential Concepts

- Depression occurs over a spectrum from normal response to usual life adversities (grief or stress reactions) to a severe and pathological psychiatric disorder.
- Major depressive disorder (MDD) is experienced as excessive, pervasive sadness associated with a clear loss of enjoyment.
  - Melancholic features may be marked by anhedonia and lack of mood reactivity.
  - Atypical features may be marked by increased appetite or weight gain, sleepiness, fatigue, mood reactivity, and rejection hypersensitivity.
  - Catatonic features also occur, such as a lack of speech and motion for extended periods.
  - Psychotic features may develop allowing for marked psychotic symptoms.
- Persistent depressive disorder (PDD) (previously known as dysthymic disorder) is characterized by chronic, low-level depression intermixed with anxious symptoms.
- Premenstrual dysphoric disorder (PMDD) involves the acute development of depressive, anxious, and somatic distress symptoms routinely occurring during the female luteal phase of the menstrual cycle.
- MDD with seasonal pattern is also known as seasonal affective disorder or seasonal depressive disorder (SDD).
- Adjustment disorder involves transient temporary depression due to stressful life events that usually passes with resolution of the stressful event.
- Secondary depression involves full MDD episodes directly from preexisting medical illness, addiction, or other psychiatric disorders.

Phenomenology, Diagnosis, Clinical Interviewing

For any new practitioner in any field, the goal is to be able to make an accurate diagnosis. All of psychiatric prescribing at this beginning level is based on regulatory findings, approvals, and indications that are psychiatric disorder specific. Psychotropics will only deliver the outcomes promised if the patient at hand actually has been accurately identified as having a bona fide DSM-5 depressive disorder. The reader should appreciate the commonalities of the genetic heritability and brain functional abnormalities that appear to be common across the DSM-5 depressive disorders, and should also understand there may be significant symptom overlap across the disorders. All of the depressive disorders are associated with a pervasive dysphoria, which may be experienced as sadness, irritability, or perhaps the absence of any positive emotional feelings. Major depressive disorder (MDD) may be further classified within itself. As this chapter focuses upon MDD, PDD, PMDD, and SDD, it shows the basic differences listed in the table above and urges the reader to appreciate that certain antidepressants may have a clinical edge depending on the precise diagnosis at hand. The reader is also urged to not downplay the significance of the more "minor" depressive disorders. For example, PDD is a low level of depression that lasts at least two years. The psychosocial dysfunction of PDD is less than that of MDD but given its chronicity, there is a "nickel and diming" effect with lower levels of suffering but over a longer period of time. Psychosocial disability findings are therefore high for both depressive states. In regard to PMDD and SDD, these patients suffer from MDD and PDD type symptoms but there is an element of specific cadence or timing to these symptoms. PMDD patients exhibit depressive type symptoms in only the luteal phase of the menstrual cycle and SDD patients exhibit their symptoms only in a specific season of the year (typically, but not always, isolated to winter months). A good interviewer will detect MDD symptoms quite readily, but an astute clinician will be able to better delineate the specific type of depression that is evident and choose a more accurate treatment.

The clinician should also be aware that MDD in particular is a highly comorbid disorder. Some patients are temporarily depressed due to a stressful event in their life, called an adjustment disorder. These transient depressive symptoms generally resolve as the life stressor improves. In these cases, the patient is expected to "bounce back," gradually improving with support. Antidepressants are generally not needed. Bolstering of social support or a referral for supportive psychotherapy is the treatment of choice. Despite this recommendation, patients who present as sad, crying, or despondent with adjustment disorder are often treated with antidepressants. Interestingly, adjustment patients may have double the response rate to antidepressants compared to MDD patients. However, this may be misleading as adjustment patients are by definition expected to get better without pharmacological management. There may be a significant placebo effect if drugs were to be utilized in these cases. Unfortunately, a pharmacological approach to the treatment of life stressors may be fraught with the same, sometimes serious, side effects that antidepressants may cause while treating MDD individuals.

Often, patients will develop a full MDD episode secondary to their lives being ruined by a pre-existing disease, illness, or other psychiatric disorder. For example, patients with deteriorating neurological conditions (Parkinson's disease or multiple sclerosis), chronic pain conditions (fibromyalgia, arthritis), or anxiety disorder have increased rates of daily suffering, loss of quality of life, etc. MDD may ensue as a result of these chronic, life-long stressors. Unlike adjustment disorder where there is a transient stressor and an expected recovery, patients with these types of secondary depression truly meet full MDD criteria and should be treated as such. There is a gray zone where a patient may convert from an adjustment disorder to a full blown MDD. This is generally determined by lack of improvement over time, as the patient should theoretically be adapting to their premorbid disorder, and by a much more severe impact on psychosocial functioning compared to that experienced by typical patients with adjustment disorder. Finally, any patient who develops suicidal or psychotic symptoms are generally considered to have moved from an adjustment disorder into full MDD.

TIP: Screening Questions for Depressive Disorders

Screening for MDD

- Have you felt predominantly sad, down, or blue over the last few weeks?
- Do you consider yourself to be depressed?
- In the last two weeks, have you had little interest or pleasure in doing things?*
- In the last two weeks, have you been feeling down, depressed, or hopeless?*

*These latter two items make up the bases for the shortest MDD screening instrument called the PHQ-2. http://www.phqscreeners.com/select-screener/111.

Screening for PDD

- Have you been depressed more often than not over two or more years continuously?
- Have you been depressed at least two years without any distinct two-month period where you were not depressed?
- Have you functioned okay despite this?

Screening for PMDD

- Do you typically only get depressed, anxious, or irritable just prior and during your period?
- Do you completely recover from these symptoms outside of this time frame?

Screening for SDD

- Do you typically function well all year and then suffer depression only during the winter months? Or a different season?

DSM-5 Diagnosis

Major Depressive Disorder (MDD)

A. Patients will have five (or more) of the following symptoms which have been present during the same two-week period and represent a change from previous functioning; at least one of the symptoms is either (1) depressed mood or (2) loss of interest or pleasure.
   1. Depressed mood most of the day, nearly every day, as indicated by either subjective report (e.g., feels sad, empty, or hopeless) or observation made by others (e.g., appears tearful).
   2. Markedly diminished interest or pleasure in all, or almost all, activities most of the day, nearly every day (as indicated by either subjective account or observation).
   3. Significant weight loss when not dieting or weight gain (e.g., a change of more than 5% of body weight in a month), or decrease or increase in appetite nearly every day.
   4. Insomnia or hypersomnia nearly every day.
   5. Psychomotor agitation or retardation nearly every day (observable by others, not merely subjective feelings of restlessness or being slowed down).
   6. Fatigue or loss of energy nearly every day.
   7. Feelings of worthlessness or excessive or inappropriate guilt (which may be delusional) nearly every day (not merely self-reproach or guilt about being sick).
   8. Diminished ability to think or concentrate, or indecisiveness, nearly every day (either by subjective account or as observed by others).
   9. Recurrent thoughts of death (not just fear of dying), recurrent suicidal ideation without a specific plan, or a suicide attempt or a specific plan for committing suicide.

B. The symptoms cause clinically significant distress or impairment in social, occupational, or other important areas of functioning.

C. The episode is not attributable to the physiological effects of a substance or to another medical condition.

Persistent Depressive Disorder (PDD)

A. Patients will have a depressed mood for most of the day, for more days than not, as indicated by either subjective account or observation by others, for at least two years.
B. Presence, while depressed, of two (or more) of the following:
   1. Poor appetite or overeating.
   2. Insomnia or hypersomnia.
   3. Low energy or fatigue.
   4. Low self-esteem.
   5. Poor concentration or difficulty making decisions.
   6. Feelings of hopelessness.
C. During the two-year period of the disturbance, the individual has never been without the symptoms in Criteria A and B for more than two months at a time.
D. Criteria for a major depressive disorder may be continuously present for two years.
E. There has never been a manic episode or a hypomanic episode, and criteria have never been met for cyclothymic disorder.
F. The disturbance is not better explained by a persistent schizoaffective disorder, schizophrenia, delusional disorder, or other specified or unspecified schizophrenia spectrum and other psychotic disorder.
G. The symptoms are not attributable to the physiological effects of a substance (e.g., a drug of abuse, a medication) or another medical condition (e.g., hypothyroidism).
H. The symptoms cause clinically significant distress or impairment in social, occupational, or other important areas of functioning.

Premenstrual Dysphoric Disorder (PMDD)

A. In the majority of menstrual cycles, at least five symptoms must be present in the final week before the onset of menses, start to *improve* within a few days after the onset of menses, and become *minimal* or absent in the week post-menses.
B. One (or more) of the following symptoms must be present:
   1. Marked affective lability (e.g., mood swings, feeling suddenly sad or tearful, or increased sensitivity to rejection).
   2. Marked irritability or anger or increased interpersonal conflicts.
   3. Marked depressed mood, feelings of hopelessness, or self-deprecating thoughts.
   4. Marked anxiety, tension, and/or feelings of being keyed up or on edge.

C. One (or more) of the following symptoms must additionally be present to reach a total of *five* symptoms when combined with symptoms from Criterion B above:
   1. Decreased interest in usual activities (e.g., work, school, friends, hobbies).
   2. Subjective difficulty in concentration.
   3. Lethargy, easy fatigability, or marked lack of energy.
   4. Marked change in appetite, overeating, or specific food cravings.
   5. Hypersomnia or insomnia.
   6. A sense of being overwhelmed or out of control.
   7. Physical symptoms such as breast tenderness or swelling, joint or muscle pain, a sensation of "bloating," or weight gain.

Note: The symptoms in Criteria A through C must have been met for most menstrual cycles that occurred in the preceding year.

D. The symptoms are associated with clinically significant distress or interference with work, school, usual social activities, or relationships with others (e.g., avoidance of social activities; decreased productivity and efficiency at work, school, or home).
E. The disturbance is not merely an exacerbation of the symptoms of another disorder, such as major depressive disorder, panic disorder, persistent depressive disorder (dysthymia), or a personality disorder (although it may co-occur with any of these disorders).
F. Criterion A should be confirmed by prospective daily ratings during at least two symptomatic cycles. (**Note:** The diagnosis may be made provisionally prior to this confirmation.)
G. The symptoms are not attributable to the physiological effects of a substance (e.g., a drug of abuse, a medication, other treatment) or another medical condition (e.g., hyperthyroidism).

Seasonal Depressive Disorder (SDD)

Patients with SDD have the exact same MDD criteria except they will experience:

A. Depression that begins during a specific season every year.
B. Depression that ends during a specific season every year.
C. No episodes of depression during the season in which they typically have normal moods.
D. Many more seasons of depression than seasons without depression over a lifetime of recurrent depressive seasonal specific episodes.

TIP: Mnemonic for MDD

SMIGECAPS may be used to inquire about **S**leep, **M**ood, **I**nterest, **E**nergy, **C**oncentration, **A**ppetite, **P**sychomotor change, and **S**uicidal thinking. It is also advised to ask about homicidal thinking. It is imperative to ask about previous manic events to rule out bipolarity and to ask about psychotic symptoms to rule out schizoaffective disorder.

Rating Scales

Patient Health Questionnaire (PHQ-9)

- This scale was adapted and validated using a DSM-based MDD symptom checklist structure.
- It is short and easy for patients to complete in office-based settings. It comes in a variety of forms (two-question, four-question, nine-question, etc.). The nine-item questionnaire is likely the most commonly employed in outpatient primary care settings. The nine-item scale assesses every one of the nine DSM-5 MDD criteria, likely saving the clinician some interviewing time in the office setting.
- A positive score of 5 or greater is likely indicative of depressive disorder. (0–9 = mild, 10–19 = moderate, 20 = severe).
- This checklist screener likely can be used to detect both PDD and SDD. The PHQ-9 will delineate the presence of depressive symptoms, but the clinician will have to assess the timing of two years or more for PDD and the localization to a season for SDD.
- It is public domain and offered free of charge via a central website (http://www.phqscreeners.com/).

Premenstrual Tension Syndrome Multiple Visual Analogue Scale (PMTS-VAS)

- This scale does not utilize a 1 to 5 Likert-type scale, instead it uses a visual analogue system where a patient places an "X along several horizontal lines to demarcate her perceived severity of symptoms. This is similar to well-adopted pain measurement scales used in hospital-based practices. It is simple and takes less than 1–2 minutes to complete.
- This scale is free for use and is in the public domain. Its reference is available at the end of this chapter.

Table 5.1 The Patient Health Questionnaire

Over the last 2 weeks, how often have you been bothered by any of the following problems? (Use "✓" to indicate your answer.)	Not at all	Several days	More than half the days	Nearly every day
1. Little interest or pleasure in doing things.	0	1	2	3
2. Feeling down, depressed, or hopeless.	0	1	2	3
3. Trouble falling or staying asleep or sleeping too much.	0	1	2	3
4. Feeling tired or having little energy.	0	1	2	3
5. Poor appetite or overeating.	0	1	2	3
6. Feeling bad about yourself—or that you are a failure or have let yourself or your family down.	0	1	2	3
7. Trouble concentrating on things, such as reading the newspaper or watching television.	0	1	2	3
8. Moving or speaking so slowly that other people have noticed? Or the opposite—being so fidgety or restless that you have been moving around a lot more than usual.	0	1	2	3
9. Thoughts that you would be better off dead or of hurting yourself in some way.	0	1	2	3

Table 5.2 Premenstrual Tension Syndrome Multiple Visual Analogue Scale

For each item, place a vertical mark on the line to indicate how you have felt during the past week.

	NOT AT ALL *VERY MUCH*
Depressed mood	______________________
Tense, restless, anxious	______________________
Emotional, mood swings	______________________
Irritable, hostile	______________________
Decreased interest in activities	______________________
Difficulty concentrating	______________________
Lethargy, easy fatigability, lack of energy	______________________
Overeating, food cravings	______________________
Change in sleep pattern:	______________________
Unable to sleep	______________________
Sleeping more	______________________
Feeling overwhelmed or out of control	______________________
Breast tenderness, bloating, water retention	______________________

Premenstrual Diaries

- There are a variety of these available online. For the greatest accuracy, women may be asked to complete a daily diary throughout 2–3 consecutive months to best delineate what PMDD symptoms they have and the timing of them as well. This approach clearly delineates the presence of depressive, anxious, and somatic PMDD symptoms only during the luteal phase. This approach helps to separate bona fide PMDD from recurrent MDD diagnoses.

Treatment Guidelines

MDD and PDD

TIP: American and European Guidelines

- Per most guidelines, an accurate diagnosis and ruling out of comorbidities is essential.
- Knowledge of the FDA indications for MDD and its subtypes and appropriate use of antidepressants is assumed.
- Generally, when MDD is diagnosed, patients may be offered psychotherapy or a safer, entry-level antidepressant, most typically a selective serotonin reuptake inhibitor (SSRI).
- For more severe depressive states, more complex psychopharmacology becomes warranted.
- A variety of medications of varying mechanisms of action are available for use at this point, where riskier medications and combinations of medications are held for later consideration.
- Typically, a single antidepressant monotherapy is escalated through its full dosing range over 2–3 months. Dose response curves may be proven factual or theoretically assumed depending on the drug.
- Successive, aggressive monotherapies should occur until a full remission of symptoms occurs. Successive agents should not utilize the same neurotransmitter mechanism of action. In other words, antidepressant classes that have failed should not be used again and again in the face of ongoing resistant depressive symptoms. If there is less than 20% measured improvement, a different antidepressant is clearly warranted.
- Sometimes, polypharmacy is warranted when two drugs of different neurotransmitter mechanisms are added together for better effectiveness and sometimes tolerability. These options are covered in greater detail in Section 2.
- Remission from symptoms is the goal, and partial responses are known to promote excessive depressive relapses later on.
- Once remission is gained, maintain the antidepressant at least one year for a single episode, 3–5 years for a second episode, and 10 years or more for a third episode. After three episodes, many patients enter a highly recurrent and refractory pattern.
- Guidelines strongly encourage the use of rating scales such as the PHQ-9.

Table 5.3 Premenstrual Diary Example

Date																															
Days of the month	1	2	3	4	5	6	7	8	9	10	11	12	13	14	15	16	17	18	19	20	21	22	23	24	25	26	27	28	29	30	31
Irritability or muscle tension																															
Anger or irritability																															
Anxiety or nervousness																															
Depression or sadness																															
Crying or tearfulness																															
Relationship problems																															
Tiredness or fatigue																															
Insomnia																															
Changes in socialization																															
Food cravings or overeating																															
Difficulty concentrating																															
Feeling overwhelmed																															
Headaches																															
Breast tenderness or swelling																															
Back or neck pain																															
Abdominal pain																															
Muscle and joint pain																															
Weight gain																															
Nausea or stomach distress																															

For the novice prescriber who attempts to treat an adult with depressive disorder, it is essential to know the basics of the available guidelines that exist to help provide a high level of care. Next, a prescriber must know what psychotropics are specifically approved for each MDD and its subtypes. This is the medico-legally sound way to prescribe and ideally obtain the outcomes that are desired for the patient. It is important to disclose to the patient that the approach being used is approved by the FDA (U.S. Food and Drug Administration).

Each DSM-5 depressive disorder will have essentially the same approach to guideline-based treatment. The safer serotonergic drugs (SSRIs) are always preferred as a first intervention. After this, a variety of medications of varying mechanisms of action are available for use. There are very few compelling guidelines for the treatment of PDD, so throughout this chapter, the recommendations for treating MDD should also be utilized for the treatment of PDD. Later in this section, there are more specific suggestions for PMDD and SDD.

There are several classes of more modern-era antidepressants that are generally considered to be safer than the older-era, tricyclic antidepressants (TCAs) and monoamine oxidase inhibitors (MAOIs). Generally, when MDD is diagnosed, patients may be offered psychotherapy or a safer, entry-level antidepressant, most typically a selective serotonin reuptake inhibitor (SSRI). The greater the severity of the MDD, the more likely an antidepressant should be utilized early on in treatment. Interestingly, some of the newer antidepressants available capitalize on the SSRI mechanism but additionally may modulate certain serotonin receptors, called SSRI-Plus antidepressants. Other authors have termed these serotonin partial agonist-reuptake inhibitors, or SPARI antidepressants for short. These multimodal drugs may actually have less sexual dysfunction and weight gain compared to the predecessor SSRI agents and certainly could be considered to be the more modern version SSRI with potentially greater tolerability in frontline management of MDD and PDD. Below are tables that describe frontline antidepressants, their mechanism of action, and purported side effects. **In regard to dosing, it is suggested that the first few days of treatment begin at slightly lower doses than those in the table below.** These doses are not more effective than placebo but likely improve compliance through minimizing initial side effects and boosting the confidence of the patient in taking the drug.

Table 5.4 SSRI Antidepressant Dosing and Side Effects

	Mechanism of Action	Dosing	Class Side Effects
SSRI			
Fluoxetine	Serotonin reuptake inhibitor (SSRI)	20–60mg/day	GI upset, headache, fatigue, anxiety, insomnia, weight gain, and sexual dysfunction More serious risk of paradoxical worsening in ages <25
Sertraline		50–200mg/day	
Paroxetine		20–50mg/day	
Citalopram		20–40mg/day	
Escitalopram		10–20mg/day	

	Mechanism of Action	Dosing	Class Side Effects
SSRI-Plus			
Vilazodone	Serotonin reuptake inhibitor and modulation of serotonin receptors (SSRI-Plus, or sometimes called serotonin partial agonist reuptake inhibitors (SPARI))	10–40 mg/day	Same as SSRIs, perhaps less weight gain and sexual dysfunction
Vortioxetine		10–20 mg/day	

	Mechanism of Action	Dosing	Class Side Effects
NDRI			
Bupropion (SR and XL)	Norepinephrine and dopamine reuptake inhibitor (NDRI)	150–450mg/day	Dry mouth, nausea, insomnia, anxiety, weight loss, subtle blood pressure increases. Risk of seizures in those with epilepsy or eating disorder. Relatively devoid of sexual side effects

	Mechanism of Action	Dosing	Class Side Effects
SNRI			
Venlafaxine	Serotonin and norepinephrine reuptake inhibitor (SNRI)	75–225mg/day	Same as SSRI but though subtle worsening of dry mouth, nausea, anxiety, insomnia, or blood pressure may be noted
Desvenlafaxine		50–400mg/day	
Duloxetine		60–120mg/day	
Levomilnacipran		40–120mg/day	

	Mechanism of Action	Dosing	Class Side Effects
Sedating Antidepressants			
Trazodone	Serotonin-2a antagonist/reuptake inhibitor (SARI)	50–600mg/day	Dizziness, sedation, hypotension. Relatively devoid of sexual dysfunction and activating side effects
Nefazodone		50–300mg/day	Same as above except rare cases of hepatitis
Mirtazapine	Noradrenergic alpha-2 antagonist and specific serotonergic agent (NaSSA)	15–45mg/day	Same as above except weight gain and metabolic syndrome

Summary for Initial MDD Treatment

In reality, any one of the above agents is remarkably safer for MDD treatment when compared to the older TCAs or MAOIs. Prescribers would have the evidence base and the standard of care to support use of any one of the above. As the SSRIs are all generic, easy to obtain from insurance carriers, and have been successfully in use since the 1980s, they are generally prescribed first. All antidepressants may worsen patients, create anxiety, insomnia, or suicidal thinking. All of the above antidepressants are relatively devoid of end-organ side effects and rarely require any blood or EKG monitoring. Most can induce mild to severe weight gain at times (those with serotonergic mechanisms). Some can induce increases in blood pressure (those with norepinephrine mechanisms). Vital sign monitoring is suggested. SSRIs and SNRIs may promote blood thinning and bruising due to increases in peripheral serotonin and lowered platelet clotting efficiency.

TIP: Some Reasons to NOT Start with an SSRI Include:

- If the patient fears weight gain, consider a non-SSRI or non-SNRI.
- If the patient prefers to lose weight, consider an NDRI.
- If the patient fears sexual dysfunction, consider a non-SSRI or non-SNRI.
- If the patient is cachectic and needs weight gain, consider a sedating antidepressant.
- If the patient is remarkably anxious or insomnic, consider a sedating antidepressant.
- If the patient suffers from neuropathic pain, consider an SNRI.
- If the patient suffers from vasomotor symptoms, consider an SNRI.

Acute Management Dosing Considerations

TIP: Acute Management Dosing Considerations

- All antidepressants have a minimum effective dose that has been shown to beat a placebo in regulatory studies. Some antidepressants start at this dose and others must be titrated to this level. Failure to reach this dose generally guarantees non-effectiveness.
- For greater tolerability, sometimes smaller doses and tablet sizes are started for a few days. This may delay the time to antidepressant effect, but the patient generally experiences the first few doses without side effects and may have greater confidence in the drug and the prescriber. Starting low is reasonable but the minimum therapeutic dose must be achieved.

- After 2–4 weeks at the initial therapeutic dose, the patient should be evaluated. If they are in remission, then this dose should be continued as is.
- If the patient does not respond partially to the minimum dose, then a middle and higher dose should be tried for 2–4 weeks each. Again, if no response then a titration to the maximal regulatory dose should occur.
- Despite language that suggests there may be no additional benefit to higher doses, more modern antidepressants do show a dose-response curve, and recent meta-analyses have shown that larger doses provide better antidepressant effects even for the older SSRIs.
- There may be a higher side effect rate at higher doses.
- A therapeutic antidepressant monotherapy trial typically involves titration from low to middle to high doses. It takes 2–4 months to complete. If a trial fails to improve a patient to remission, then a cross titration to a new monotherapy is suggested.
- When switching from one failed antidepressant trial to another, the failed medication should be gradually lowered while the new antidepressant is again raised through the same low to high dose protocol.
- Generally, if a patient fails to respond to an initial antidepressant, then the next antidepressant to be tried should be from a different antidepressant class.
- For example, if a patient failed an SSRI, the next antidepressant might be an SSRI-Plus, or an NDRI, an SNRI, or a sedating antidepressant, not another SSRI as this just replicates a mechanism that biologically has just failed the patient.
- If a patient cannot tolerate the initial SSRI due to activating insomnia or anxiety side effects, then generally a much lower dose and much lower titration strategy can be tried on the next antidepressant, or the patient should be tried on a sedating antidepressant which tends to avoid this side effect profile overall.

TIP: Remission

- A response to an antidepressant trial per the trial literature is considered to be when a patient has at least 50% improvement in regard to DSM-5 depressive symptom severity.
- Unfortunately, partially better usually results in greater depressive relapses. The goal of treatment is remission. At the highest level, this means a complete resolution of every depressive symptom.

- Sometimes this is achieved with aggressive monotherapy trials as outlined above. Sometimes addition of psychotherapy, hypnotics, anxiolytics, antipsychotics, nutraceuticals, or multiple antidepressants is needed to gain a full remission.
- More realistically, a remission could be defined as the patient becomes 80–90% better compared to their baseline evaluation or rating scale findings. For example, a PHQ-9 score of less than five would suggest no depression.
- Oftentimes, patients will become less sad and be less visibly depressed but still have fatigue, insomnia, and poor concentration. These three symptoms may be residual enough to trigger more depressive relapses later. Repeating a depression interview or rating scale is needed at each visit to best determine if remission has occurred.
- Once remission is achieved, it is imperative to monitor for pending relapses at each visit. If the depression is returning, typically the monotherapy dose is subtly increased to abort the pending relapse. If that fails, a new antidepressant can be cross titrated.

TIP: Long-Term Maintenance

- MDD and PDD are considered more often to be chronic and recurring disorders. It is often better to err on the side of over-treating regarding dosing and consecutive months of treatment to avoid depressive recurrences.
- Once a remission is achieved for the patient's first ever depressive episode, then the drug and dosing should continue for 6–12 months to ensure a long period of remission. After this, the antidepressant can be tapered off over several weeks.
- If the patient is in a second lifetime depressive episode and has achieved remission, he/she should be maintained 3–5 years prior to a slow tapering over a few months. If the patient is in a third episode, perhaps a decade to lifetime of treatment is warranted.
- Longer maintenance may be warranted if the patient is geriatric (recurrence rates are very high), if the current depressive episode was very severe with frequent suicidality, or if the episode was very refractory and remission was hard to achieve.
- It is generally accepted that antidepressants and augmentations needed to achieve a depressive remission should continue throughout treatment to ensure a lengthy remission unless side effects and tolerability interfere.

PMDD

- There are only two treatments approved for PMDD currently. They are the SSRIs fluoxetine and sertraline.
- Fluoxetine is dosed for the luteal two weeks of every menstrual cycle, and the patient is off medication the other two weeks.
- Sertraline is dosed daily, every day of the month. Dosing and side effects are similar to those outlined for MDD and PDD.

SDD

- There is currently only one approved antidepressant: bupropion XL. It is started in the early fall for winter-based depressions and tapered in the spring.
- Bright light therapy of 10,000 lux broad spectrum white light or 5,000 lux of blue light have been shown to alleviate this depression if used every morning for 30–60 minutes.

SECTION 2 Advanced Prescribing Practices

Introduction

In Section 1, the premise was to convince the reader that they must make an accurate diagnosis and pick an approved agent with well-defined dosing guidelines and expected clinical outcomes. This approach is largely one of pattern recognition: (1) identify the pattern of phenotypic symptoms, (2) choose from a finite list of available, proven effective drugs, (3) start dosing low and escalate through an approved dosing range, (4) assess for effectiveness, and (5) continue medication if effective, and cross-titrate to a new drug if ineffective or not tolerated. This is a methodical, mathematical approach that can improve the standard of care and, ideally, patient outcomes when treated by the novice psychopharmacologist.

Section 2 again is designed to provide a greater depth of neuroscience and pharmacodynamic knowledge to the reader. It is written for prescribers who are knowledgeable and competent in those skills outlined in Section 1. It is also written for those clinicians who treat patients who fail to respond to first-level treatments. The section is generally intended for those patients felt to be treatment resistant. This means that the depressive-disordered patient has failed to respond to serotonergic only (SSRI) monotherapy or two successive monotherapy trials. Section 2 will also teach more about depression psychopharmacology when treating complicated, comorbid conditions (addiction, bipolarity, anxiety, etc.).

This section will address appropriate combinations of medications and augmentations of medications, which are usually reserved for those patients who have failed more easy and typical pharmacological approaches. A *combination* occurs when a prescriber adds one approved antidepressant medication to a second approved antidepressant medication in hopes of gaining additive effects and further aiming for a full remission after a monotherapy has failed. An augmentation occurs when a non-approved, or off-label medication is added to an approved antidepressant medication that failed to produce a full remission of symptoms. Off-label prescribing is not *experimental.* These medications are often approved for other medical disorders (Parkinson's disease, schizophrenia, ADHD, etc.) and have efficacy and safety data available in the literature for these indicated conditions but are repurposed for use in adult depressive disorders. Augmentations may have a wide variety of data available in the evidence base. In Section 2, the drugs reviewed are felt to have at least a moderate amount of effectiveness and safety data to support their use in the treatment of MDD and PDD (there is much less supportive data for PMDD and SDD), have solid neuroscience and pharmacodynamic theory to support their use, and are felt to be commonly deployed in clinical practice and considered to be within the standard of care in treating adults with DSM-5 described MDD. While following suggestions from this section in your clinical work, it would make sense to document that initial, approved treatments have failed and that the rationale to use a combination or augmentation is warranted due to the MDD's resistance to treatment and support within the literature, and is evident in the standard of care for your geographic area.

Epidemiology

- Depression runs the spectrum from normal response to usual life adversities (grief) to severe and pathological psychiatric disorders. Over the course of development of the DSM system, there is ongoing refinement in the classification and diagnosis of the depressive disorders.
- Major depressive disorder (MDD) is experienced as excessive, nonstop, pervasive sadness and loss of enjoyment.
- Persistent depressive disorder (PDD) is characterized by chronic, low-level depression intermixed with anxious symptoms. It used to be called dysthymic disorder in previous DSM versions.
- Premenstrual dysphoric disorder (PMDD) involves the acute development of depressive, anxious, and somatic distress symptoms that occur regularly during the female luteal phase of the menstrual cycle.
- MDD with seasonal pattern is also known as seasonal affective disorder (SAD) or seasonal depressive disorder (SDD). This occurs when major depressive episodes (MDEs) regularly occur only on a particular part of the calendar year (ex. winter-only depression).

Table 5.5 Depressive Disorder Lifetime Prevalences

DEPRESSIVE DISORDER LIFETIME PREVALENCES	
MDD	16%
PDD	3%
PMDD	6.4%
SDD	1.4–9.7%*

*Highest prevalence rates likely occur at higher latitudes.

Genetics

- The heritability of depressive disorders may be comparable to that of many of the anxiety disorders. Perhaps 20–40% of depressive disorder onset may be attributable to genetic causes.
- ADHD, bipolar disorder, and schizophrenia likely have greater heritability. This would suggest that depressive disorder may occur as a result of greater environmental impact or by way of gene/environment interactions (epigenetics).

TIP: Genetics of MDD

- MDD is felt to be 36–44% heritable based upon twin studies.
- PDD has very little data but is considered to be similar to that of MDD.
- Meta-analyses of genome-wide association studies (GWAS) suggest no clear single genetic link to MDD. Researchers feel that study sample sizes may have to be three-fold higher than those used in bipolar or schizophrenia genome-wide association studies, suggesting much less heritability for MDD.
- Adenylate cyclase-3 and galanin genes have been subtly implicated and both tied to errors in serotonergic transmission.
- CACNA1C gene has been implicated in cyclical depressive states.
- At times, positive findings suggest that mutations in the serotonin transporter (SERT), or reuptake pump, may lead to depressive risks. Those with the short S-alleles tend to experience greater depression and suicidality in response to social stress.
- Other implicated genes may include tryptophan hydroxylase, brain-derived neurotrophic factor (BNDF), catechol-O-methyl transferase (COMT), monoamine oxidase A/B (MAO), phospholipase A2, the glucocorticoid receptor methylenetetrahydrofolate reductase (MTHFR), and the serotonin receptor 1A gene.
- Generally, target genes are those felt to impede or alter monoaminergic (serotonin-norepinephrine, dopamine) neurotransmission.

TIP: Genetics of PMDD

- Mutations in estrogen receptor alpha (ER1) have been found to be related to development of PMDD.
- There may be an epistasis with the catechol-O-methyltransferase (COMT) Val alleles that may amplify risk. COMT generally degrades monoamines such as serotonin, dopamine, and norepineprhine. The Val alleles may allow for aggressive COMT subtypes, thus lowering CNS monoamines.
- The 5-HTTLPR serotonin transporter gene may be implicated as a risk to the development of both PMDD and SDD. Even having one short S-allele may convey this risk based on smaller studies.
- Other efforts regarding serotonin metabolism have shown no gene influence on PMDD. MAO-A is another CNS enzyme that degrades monoamines. It likewise has shown no association in smaller studies.

TIP: Genetics of SDD

- Some genetic research has investigated the "clock genes" which create proteins that cycle in counterphase to help the brain determine daytime versus nighttime. This may be the biological basis of the 24-hour circadian clock.
- SDD patients more often may have mutations in some of these clock genes. CLOCK, Period2, Period3, and NPAS2 genes have been studied, and the NPAS2 leucine allele may convey the greatest risk for SDD development.
- Period3 heterozygous alleles (VAL/GLY) were associated with self-reported morningness–eveningness, suggesting genetic vulnerability here as well.

Neuroanatomy

- There are several key neuroanatomic structures in the brain responsible for promoting good mental health, and when any of these structures function abnormally, becoming hyperactive or hypoactive, psychiatric symptoms may develop.
- Generally, many functional imaging studies tend to show a hyperactive limbic system and ventromedial prefrontal cortex (VMPFC) while showing an underactive dorsolateral prefrontal cortex (DLPFC).

TIP: Functional Neuroanatomical Findings in Depressive Disorder

- **VMPFC**—increased activity representing emotional processing.
- **Amygdala**—increased activity representing fear processing.
- **Subcallosal Cingulate**—increased activity representing sadness.
- **Anterior Cingulate and Insular Cortex**—increased activity representing emotional recall and social cues.

Neuroscientific Background and Rationale for Medication Use

In treating MDD, there are several classes of frequently-used medications (SSRIs, SNRIs, SSRI-Plus, sedating antidepressants, and NDRIs as discussed in Section 1). Additionally, the approved TCA and MAOI classes tend to be used in more treatment-resistant depressive disorders. All antidepressants seem to increase the availability of the monoamine neurotransmitters dopamine, norepinephrine, or serotonin. Off-label (non-antidepressant medications) agents that have antidepressant potential also most often work through these transmitter systems.

1) The SSRI (Selective Serotonin Reuptake Inhibitors)

MECHANISM OF ACTION

Fluoxetine (Prozac), sertraline (Zoloft), paroxetine (Paxil), citalopram (Celexa), escitalopram (Lexapro)

- All SSRIs are similar in that they block serotonin reuptake pumps. More scientifically, this is called inhibition of the serotonin transporter (SERT). The net effect is an increase in serotonin (SR or sometimes abbreviated "5HT") availability in BOTH the frontal cortex and the limbic system.
- The frontal cortex may govern higher levels of emotional processing and emotional thinking, especially in the ventromedial prefrontal cortex (VMPFC). The limbic system is likely in charge of more primitive functions, such as threat assessment, fight or flight responses, etc. This system evolutionarily functions to provide enjoyment and reward emotionally as well. SSRI use may restore abnormal functioning.
- Interestingly, the SSRI increases SR immediately, with an increase in SR neuronal circuitry firing, though these agents often take a few weeks to become effective. Increasing SR likely creates a more toxic or unusual environment for SR neurons in the brain. Each neuron likely registers this increased SR concentration as foreign and responds by activating transcription factors within said neurons. These factors will

interact with neuronal DNA and create new proteins. Some of these proteins may migrate to the neuronal surface and engulf the SR receptors. This is called downregulation, which may take a few weeks to occur as this is the length of time it takes for DNA to RNA to protein synthesis (transcription and translation) to occur in a great enough volume to see enough receptors downregulate to create a clinical antidepressant effect. Other proteins may be new transcription factors that turn other neuronal DNA genes on or off.

- Sometimes brain or neuronal health proteins are turned on, such as brain derived neurotrophic factors (BDNF). These factors may improve neuronal connectivity and allow different brain areas to communicate more effectively, thus lowering depressive symptoms.

2) The SNRI (Serotonin-Norepinephrine Reuptake Inhibitors)

MECHANISM OF ACTION

Venlafaxine XR (Effexor XR), desvenlafaxine (Pristiq), duloxetine (Cymbalta), levomilnacipran (Fetzima)

- All SNRIs are similar in that they block serotonin reuptake pumps. (Des) venlafaxine and duloxetine, even at lower doses, are as effective as the SSRI class in regard to serotonin reuptake inhibition (SRI). They essentially have the same ability as an SSRI. Norepinephrine reuptake inhibition (NRI) is also accomplished by these agents. Levomilnacipran may have the greatest noradrenergic potential even at lower doses, where venlafaxine XR may have the least until maximal doses are reached.
- SNRIs have two mechanisms in place to treat MDD: SRI and NRI properties. The net effect of SERT and NET reuptake inhibition with the SNRI antidepressants is an increase in SR and NE availability in BOTH the frontal cortex and the limbic system.
- The downstream effects of increasing NE may lead to receptor downregulation, etc. comparable to those described in the SSRI mechanism section.

3) SSRI-Plus Antidepressants

MECHANISM OF ACTION

Vilazodone (Viibryd), vortioxetine (Trintellix)

- Vilazodone is a unique antidepressant as it is felt to be a weak to moderate SSRI affording it a more benign side effect profile. It also has the ability to partially agonize the serotonin 5HT-1a receptor *both* at pre- and postsynaptic receptors, which is different from buspirone and other psychotropics' presynaptic-only activity. This dual mechanism facilitates greater synaptic serotonin activity through SERT inhibition and ultimately the serotonin neuron outputs greater serotonin as the 5HT-1a receptors gradually are over-stimulated and downregulated and the inhibiting autoreceptor effect is lost.

- Vortioxetine is more fully an SSRI at usual therapeutic doses. It also affects 5HT-1a receptors presynaptically via partial agonism. Additionally it antagonizes 5HT-1d (circadian rhythm improvement theoretically), 5HT-3 (increases monoamine release from the midbrain), and 5HT-7 (likely improves cognition).
- Side effects: comparable to the SSRI as both of these SSRI-Plus antidepressants use the SRI mechanism (described in Section 1 and the Prescribing Table). Interestingly, by facilitating 5HT-1a partial agonism, more dopamine may be available in spinal cord tracts, thus lowering the rate of sexual dysfunction. Weight gain side effects may also be less with these agents, but the supporting data is less stringent.

4) TCA (Tricyclic Antidepressants)

MECHANISM OF ACTION

Imipramine (Tofranil), desipramine (Norpramin), amitriptyline (Elavil), nortriptyline (Pamelor), etc.

- This class of antidepressant is placed here in the discussion as it uses the same type of reuptake inhibition as those drug families noted above. These agrents are clearly second or third line as their tolerability is generally much worse and safety profile more risky.
- TCAs share a similar mechanism to that of SNRIs. SNRIs are called selective as they mainly act at SERT and NET but avoid anticholinergic, anti-alpha-adrenergic, and antihistaminergic side effects. Essentially, TCAs can provide SRI and NRI properties to treat depression, but unfortunately block, or antagonize, cholinergic muscarinic (ACHm) and alpha-1 (A1) and histamine-1 (H1) receptors causing more remarkable side effects when compared to SSRI, SNRI, and SPA classes of antidepressants.
- TCAs can be separated and divided in many ways. It may be useful to consider each TCA's unique ability to provide either more or less NRI as a simple, delineating factor.
  - **Desipramine and nortriptyline** are actually metabolites of imipramine and amitriptyline, respectively. Desipramine and nortriptyline are NRI predominant. Add protriptyline as the third NE robust TCA and this makes a sub-class within the TCA family. If a

prescriber is looking for NE tone activity in order to treat ADHD-like symptoms or improve frontal lobe functioning (change fatigue to alertness, inattention to vigilance, improve cortical control of limbic anxiety, etc.), then these may be the more select TCA to use. However, it should be noted that drugs with primary NRI property may iatrogenically increase anxiety or insomnia at first. On the positive side, these NRI-based TCAs often have less anticholinergic, histaminergic, and alpha adrenergic side effects.
    - **Imipramine, amitriptyline, clomipramine, and doxepin** all start as potent SRI-based anxiolytic antidepressants. Clomipramine is only approved for anxiety treatment (OCD). All of these agents are converted by the liver into metabolites that possess NRI properties (desipramine, nortriptyline, norclomipramine, and nordoxepin). Essentially, after first-pass hepatic metabolism these drugs now possess SRI and NRI properties.
- If prescribers divide TCAs into the NRI predominant versus SRI/NRI balanced, then clinical application can be considered as follows: for patients who are currently taking an SSRI, an NRI predominant TCA can be added essentially to create an SNRI situation. For those patients who have failed SSRIs and need to move to an SNRI, then a balanced TCA may be an option. The dropout rate is much higher for TCAs over SNRIs, so that the SNRI class should be considered first. If the SNRI fails, then a cross-titration to a balanced TCA may be warranted.

Table 5.6 Common Side Effects Associated with Receptor Blockade of Tricyclic Antidepressants

	Receptor Blockade		
	Anticholinergic	**Antiadrenergic**	**Antihistaminergic**
Side Effects	Dry mouth, blurred vision, constipation, urinary retention, memory problems.	Dizziness, orthostasis syncope, fatigue.	Fatigue, sedation, appetite and weight gain.

Side Effects

- TCAs, as noted above, are often associated with greater amounts of fatigue, weight gain, dizziness, orthostasis, dry mouth, blurred vision, and constipation. The elderly are much more prone to these side effects and have higher TCA cessation rates. In addition, as these drugs are SRI-based, patients can experience all of the SSRI side effects that are attributable to SR excess (headaches, GI upset, activating side effects, sexual dysfunction, and weight gain).
- The NRI-predominant TCAs will have side effects similar to SNRIs, with elevated chances of developing dry mouth, activating side effects

including insomnia and anxiety, palpitations, tremors, and mild increases in blood pressure. The TCA class is the most likely class to activate and escalate bipolar depressives into manic states. TCAs have narrow therapeutic windows where low doses are ineffective and high doses may cause cardiac conduction abnormalities. The latter often include an increase in EKG QTc measurements and may result in ventricular arrhythmia and myocardial infarction.

- A 1500mg purposeful overdose may be enough in some patients to cause this to occur. As such, these drugs are often avoided or used in weekly supplies with suicidal patients.
- Middle aged and older patients likely should have an initial EKG completed, again after TCA titration, and then annually. Blood may be drawn for many of the TCAs to determine if blood plasma levels are therapeutic and not toxic. (**See Prescribing Table.**) These are drawn after steady state, approximately one week of treatment at moderate dose and in the morning prior to any TCA use (trough level).
- Prescribers also must be advised that TCAs are highly dependent on the hepatic CYP4502D6 metabolic pathway to be cleared. The SSRIs paroxetine and fluoxetine, being strong inhibitors here, may triple TCA levels and risk rapid toxicity as a result. Citalopram is a moderate inhibitor and may double levels. The SSRIs with the least interaction would include sertraline and escitalopram, and the safest SNRIs would be venlafaxine and desvenlafaxine.

5) MAOI (Monoamine Oxidase Inhibitors)

MECHANISM OF ACTION

Tranylcypromine (Parnate), phenelzine (Nardil), isocarboxazid (Marplan), selegeline (EMSAM Patch)

- MAOIs are one of the original antidepressant treatments approved for use in MDD. They have a unique mechanism where these drugs irreversibly inhibit and render ineffective monoamine oxidase A and B enzymes, which serve to destroy serotonin, norepinephrine, and dopamine simultaneously, increasing the levels of these monoamines in the central nervous system (CNS). Inhibiting MAO robustly increases all three transmitters at once.
- These are used primarily for MDD, but MAOIs do have a niche in treating certain refractory anxiety disorders. Social anxiety disorder (SAD) has many similarities to atypical depressive states (rejection sensitivity) and may be used for more treatment-resistant SAD when SSRIs, SNRIs, and BZs fail to remit symptoms. Sometimes MAOIs are used in the treatment of OCD as well.

Side Effects

Drug-Drug Interactions:

- MAOI agents have major *synergistic* interactions if combined with other agents that are effective at increasing serotonin in the CNS. Classically, most antidepressants with serotonin reuptake inhibition (SRI) and, theoretically, some with serotonin receptor modulation (5HT-1A agonism) may create serotonin toxicity or syndrome. This adverse effect can be lethal as a result of hyperthermia and cardiovascular instability.
- MAOIs may have *additive* drug interactions when combined with other agents that facilitate or increase norepinephrine activity and may be associated with gradual increases in blood pressure. Generally, these are not hypertensive crises.

Drug-Dietary Interactions:

- MAOI agents have a *synergistic* interaction when combined with foods that contain tyramine. Tyramine in food reacts in the GI tract and creates a robust release of norepinephrine (NE) in the periphery. This causes constriction of blood vessels and an acute, extreme increase in blood pressure may occur. This may lead to heart attack or stroke. Tyramine rich foods should be avoided if MAOIs are prescribed. The only exception is the use of the MAOI transdermal skin patch, selegiline. At the low, 6mg/day dose, the MAOI diet is not necessary.

TIP: Serotonin Syndrome

- Serotonin syndrome may be caused by adding any antidepressant except for bupropion to an MAOI. Certain controlled pain medication (meperidine, fentanyl, tramadol, etc.) may contain SRI properties and cause this lethal side effect. Certain antihistamines and cough suppressants (brompheniramine, chlorpheniramine, dextromethorphan, etc.) may as well. Certain antipsychotics theoretically possess higher serotonergic activity (ziprasidone, aripiprazole, brexpiprazole, cariprazine, etc.) and may become problematic.
- Serotonin syndrome consists of confusion, agitation, headache, blood pressure changes, fever, nausea, diarrhea, palpitations, tremors, loss of coordination or balance, and diaphoresis. Vital sign instability may cause death.

TIP: Drugs That May Gradually Increase Blood Pressure

- ADHD stimulants
- Nasal decongestants
- Noradrenergic antidepressants

TIP: Dietary Foods That May Create a Hypertensive Crisis

- Aged cheeses, such as cheddar, blue, gorgonzola, camembert, and brie.
- Aged, fermented, smoked, air dried, and pickled meats, such as mortadella, pepperoni, salami, summer sausage, and jerky.
- Fermented soybeans and soybean paste (such as miso), tofu, and soy sauce; kimchi (fermented cabbage), and sauerkraut.
- Fermented or spoiled fruits or vegetables.
- Yeast extracts, such as brewer's yeast pills or liquid; bottled or canned beer, including non-alcoholic beer (drink only one 12-ounce bottle per day); red and white wine (drink only four ounces per day).

6) NDRI (norepinephrine-dopamine reuptake inhibitors)

MECHANISM OF ACTION

Bupropion (Wellbutrin XL)

- Bupropion is the only agent in this class and it comes in once, twice, and three times daily preparations (IR, SR, XL).
- It is an NRI that inhibits NET, and this elevates NE tone to treat depression. This is also a dopamine reuptake inhibitor (DRI) that blocks the dopamine transporter (DAT).
- This is the only antidepressant with this mechanism and is devoid of serotonergic activity. This offers the unique side effect profile of a relative absence of sexual dysfunction and often provides for weight loss.

Side Effects

- Bupropion products are generally well tolerated. Dry mouth, anxiety, agitation, insomnia, and diaphoresis may be noted. Upon release of the original bupropion preparation, which was often utilized at high doses, some patients suffered from seizures. This drug has been reformulated and dosed lower, and induction of seizures theoretically only occurs in those with previous seizure or eating disorder history.

7) Sedating Antidepressants

MECHANISM OF ACTION

Trazodone (Desyrel), nefazodone (Serzone), mirtazapine (Remeron)

- These three drugs all share a similar side effect. Antihistamine properties make them sedating in nature. Anti-alpha1 receptor activity also provides for a sedating profile. They are sometimes used as hypnotics or anxiolytics as such. Lowering insomnia and agitation may alleviate two core depressive symptoms very quickly.
- All of these agents antagonize the 5HT-2a and 2c receptor. Mechanistically, this property allows for cortical increases in NE and DA, which are felt to lower depressive symptoms.
- Trazodone and nefazodone are weaker SRI agents as well. This property likely becomes more effective at higher doses. These two agents are sometimes termed serotonin antagonist-reuptake inhibitors (SARI).
- Mirtazapine is different and unique within this class and among all antidepressants, and is sometimes called a norepinephrine antagonist-specific serotonin antagonist (NASSA). In addition to H1, 5HT-2a, 5HT-2c antagonism, it blocks the 5HT-3 receptor which may stimulate mid-brain release of NE, DA, and SR to the cortex. Additionally, it antagonizes noradrenergic alpha-2 receptors. By inhibiting these autoreceptors, cortical NE neurons are forced to release excess NE, yielding yet another antidepressant effect.

Side Effects

- These agents often create fatigue, sedation, or somnolence. Occasionally dizziness or syncope may be noted. Specifically, trazodone is noted for inducing priapism, nefazodone for hepatotoxicity, and mirtazapine for weight gain and metabolic disorder.
- These drugs may also be considered frontline treatments for MDD along with the NDRI, SSRI, SNRI, and SSRI-Plus medications as they do not carry the major risks associated with MAOIs or TCAs.
- These drugs are ideal for patients who cannot tolerate SSRIs, SSRI-Plus, or SNRIs. These drugs are not activating, and do not create insomnia or panic. They do not often induce sexual dysfunction. They seem to have the opposite side effect profile of SSRIs and SNRIs. In fact, these drugs are sometimes added to SSRI/SNRIs not only as a combination strategy to further treat MDD, but may be used to lower initial side effects from the SSRI/SNRIs as well. This is a win-win situation, as effectiveness may increase and adverse effects decrease as two meds are combined.

Augmentation/Combination Strategies and Off-Label Antidepressants

The above listing of antidepressants are all approved for use in the U.S. and have largely been described in successive monotherapy strategies. This next subsection will discuss approved augmentation strategies and their mechanisms of action, as well as some off-label pharmacological approaches used to treat depression.

1) Olanzapine-Fluoxetine Combination (Symbyax)

MECHANISM OF ACTION

- Olanzapine (Zyprexa) is an atypical antipsychotic (SGA) and as such may treat psychomotor agitation via D2 receptor antagonism. 5HT-2a receptor antagonism may have properties similar to the sedating antidepressants nefazodone and trazodone. Additionally, the SSRI fluoxetine (Prozac) is combined for further antidepressant activity.

Side Effects

- Olanzapine (SGA) and fluoxetine (SSRI) have been discussed extensively in prior sections. Major side effects to monitor for include TD, EPS, metabolic syndrome, agranulocytosis, and increased lethality symptoms (those under age 25). Typically, patients may also suffer from sedation and somnolence.

2) Aripiprazole (Abilify) or Brexpiprazole (Rexulti) Augmentation

MECHANISM OF ACTION

- These are both SGAs and block 5HT-2a receptors as a possible antidepressant property. This novel class of SGAs are known to partially agonize D2 and D3 receptors. As such, brain areas low in DA activity may be stimulated, theoretically providing an antidepressant effect. Furthermore, both agents partially agonize 5HT-1a receptors in a mechanism similar to the anxiolytic buspirone.

Side Effects

- Similar to all SGAs there is risk of TD, EPS, metabolic disorder, and agranulocytosis. Increased lethality may be seen initially in those under

the age of 25. Aripiprazole may have double the akathisia risk but brexpiprazole may allow for more sedation and weight gain.
- Readers are referred to the bipolar and schizophrenia chapters for further discussion.

3) Quetiapine (Seroquel XR)

MECHANISM OF ACTION

- This is another SGA which commonly blocks 5HT-2a receptors as a possible antidepressant property. This SGA has a known metabolite, norquetiapine, which is a potent NRI, blocks 5HT-2c/5HT-3 similar to vortioxetine (Trintellix), and also partially agonizes 5HT-1a receptors. It is a multimodal SGA with many antidepressant properties.

Side Effects

- Similar to all SGAs there is risk of TD, EPS, metabolic disorder, and agranulocytosis. Increased lethality may be seen initially in those under the age of 25. Quetiapine has a fair amount of sedation, weight gain, and other metabolic symptoms. It also carries a warning for cataracts.
- Readers are referred to the bipolar and schizophrenia chapters for further discussion.

Evidence-Based, Off-Label Strategies for MDD

1) Bupropion + SSRI/SNRI/SSRI-Plus/Sedating Antidepressant

MECHANISM OF ACTION

- Bupropion (Wellbutrin XL) is an NDRI and is novel in that it increases synaptic levels of NE and DA given its DRI (DAT inhibition) and NRI (NET inhibition) without affecting serotonin (5HT). This makes it an ideal combination agent where it can be safely mixed with other more predominantly serotonergic drugs. It can be added to other noradrenergic or dopaminergic agents (SNRI, TCA) but additive side effects should be considered (ex. gradual blood pressure increases, insomnia, etc.).

Side Effects

- As previously discussed, bupropion generally is an activating drug (causing insomnia and agitation) and if added to other activating drugs (SNRI) then these side effects may increase. Interestingly, if added to a more sedating agent, those side effects may be nicely countered and alleviated.

2. Mirtazapine + SSRI/SNRI/SSRI-Plus

MECHANISM OF ACTION

- As noted previously, mirtazapine (Remeron) increases NE tone by inhibiting alpha-2 autoreceptors. This drug also antagonizes 5HT-2a, 5HT-2c, and 5HT-3 receptors, all of which have theoretical antidepressant properties. As this drug is not an SSRI/SNRI, it can be safely added to almost any other antidepressant. The serotonergic properties of mirtazapine are fairly weak, making serotonin syndrome risk minimal.
- This combination has clear, randomized control trials to support its use.

Side Effects

- As a sedating antidepressant, it may cause fatigue and somnolence. Interestingly, if this drug is combined with an activating SSRI, SNRI, or NDRI it may counteract these side effects nicely. This drug also has a propensity for inducing remarkable weight gain. Again, this is sometimes counteracted by noradrenergic antidepressants in combination or may increase weight gain if combined with more serotonergic agents.

3. Trazodone + SSRI/SNRI/SSRI-Plus

MECHANISM OF ACTION

- Blockade of 5HT-2a and weak SSRI properties allow for antidepressant effects of trazodone (Desyrel). This drug is often combined with SSRI, SNRI, NDRI, NASSA, SARI, and SSRI-Plus agents. Its SRI effects are weak and there is minimal risk for serotonin syndrome. Trazodone is quite sedating and often is used in sub-therapeutic antidepressant doses which improve insomnia.

Side Effects

- Sedation and lightheadedness are the most common side effects and thought to occur due to alpha-1 noradrenergic receptor activity. Antihistamine properties may also exist. Orthostasis and priapism are concerning as well but fairly rare in practice.

4. Buspirone + SSRI/SNRI/SSRI-Plus/Sedating antidepressants

MECHANISM OF ACTION

- Buspirone (BuSpar) works via partial agonism at presynaptic 5HT-1a receptors. Initially this dampens 5HT neuronal firing but after prolonged (2–3 weeks) use, these autoreceptors are downregulated, thus allowing for net increases in 5HT firing rates.

Side Effects

- Very similar to the SSRI (headache, GI side effects) but relatively lacking in sexual dysfunction or weight gain. Minimal risks of serotonin syndrome when mixed with SSRI, SNRI, or sedating antidepressants

5. BZRA + SSRI/SNRI/SSRI-Plus

MECHANISM OF ACTION

- The benzodiazepine receptor agonist (BZRA) hypnotic agents are very similar to true BZ anxiolytics and are discussed in greater detail in the insomnia chapter.
- These bind to the GABA-A receptor complex and facilitate chloride channel activity and neuronal hyperpolarization. When this occurs in the sleep-inducing centers in the ventrolateral preoptic area (VLPO), specifically via BZ1 subreceptors, sleep is facilitated.
- Within a single dose, sleep may improve in depressed patients. With better sleep, patients may have improved energy and concentration, and it is suspected that these three MDD criteria may preferentially respond in this augmentation strategy.

Side Effects

- Like the BZ anxiolytics, sedation, somnolence, ataxia, dysarthria, and the potential for addiction must be considered.
- Parasomnias are also possible.

6. Lithium + SSRI/SNRI/SSRI-Plus/Sedating Antidepressant

MECHANISM OF ACTION

- As noted in the bipolar disorder chapter, it is difficult to elucidate the exact mechanism of lithium's antidepressant action. Theoretically, it is thought to stimulate the mid-brain nuclei consisting of the ventral tegmental area (VTA), locus coeruleus (LC), and raphe nuclei (RN), which promote and release DA, NE, and SR throughout the rest of the brain. This has been called a tri-monoamine modulator in effect. Lithium may be neuroprotective and facilitate neuronal growth and plasticity as another antidepressant mechanism.

Side Effects

- Polydipsia, polyurea, and diarrhea are side effects initially noted in some patients. More serious side effects of psoriasis, QTc prolongation, hypothyroidism, hyperparathyroidism, lymphocytosis, and renal dysfunction may occur.

7. Thyroid + SSRI/SNRI/SSRI-Plus/Sedating Antidepressant

MECHANISM OF ACTION

- Tri-iodothyronine (Cytomel) has slightly better effectiveness data than levothyroxine (Synthroid) products. Similar to lithium, this drug may increase metabolic production of the three monoamines.

Side Effects

- Hyperthyroidism may be induced and levels must be monitored. Patients may suffer from diaphoresis, heat intolerance, tremor, diarrhea, weight loss, palpitations, or atrial arrhythmia.

8. Noradrenergic TCA + SSRI/SSRI-Plus/Sedating Antidepressant

MECHANISM OF ACTION

- TCAs have been discussed as a monotherapy in Section 1. Typically a noradrenergic only TCA (desipramine (Norpramin), nortriptyline (Pamelor), protriptyline (Vivactil)) is added to a therapeutically-dosed initial SSRI. This creates an SNRI-like profile but avoids two SERT inhibitors together and risk of serotonin syndrome. This approach could be used with SSRI-Plus agents effectively as well. Use of TCAs with SNRIs is generally frowned upon as they often duplicate mechanism of action and may promote serotonin syndrome as if adding two SSRIs together. TCAs could be added to sedating antidepressants if needed.

Side Effects

- Sedation, orthostasis, blurred vision, dry mouth, constipation, and weight gain are often noted with TCAs. TCAs also risk QTc prolongation and ventricular arrhythmia if over-dosed clinically or purposefully.
- Also, TCA combinations must have dose reductions and more stringent EKG and trough blood level monitoring if these are added to a known CYP4502D6 inhibiting antidepressant (ex. fluoxetine, paroxetine, sertraline, citalopram, venlafaxine).

9. Pramipexole + SSRI/SNRI/SSRI-Plus/Sedating Antidepressant

MECHANISM OF ACTION

- Pramipexole (Mirapex) agonizes D2 and D3 receptors (similar to the possible mechanism of SGA aripiprazole/brexpiprazole) increasing DA neuronal firing and is approved for use in Parkinson's disease and restless legs syndrome (RLS). Studies support its use in more refractory depressive episodes in doses up to 5mg/day. As it uniquely solely affects DA transmission, it can be safely added to any antidepressant.

Side Effects

- Hypotension, fatigue, nausea, insomnia, and mania induction have been reported

10. Stimulant + SSRI/SNRI/SSRI-Plus/Sedating Antidepressants

MECHANISM OF ACTION

- As discussed in the ADHD chapter, these drugs aggressively inhibit DAT (DRI) and elevate DA neuronal firing. They likely operate similarly with NET inhibition. The amphetamine products may actually reverse the DAT and at very high doses act as an MAOI.
- Data suggests these may have a niche in geriatric depression.

Side Effects

- Anxiety, agitation, insomnia, dry mouth, and nausea are common. Abnormal weight loss, tachyarrhythmias, hypertension, and addiction are also complicating side effects.

11. Wakefulness Promoting Agents + SSRI/SNRI/SSRI-Plus/Sedating Antidepressants

MECHANISM OF ACTION

- Modafinil (Provigil) and armodafinil (Nuvigil) are approved for the treatment of narcolepsy, obstructive sleep apnea fatigue, and shift work sleep disorder. They are felt to work through DAT and possibly downstream via noradrenergic facilitation. These are not true stimulants but do increase wakefulness.

Side Effects

- Addiction rates and cardiac side effects are likely less than true stimulants, but possible. Insomnia, anxiety, agitation, nausea, and headache may be reported.

12. Lamotrigine + SSRI/SNRI/SSRI-Plus/Sedating Antidepressants

MECHANISM OF ACTION

- Lamotrigine (Lamictal) is approved for maintenance treatment of bipolar disorder. It is known to inhibit NMDA glutamate receptors as a potential mechanism of action. Its data as an antidepressant is limited and often has been found to be negative, but it is often used in practice.

Side Effects

- Headache, nausea, ataxia, or tremor may be reported. Risks of serious rashes must be considered and monitored.

13. SGA + SSRI/SNRI/SSRI-Plus/Sedating Antidepressants

MECHANISM OF ACTION

- SGAs have been discussed as having antidepressant potential due to the following properties (5HT-1a partial agonism, 5HT2a, 2c, 3, 7 antagonism, NET inhibition, and/or D2 and D3 partial agonism) depending on the specific SGA. Further discussion about their specific pharmacodynamic profiles may be found in the schizophrenia chapter.
- It was noted above that olanzapine, quetiapine, aripiprazole, and brexpiprazole have approvals for MDD. Risperidone (Risperdal), lurasidone (Latuda), and ziprasidone (Geodon) have positive findings also in unipolar or bipolar depression.

Side Effects

- As discussed in prior sections, these drugs often promote fatigue and somnolence, and as serotonergic facilitators may create headaches and GI side effects. More significant is their ability to cause EPS, TD, and metabolic disorder.

Nutraceutical Augmentation Strategies:

1. L-methylfolate + Antidepressant

MECHANISM OF ACTION

- L-methylfolate (Deplin) is an important part of the metabolic one-carbon cycle where it specifically acts to improve the activity of the biopterin cycle. Adding l-methylfolate enhances this cycle which increases the conversion of tyrosine to dopamine and norepinephrine and tryptophan to serotonin.

- Effectively, this increases the three monoamines known to alleviate depressive symptoms. This may be considered a tri-monoamine modulator similar to lithium and thyroid hormone augmentation.

Side Effects

- Generally are minimal to absent. GI side effects are most commonly reported.

2) SAMe + Antidepressant

MECHANISM OF ACTION

- S-adenosylmethionine (SAMe) also works in the one-carbon cycle.

Side Effects

- Generally are minimal to absent. GI side effects and sedation are most commonly reported.

3) NAC + Antidepressant

MECHANISM OF ACTION

- N-acetylcysteine (NAC) is available over the counter and is also approved for use in infantile respiratory distress and for acetaminophen overdose. It is felt to be an NMDA glutamate receptor antagonist.

Side Effects

- Generally are minimal to absent.

Table 5.7 Prescribing Table for Depressive Disorders

Drugs listed in BOLD are approved agents. Dosing is based upon clinical application. Approved dosing guidelines should be further referenced by the prescriber.						
Brand	Generic	Indication (Bold for FDA Approved)	Drug Mechanism	Dosing Tips	Monitoring Tips	Medicolegal Tips
SSRIs						
Prozac	**Fluoxetine**	• **Major depressive disorder (MDD)** • **Premenstrual dysphoric disorder (PMDD)** • **Treatment-resistant depression (in combination with olanzapine)** • Persistent depressive disorder (PDD) • Seasonal depressive disorder (SDD)	• Serotonin reuptake inhibitor	• Usual dose is 10–60mg/day • Increase 10–20mg every few weeks	• Common side effects include GI, headache, fatigue, anxiety, insomnia, weight gain, and sexual dysfunction • Serious side effects include (hypo)mania, increased suicidal ideation, easy bruising • Drug interactions as this is a major inhibitor of CYP4502D6	• In those age <25 there is increased risk of lethality, more frequent monitoring, and safety planning is warranted
Zoloft	**Sertraline**	• **MDD** • **PMDD** • PDD • SDD	• Serotonin reuptake inhibitor	• Usual dose is 25–200mg/day • Increase 50mg every few weeks	• Same as above except higher possible rate of GI side effects • Drug interactions are minimal	• Same as above • Do not stop abruptly

Paxil **Paxil CR**	**Paroxetine**	• **MDD** • **PMDD** • PDD • SDD	• Serotonin reuptake inhibitor	• Usual dose is 10–50mg/day • Increase 10–20mg every few weeks	• Same as above except higher rates of mild anticholinergic effects and greater chance of serotonin withdrawal upon cessation • Drug interactions as this is a major inhibitor of CYP4502D6	• Same as above except category D for pregnancy (evidence of increased risk of cardiovascular malformations in infants) • Do not stop abruptly
Celexa	**Citalopram**	• **MDD** • PMDD • PDD • SDD	• Serotonin reuptake inhibitor	• Usual dose is 10–40mg/day • Increase every few weeks • Do not exceed 40mg/day (or 20mg in elderly) due to cardiac QTc prolongation risks	• Same as above except for cardiac risks as this drugs increases QTc • Drug interaction is for moderate inhibition at CYP4502D6	• Same as above • If dosing at higher levels for better efficacy, consider obtaining EKG and trough blood levels as a precaution
Lexapro	**Escitalopram**	• **MDD** • PMDD • PDD • SDD	• Serotonin reuptake inhibitor	• Usual dose is 5–20mg/day • Increase 5–10 mg every few weeks	• Common side effects include GI, headache, fatigue, anxiety, insomnia, weight gain, and sexual dysfunction • Serious side effects include (hypo)mania, increased suicidal ideation, easy bruising	• Same as above but no cardiac warnings

(*Continued*)

Table 5.7 (Continued)

Brand	Generic	Indication (Bold for FDA Approved)	Drug Mechanism	Dosing Tips	Monitoring Tips	Medicolegal Tips
SNRI						
Effexor XR	**Venlafaxine**	• **MDD** • PMDD • PDD • SAD	• Serotonin and norepinephrine reuptake inhibitor • May be weakest in norepinephrine in class	• Usual dose is 37.5–225mg/day • Increase 37.5–75mg every few weeks. • Maximal dose up to 375mg/day	• Common side effects same as SSRI but additional dry mouth, nausea, insomnia, anxiety may be experienced • Serious side effects same as SSRI but may include hypertension • Higher risk of serotonin withdrawal upon cessation	• Same as SSRI • Do not stop abruptly • Monitor blood pressure for subtle increases.
Pristiq	**Desvenlafaxine**	• **MDD** • PMDD • PDD • SAD	• Serotonin and stronger norepinephrine reuptake inhibitor	• Usual dose is 50–400mg/day • Increase by 50mg every 2–3 weeks	• Same as above • May have least P4502D6 inhibition, and some patients who fail to respond to parent drug venlafaxine will to this metabolite as such	• Same as above

Cymbalta	**Duloxetine**	• **MDD** • PMDD • PDD • SDD	• Serotonin and norepinephrine reuptake inhibitor	• Usual dose is 30–120mg/day • Increase 30–60mg every few weeks	• Same as above but carries risk of liver damage in alcohol use disorder (AUD) patients	• Same as above
Fetzima	**Levomilnacipran**	• **MDD** • PMDD • PDD • SAD	• Weak serotonin and strong norepinephrine reuptake inhibitor	• Usual dose is 20–120mg once daily • Start at 20mg once daily for 2 days then increase to 40mg once daily then increase by 40mg/day every 2 or more days to therapeutic effect	• Same as above but without liver issues	• Same as above

Brand	Generic	Indication (Bold for FDA Approved)	Drug Mechanism	Dosing Tips	Monitoring Tips	Medicolegal Tips
SSRI-Plus (sometimes called serotonin partial agonist-reuptake inhibitor (SPARI))						
Viibryd	**Vilazodone**	• **MDD** • PMDD • PDD • SDD	• Weak serotonin reuptake inhibitor • Partial agonist action at serotonin-1A pre/postsynaptic receptor	• Usual dose is 10–40mg/day • Start at 10mg/day and increase to 20mg/day after one or more weeks • Must take with food for absorption	• Common side effects same as SSRI but perhaps greater GI upset but less weight gain and sexual dysfunction	• Same as SSRI

(*Continued*)

Table 5.7 (Continued)

Trintellix	**Vortioxetine**	• **MDD** • PMDD • PDD • SAD	• Serotonin reuptake inhibitor • Partial agonist action at serotonin 1A autoreceptor • Antagonist at serotonin 1b/d, 3, 7 receptors	• Usual dose is 5–20 mg/day • Increase by 5–10mg every few weeks	• Same as above and may improve cognition in depressed states	• Same as SSRI

Brand	Generic	Indication (Bold for FDA Approved)	Drug Mechanism	Dosing Tips	Monitoring Tips	Medicolegal Tips
TCAs						
Tofranil	**Imipramine**	• **MDD** • PMDD • PDD • SDD	• Norepinephrine and serotonin reuptake inhibitor (predominantly serotonin reuptake inhibitor)	• Usual dose is 25–300mg/day • Start at 25mg/day at bedtime and increase by 25mg every 3–7 days Maximum daily dose is 300mg/day	• Common side effects include sedation, weight gain, anticholinergic side effects, alpha adrenergic side effects (dizziness, orthostasis) • Serious side effects include, QTc prolongation, activation of mania and suicidality • Monitor EKG prior to and periodically during use and obtain trough blood levels periodically	• Use in limited doses in those with suicidal symptoms • Use with caution in cardiac patients • Avoid use with strong CYP4502D6 inhibitors, such as fluoxetine/ paroxetine/ citalopram

Elavil	**Amitriptyline**	• **MDD** • PMDD • PDD • SDD	• Norepinephrine and serotonin reuptake inhibitor (predominantly serotonin reuptake inhibitor)	• Usual dose is 25–300mg/day • Start at 25mg/day at bedtime and increase by 25mg every 3–7 days	• Same as above	• Same as above
Sinequan	**Doxepin**	• **MDD** • PMDD • PDD • SDD	• Norepinephrine and serotonin reuptake inhibitor (predominantly serotonin reuptake inhibitor)	• Usual dose is 10–300mg/day • Start at 10–25mg/day and increase by 25mg every 3–7 days. Maximum daily dose is 300mg/day	• Same as above	• Same as above
Norpramin	**Desipramine**	• **MDD** • PMDD • PDD • SAD	• Norepinephrine and serotonin reuptake inhibitor (predominantly norepinephrine reuptake inhibitor)	• Usual dose is 25–300mg/day • Increase by 25–75mg every 3–7 days	• Same as above	• Same as above but may have less anticholinergic effects
Pamelor	**Nortriptyline**	• **MDD** • PMDD • PDD • SDD	• Norepinephrine and serotonin reuptake inhibitor (predominantly norepinephrine reuptake inhibitor)	• Usual dose is 25–150mg/day • Increase by 25mg every 3–7 days	• Same as above	• Same as above but may have less anticholinergic effects

(*Continued*)

Table 5.7 (Continued)

Brand	Generic	Indication (Bold for FDA Approved)	Drug Mechanism	Dosing Tips	Monitoring Tips	Medicolegal Tips
MAO Inhibitors						
EMSAM	**Selegiline**	• **MDD** • PMDD • PDD • SDD	• Irreversibly inhibits MAO-A and MAO-B enzymes, increasing norepinephrine, serotonin, and dopamine	• Usual dose is 6–12mg/24 hrs for transdermal patch • Start at 6mg/24 hrs and increase by 3mg/24 hrs every few weeks	• Common side effects include application site reactions, insomnia, anxiety • Serious side effects include hypertensive crisis, serotonin syndrome, induction of mania and suicidality • Monitor for blood pressure changes	• Provide diet card and suggest patient use one pharmacy for all Rx and OTC medications • Document this and capacity to (1) follow diet and (2) patient ability to speak to pharmacist about every med utilized • This agent alone may create a false positive urine screen for methamphetamine
Marplan	**Isocarboxazid**	• **MDD** • PMDD • PDD • SDD	• Same as above	• Usual dose is 10–30mg twice a day • Increase by 10mg/day every 7 days	• Same as above but additionally may have greater weight gain and hypotension	• Same as above but no urine screen issues
Nardil	**Phenelzine**	• **MDD** • PMDD • PDD • SDD	• Same as above	• Usual dose is 15–30mg three times a day • Increase by 45mg every week	• Same as above	• Same as above

Parnate	**Tranylcypromine**	• **MDD** • PMDD • PDD • SDD	• Same as above	• Usual dose is 10mg–20mg three times a day • Increase by 10mg/day every week	• Same as above	• Same as above

Brand	Generic	Indication (Bold for FDA Approved)	Drug Mechanism	Dosing Tips	Monitoring Tips	Medicolegal Tips
NDRIs						
Wellbutrin XL	**Bupropion**	• **MDD** • **SDD** • PMDD • PDD	• Norepinephrine and dopamine reuptake inhibitor	• Usual dose is 150–450mg daily • Start at 150mg once daily and increase by 150mg every week. Maximum daily dose is 450mg once daily	• Common side effects include dry mouth, constipation, nausea, anorexia, sweating, insomnia, tremor, headache • Serious side effects include seizures, induction of mania and suicidality	• Do not use in patients with eating disorders or history of seizures

(*Continued*)

Table 5.7 (Continued)

Brand	Generic	Indication (Bold for FDA Approved)	Drug Mechanism	Dosing Tips	Monitoring Tips	Medicolegal Tips
Sedating Antidepressants						
Desyrel	**Trazodone**	• **MDD** • PMDD • PDD • SAD • Insomnia	• SARI (serotonin 2 antagonist/reuptake inhibitor) • May provide for somnolence by alpha-1 adrenergic blockade or H-1 histaminergic blockade to a lesser degree	• Usual dose is 25–600 mg/day • May be dosed at night for insomnia 50–300mg • For depression is generally dosed 50–300mg twice daily	• Common side effects include dizziness, sedation, hypotension • Serious side effects include priapism, arrhythmia, induction of (hypo) mania, and suicidal ideation	• In those age <25 there is increased risk of lethality, more frequent monitoring and safety planning is warranted • Warn of psychomotor impairment
Serzone	**Nefazodone**	• **MDD** • PMDD • PDD • SDD • Insomnia	• SARI (serotonin 2 antagonist/reuptake inhibitor) • H-1 reuptake inhibitor	• Usual dose is 50–600 mg/day • Start at 50mg twice a day and increase by 100–200mg/day weekly	• Same as above • Monitor liver functions as rare cases of hepatitis occur. Obtain AST, ALT at baseline, after titration, and annually	• Same as above • Clearly explain life-threatening or serious side effects (e.g., hepatotoxicity)

Remeron	**Mirtazapine**	• **MDD** • PMDD • PDD • SAD • Insomnia	• Blocks alpha 2 adrenergic presynaptic receptor and increases norepinephrine and serotonin in the cortex vis serotonin-2c, 3 receptor blockade • H-1 reuptake inhibitor	• Usual dose is 7.5–45 mg/day at nighttime • Increase by 7.5–15mg weekly. Maximum daily dose is 45mg/day	• Common side effects include dizziness, sedation, hypotension, weight gain • Serious side effects include excessive weight gain and metabolic syndrome, priapism, induction of (hypo)mania and suicidal ideation • Monitor at baseline and at least annually with BMP, Lipid Panel. Also conduct more routine weight and vital sign assessment	• Clearly explain life-threatening or serious side effects (e.g., weight gain, metabolic side effects)

(*Continued*)

Table 5.7 (Continued)

Brand	Generic	Indication (Bold for FDA Approved)	Drug Mechanism	Dosing Tips	Monitoring Tips	Medicolegal Tips
Thyroid Hormone						
Cytomel	Triiodothyronine	• MDD augmentation	• Increases metabolic products of three monoamines, increases metabolism, energy, and possibly corrects circadian function	• Usual dose is 5–50mcg/day • Start at 5–10mcg/day and increase to 50mcg over several weeks	• Common side effects include diaphoresis, heat intolerance, tremor, diarrhea, weight loss, palpitations • Serious side effects include atrial arrhythmia • Monitor with EKG and thyroid functions at baseline, after titration and then annually	• Do not use in patients with untreated cardiac conditions, abnormal weight loss, thyrotoxicosis, or adrenal insufficiency

Brand	Generic	Indication (Bold for FDA Approved)	Drug Mechanism	Dosing Tips	Monitoring Tips	Medicolegal Tips
Nutraceutical Agents						
Deplin	**L-methylfolate**	• **MDD augmentation**	• Increases three monoamines by enhancing one-carbon and biopterin cycle	• Usual dose is 15mg/day.	• Side effects are generally minimal to absent	• Relatively safe medication

SAMe	S-adenosyl-methionine (SAMe)	• MDD augmentation	• Increases three monoamines by enhancing one-carbon and biopterin cycle	• Usual dose is 400–800mg twice daily	• Same as above	• Same as above
NAC	N-acetylcysteine (NAC)	• MDD augmentation	• Theoretically antioxidant and NMDA glutamate receptor antagonist	• Usual dose is 1000–1200mg twice daily	• Same as above	• Same as above
Second-Generation Antipsychotics (SGA)						
Symbyax (Zyprexa + Prozac)	**Olanzapine/ fluoxetine combination**	• **Treatment-resistant depression** • **Bipolar depression**	• Blocks dopamine 2 receptors reducing psychosis and stabilizing mania. May provide calming effect • Blocks serotonin 2A receptors which may improve depression • Blocks H1 receptors which may provide sedation and anxiolysis • SSRI effects	• Usual dose is 3/25mg–12/50mg/day • Increase by 3/25mg/day every few weeks	• Common initial side effects include dizziness, sedation, headache, GI side effects • Serious side effects include risk of diabetes, hyperlipidemia, hypertension, weight gain, transient and permanent neuromuscular side effects, hyperlipidemia, gynecomastia, agranulocytosis, increased risk of death in demented elderly, increased suicidality and severe rash	• Clearly explain life-threatening or serious side effects (e.g., TD/EPS, metabolic side effects) • Provide treatments if side effects occur (e.g., weight loss agents, antiparkinson agents) • Considered one of the most metabolic syndrome inducing agents • Sedation risk is moderate • Risk of EPS is high.

(*Continued*)

Table 5.7 (Continued)

					• Monitor at baseline and at least annually with CBC Diff, BMP, Lipid Panel. Also conduct more routine weight and vital signs, AIMS tests or physical exam for EPS/TD neuromuscular symptoms	
Seroquel (XR)	**Quetiapine**	• **Major depressive disorder augmentation** • **Bipolar depression** • Agitation/ anxiety	• Blocks dopamine 2 receptors reducing psychosis and stabilizing mania. May provide calming effect • Blocks serotonin 2A receptors which may improve depression • Blocks H1 receptors which may provide sedation and anxiolysis • Has potent NRI and 5HT-1a agonism as antidepressant properties which have been shown in other agents (SPA, SNRI) to lower anxiety	• Depression dosing is 25–600mg or 50–600mg, respectively, and both can be given once nightly	• Same as above	• Clearly explain life-threatening or serious side effects (e.g., TD/ EPS, metabolic side effects) • Provide treatment if side effects occur (e.g., weight loss agents, antiparkinson agents) • Considered one of the most metabolic syndrome inducing agents • Risk of weight gain and metabolics is high • Risk of sedation is high • Risk of EPS/TD is lowest in SGA class

Abilify	**Aripiprazole**	• **Major depressive disorder augmentation** • Agitation/ anxiety	• Partially agonizes D2 and D3 receptors which may improve affect • Net effect may also block dopamine 2 receptors reducing psychosis, stabilizing mania, and allowing a calming effect • Blocks serotonin 2A receptors which may improve depression • Has 5HT-1a agonism similar to SPA anxiolytics (buspirone)	• Usual dose is 2–30mg/day • May increase 2–5mg every few days • Drug is a substrate for CYP2D6 and must be halved if 2D6 inhibitor concomitantly taken	• Same as above	• Clearly explain life-threatening or serious side effects (e.g., TD/ EPS, metabolic side effects) • Provide treatment if side effects occur (e.g., weight loss agents, antiparkinson agents) • Risk of weight gain and metabolics is moderate • Risk of sedation is moderate • Risk of akathisia is high
Rexulti	**Brexpiprazole**	• **Major depressive disorder augmentation** • Agitation/ anxiety	• Partially agonizes D2 and D3 receptors which may improve affect • Net effect may also block dopamine 2 receptors reducing psychosis, stabilizing mania, and allowing a calming effect • Blocks serotonin 2A receptors which may improve depression	• Usual dose is 0.25–3mg/day • May increase 0.5–1mg every few weeks • Drug is a substrate for CYP2D6 and must be halved if 2D6 inhibitor concomitantly taken	• Same as above	• Clearly explain life-threatening or serious side effects (e.g., TD/ EPS, metabolic side effects) • Provide treatment if side effects occur (e.g., weight loss agents, antiparkinson agents)

(*Continued*)

Table 5.7 (Continued)

			• Has 5HT-1a agonism similar to SPA anxiolytics (buspirone)			• Risk of weight gain and metabolics is moderate • Risk of sedation is moderate • Risk of akathisia is moderate
Vraylar	Cariprazine	• Acute mania/ mixed mania • Maintenance • Agitation/ anxiety	• Partially agonizes D2 and D3 receptors which may improve affect • Net effect may also block dopamine 2 receptors reducing psychosis, stabilizing mania, and allowing a calming effect • Blocks serotonin 2A receptors which may improve depression • Has 5HT-1a agonism similar to SPA anxiolytics (buspirone)	• Usual dose is 1.5–6mg/day • May increase 1.5mg every few weeks	• Same as above	• Clearly explain life-threatening or serious side effects (e.g., TD/ EPS, metabolic side effects) • Provide treatment if side effects occur (e.g., weight loss agents, antiparkinson agents) • Risk of weight gain and metabolics is moderate • Risk of sedation is moderate • Risk of akathisia is high

Saphris	Asenapine	• Acute mania/ mixed mania • Agitation/ anxiety	• Blocks D2 receptors reducing psychosis, stabilizing mania, and allowing a calming effect • Blocks serotonin 2A receptors which may improve depression • Has 5HT-1a agonism similar to SPA anxiolytics (buspirone) • Blocks H1 receptors which may provide sedation and anxiolysis • Has similar antidepressant theoretical properties to mirtazapine (alpha-2 antagonism, 5HT-2c,3 antagonism)	• Usual dose is 5–10 mg twice daily • It is taken SL or will not be absorbed	• Same as above	• Clearly explain life-threatening or serious side effects (e.g., TD/EPS, metabolic side effects) • Provide treatment if side effects occur (e.g., weight loss agents, antiparkinson agents) • Risk of weight gain and metabolics is moderate • Risk of sedation is moderate

(*Continued*)

Table 5.7 (Continued)

Latuda	Lurasidone	• **Bipolar depression**	• Blocks dopamine 2 receptors reducing psychosis and stabilizing affective symptoms • Blocks serotonin 2A receptors and 7 receptors which may improve cognitive and affective symptoms without marked EPS	• Usual dose is 40–80mg/day for schizophrenia • Start at 40–80mg/day once daily with food and increase to therapeutic dose. Maximum daily dose is 160mg/day	• Same as above	• Clearly explain life-threatening or serious side effects (e.g., NMS, metabolic side effects, tardive dyskinesia) • Should be discontinued before pregnancies (risk category B) • Weigh and track weight and BMI • Before starting obtain waist circumference, blood pressure, fasting plasma glucose, fasting lipid profile
Geodon	Ziprasidone	• Bipolar depression	• Blocks dopamine 2 receptors reducing psychosis and stabilizing affective symptoms • Blocks serotonin 2A receptors • Has SNRI properties	• Usual dose is 80–160mg/day in divided doses • Start 40mg twice a day, increase to 60–80mg twice a day on day 2. Maximum daily dose is 100mg twice a day	• Same as above but known for QTc prolongation	• Clearly explain life-threatening or serious side effects (e.g., NMS, metabolic side effects, tardive dyskinesia) • Should be discontinued before pregnancies (risk category C) • Weigh and track weight and BMI

						• Before starting obtain waist circumference, blood pressure, fasting plasma glucose, fasting lipid profile
Risperdal	Risperidone	• Major depressive disorder augmentation	• Blocks dopamine 2 receptors reducing psychosis and stabilizing affective symptoms • Blocks serotonin 2A receptors	• Usual dose is 2–8mg/day. Usual dose for depot injection is 25–50mg every 2 weeks • Start at 1mg/day orally in 2 divided doses and increase daily by 1mg/day to therapeutic dose. Maximum daily dose is 16mg/day	• Same as above	• Clearly explain life-threatening or serious side effects (e.g., NMS, metabolic side effects, tardive dyskinesia) • Should be discontinued before pregnancies (risk category C) • Weigh and track weight and BMI • Before starting obtain waist circumference, blood pressure, fasting plasma glucose, fasting lipid profile

(*Continued*)

Table 5.7 (Continued)

Brand	Generic	Indication (Bold for FDA Approved)	Drug Mechanism	Dosing Tips	Monitoring Tips	Medicolegal Tips
The Serotonin Partial Agonists (SPAs)						
BuSpar	Buspirone	• Major depressive disorder augmentation • **Generalized anxiety disorder (GAD)**	• Partial agonist at presynaptic serotonin type 1A receptors	• Usual dose is 5–22.5mg twice a day • Increase 5mg twice daily every few weeks	• Common initial side effects include dizziness, headache, nervousness • Generally is felt to be least risky for sexual dysfunction or weight gain compared to SSRI, SNRI, TCA	

Brand	Generic	Indication (Bold for FDA Approved)	Drug Mechanism	Dosing Tips	Monitoring Tips	Medicolegal Tips
Lithium						
Eskalith Lithobid Lithostat	Lithium carbonate	• Major depressive disorder augmentation • Bipolar depression	• May stabilize neuronal membranes reducing limbic firing rates • Downregulates serotonin-5HT-1a receptors • Improves neuronal health, growth factors, and connectivity	• Usual dose is 1800mg/day in divided doses • Maintenance: usual dose is 300–1200mg/day in divided doses • Therapeutic trough plasma lithium levels should be 0.8–1.2mEq/l for acute mania and 0.6–1.2mEq/l for maintenance • Use of concomitant NSAIDS or diuretics may increase lithium levels	• Common initial side effects include increased thirst and urination, tremor, GI side effects • Other notable side effects include acne, psoriasis, weight gain • Serious side effects include lithium toxicity, thyroid and kidney dysfunction, lymphocytosis, arrhythmia • Monitor blood levels 4–5 days after dose increases and after steady state, then annually • Monitor EKG, CBC, TSH, CRE at baseline, after titration, and then annually	• Clearly explain life-threatening toxicity, drug interactions, and side effects • Should be discontinued before pregnancies (risk category D) due to evidence of increased risk of birth defects and cardiac anomalies (Ebstein's anomaly)

(Continued)

Table 5.7 (Continued)

Amphetamine Stimulant Products (Slow Release)						
Adderall XR	d/l -Mixed amphetamine extended release	• Major depressive disorder augmentation	• Both amphetamine and methylphenidate stimulants block dopamine and norepinephrine reuptake • Amphetamine class differs from methylphenidate class in that it blocks and then reverses dopamine reuptake pumps causing greater amounts of dopamine release	• Usual dosing is 5–60mg/day • Increase by 5–10mg every week	• Common side effects include anxiety, insomnia, weight loss, nausea, palpitations, dry mouth, or diaphoresis • Serious side effects include psychosis, seizures, hypertension, activation of (hypo)mania and suicidal ideation, addiction, hypertension and cardiovascular events • Monitor vital signs and consider urine drug screening	• Stimulants carry classic warnings of drug dependency and in younger adults activation of suicidal ideation • Avoid stimulants in those with cardiac structural abnormalities, arrhythmia, history of myocardial infarction
Vyvanse	Lisdexamfetamine dimesylate	• Same as above	• Same as above	• Usual dosing is 10–70mg/day • Increase by 10–20mg every week	• Same as above	• Same as above
Concerta	Methylphenidate OROS extended release	• Same as above	• Same as above	• Usual dosing is 18–72mg/day • Up to 12 hrs of duration • Increase by 18mg every week	• Same as above	• Same as above
Focalin XR	D–methylphenidate extended release	• Same as above	• Same as above	• Usual dosing is 5–40mg/day • Increase by 10mg every week	• Same as above	• Same as above
Metadate ER/CD, Ritalin SR/LA	Methylphenidate	• Same as above	• Same as above	• Usual dosing is 10–60 mg/day • Up to 4–6 hrs of duration • Increase by 10mg	• Same as above	• Same as above

Good Polypharmacy for Reaching Remission in Resistant Patients

DO

- Start low dose to minimize side effects.
- Escalate dosing within full range for optimal effectiveness.
- Aim for aggressive monotherapy as treatment of choice.
- Combine medications that affect complementary neurotransmitter systems instead of those that duplicate mechanisms of action.
- If remarkable dysphoria, guilt, anxiety, or suicidality occurs, consider combining more serotonergic complementary mechanistic medications.
- If remarkable vegetative, cognitive, or anhedonic symptoms occur, consider using or adding medications that preferentially utilize pro-norepinephrine or dopaminergic mechanisms.
- When switching drugs due to inefficacy, change from one class of antidepressant to a different class that uses a different mechanism of action.

DON'T

- Use successive monotherapies that use the same mechanism (use of three SSRIs in a row).
- Combine identical mechanistic drugs together (SSRI + SSRI, SSRI + SNRI, TCA + SNRI).

Good Polypharmacy to Be Used to Gain Remission in Comorbid Patients

MDD + ADHD

- **Use of NDRI:** bupropion XL (Wellbutrin XL) monotherapy.
- **Use of SNRI:** venlafaxine XR (Effexor XR), duloxetine (Cymbalta), desvenlafaxine (Pristiq), levomilnacipran (Fetzima) monotherapy.
- **Use norepinephrine based TCA:** desipramine (Norpramin), nortriptyline (Pamelor), protriptyline (Vivactil).
- **Use MAOI:** selegiline transdermal patch (Emsam), actually has amphetamine derivatives.
- **Use second-generation antipsychotic (SGA) augmentation:** aripiprazole (Abilify)/brexpiprazole(Rexulti) have partial dopamine receptor 2/3 agonism, quetiapine (Seroquel XR) has potent NRI.

MDD + Anxiety Disorder

- Use of SSRI, SNRI, or SSRI-Plus monotherapies.
- Combination of any of the above with lower dose SGAs, buspirone, sedating antidepressants, benzodiazepines.
- Use alpha-2 agonists, guanfacine (Tenex) or clonidine (Catapres), as they often dampen agitation.

MDD + Schizophrenia

- Use second-generation antipsychotic (SGA) monotherapy (quetiapine XR (Seroquel XR), lurasidone (Latuda)).
- Use of combination olanzapine-fluoxetine (Symbyax), SSRI/SNRI Plus aripiprazole (Abilify), brexpiprazole (Rexulti), ziprasidone (Geodon), asenapine (Saphris), cariprazine (Vraylar) as all agents have some anti-depression data or at least theoretical capacity based on their purported mechanisms of action.

MDD + Borderline Personality

- Use second-generation antipsychotic (SGA) monotherapy or combination strategy.

Bibliography

Alpert, J. E., et al. (2004) "S-adenosyl-L-methionine (SAMe) as an adjunct for resistant major depressive disorder: an open trial following partial or nonresponse to selective serotonin reuptake inhibitors or venlafaxine." *Journal of Clinical Psychopharmacology* 24(6), 661–664.

American Psychiatric Association. (2013) *Diagnostic and Statistical Manual of Mental Disorders: DSM-5.* (5th ed.). Washington, D.C.: American Psychiatric Association.

Arroll, B., Goodyear-Smith, F., Crengle, S., Gunn, J., Kerse, N., Fishman, T., & Hatcher, S. (2010) "Validation of PHQ-2 and PHQ-9 to screen for major depression in the primary care population." *The Annals of Family Medicine* 8(4), 348–353.

Berk, M., et al. (2008) "N-acetyl cysteine for depressive symptoms in bipolar disorder—a double-blind randomized placebo-controlled trial." *Biological Psychiatry* 64(6), 468–475.

Bierut, L. J., et al. (1999) "Major depressive disorder in a community-based twin sample: are there different genetic and environmental contributions for men and women?" *Archives of General Psychiatry* 56(6), 557–563.

Broadhead, W. E., Blazer, D. G., George, L. K., & Tse, C. K. (1990) "Depression, disability days, and days lost from work in a prospective epidemiologic survey." *Jama* 264(19), 2524–2528.

Campbell, S., Marriott, M., Nahmias, C., & MacQueen, G. M. (2014) "Lower hippocampal volume in patients suffering from depression: a meta-analysis." *American Journal of Psychiatry* 161(4), 598–607.

Carpenter, L. L., Yasmin, S., & Price, L. H. (2002) "A double-blind, placebo-controlled study of antidepressant augmentation with mirtazapine." *Biological Psychiatry* 51(2), 183–188.

Cohen, L. S., Soares, C. N., Otto, M. W., Sweeney, B. H., Liberman, R. F., & Harlow, B. L. (2002) "Prevalence and predictors of premenstrual dysphoric disorder (PMDD) in older premenopausal women: the Harvard study of moods and cycles." *Journal of Affective Disorders* 70(2), 125–132.

Cusin, C., Iovieno, N., Iosifescu, D. V., Nierenberg, A. A., Fava, M., Rush, A. J., & Perlis, R. H. (2013) "A randomized, double-blind, placebo-controlled trial of pramipexole

augmentation in treatment-resistant major depressive disorder." *The Journal of Clinical Psychiatry* 74(7), 1–478.
Davidson, J. R. (2010) "Major depressive disorder treatment guidelines in America and Europe." *The Journal of Clinical Psychiatry* 71(suppl E1), 1–478.
DeBattista, C., Solvason, H. B., Poirier, J., Kendrick, E., & Schatzberg, A. F. (2003) "A prospective trial of bupropion SR augmentation of partial and non-responders to serotonergic antidepressants." *Journal of Clinical Psychopharmacology* 23(1), 27–30.
Dhingra, V., Magnay, J. L., O'Brien, P. M. S., Chapman, G., Fryer, A. A., & Ismail, K. M. (2007) "Serotonin receptor 1A C (-1019) G polymorphism associated with premenstrual dysphoric disorder." *Obstetrics & Gynecology* 110(4), 788–792.
Douglas, J. (1995) "MRI-based measurement of hippocampal volume in patients with combat-related posttraumatic stress disorder." *American Journal of Psychiatry* 152, 973–98.
Fava, M., & Rush, A. J. (2006) "Current status of augmentation and combination treatments for major depressive disorder: a literature review and a proposal for a novel approach to improve practice." *Psychotherapy and Psychosomatics* 75(3), 139–153.
Fava, M., et al. (2006) "Eszopiclone co-administered with fluoxetine in patients with insomnia coexisting with major depressive disorder." *Biological Psychiatry* 59(11), 1052–1060.
Fava, M., Thase, M. E., & DeBattista, C. (2005) "A multicenter, placebo-controlled study of modafinil augmentation in partial responders to selective serotonin reuptake inhibitors with persistent fatigue and sleepiness." *The Journal of Clinical Psychiatry* 66(1), 1–478.
Gitlin, M. J., & Altshuler, L. L. (2014) "A review of the use of stimulants and stimulant alternatives in treating bipolar depression and major depressive disorder." *The Journal of Clinical Psychiatry* 75(9), 1–478.
Grady, M. M., & Stahl, S. M. (2012) "Practical guide for prescribing MAOIs: debunking myths and removing barriers." *CNS Spectrums* 17(1), 2–10.
Hameed, U., Schwartz, T.L., & Malhotra, K. (2005) "Antidepressant treatment in the primary care office: outcomes for adjustment disorder versus major depression?" *Annals of Clinical Psychiatry* 17(2), 1–5.
Horst, W. D., & Preskorn, S. H. (1998) "Mechanisms of action and clinical characteristics of three atypical antidepressants: venlafaxine, nefazodone, bupropion." *Journal of Affective Disorders* 51(3), 237–254.
Huo, L., et al. (2007) "Risk for premenstrual dysphoric disorder is associated with genetic variation in ESR1, the estrogen receptor alpha gene." *Biological Psychiatry* 62(8), 925–933.
Johansson, C., et al. (2003) "Circadian clock-related polymorphisms in seasonal affective disorder and their relevance to diurnal preference." *Neuropsychopharmacology* 28(4), 743–739.
Kessler, R. C., et al. (2003) "The epidemiology of major depressive disorder: results from the National Comorbidity Survey Replication (NCS-R)." *JAMA* 289(23), 3095–3105.
Kroenke, K., Spitzer, R. L., & Williams, J. B. (2003) "The Patient Health Questionnaire-2: validity of a two-item depression screener." *Medical Care* 41(11), 1284–1292.
Marchesi, C. (2008) "Pharmocologic management of panic disorder." *Neuropsychiatric Disease and Treatment* 4(1): 93–106.
McCall, C., & McCall, W. V. (2012) "What is the role of sedating antidepressants, antipsychotics, and anticonvulsants in the management of insomnia?" *Current Psychiatry Reports* 14(5), 494–502.
Mill, J., & Petronis, A. (2007) "Molecular studies of major depressive disorder: the epigenetic perspective." *Molecular Psychiatry* 12(9), 799–814.
Nelson, J. C., Mazure, C. M., Bowers, M. B., & Jatlow, P. I. (1991) "A preliminary, open study of the combination of fluoxetine and desipramine for rapid treatment of major depression." *Archives of General Psychiatry* 48(4), 303–307.

Phan, K. L., Wager, T., Taylor, S. F., & Liberzon, I. (2002) "Functional neuroanatomy of emotion: a meta-analysis of emotion activation studies in PET and fMRI." *Neuroimage* 16(2), 331–348.

Praschak-Rieder, N., et al. (2002) "Role of family history and 5-HTTLPR polymorphism in female seasonal affective disorder patients with and without premenstrual dysphoric disorder." *European Neuropsychopharmacology* 12(2), 129–134.

Rosen, L. N., et al. (1990) "Prevalence of seasonal affective disorder at four latitudes." *Psychiatry Research 31*(2), 131–144.

Sanchez, C., Asin, K. E., & Artigas, F. (2015) "Vortioxetine, a novel antidepressant with multimodal activity: review of preclinical and clinical data." *Pharmacology & Therapeutics* 145, 43-57.

Schwartz, T. L., & Petersen, T. (eds.). (2006) *Depression: Treatment Strategies and Management.* New York: Taylor & Francis.

Schwartz, T.L., & Stahl, S.M. (2011) "Vilazodone: a brief pharmacologic and clinical review of the novel SPARI (Serotonin Partial Agonist and Reuptake Inhibitor)." *Therapeutic Advances in Psychopharmacology* 1(3), 81–87.

Stahl, S.M. (2003) "Symptoms to circuits part 2: anxiety disorders." *Journal of Clinical Psychology* 64(12), 1408–1409.

Stahl, S. M. (2007) "Novel therapeutics for depression: L-methylfolate as a trimonoamine modulator and antidepressant-augmenting agent." *CNS Spectrums* 12(10), 739–744.

Stahl, S. M., & Felker, A. (2008) "Monoamine oxidase inhibitors: a modern guide to an unrequited class of antidepressants." *CNS Spectrums* 13(10), 855–871.

Stahl, S. M. (2013) *Stahl's Essential Psychopharmacology: Neuroscientific Basis and Practical Applications.* Cambridge, UK: Cambridge University Press.

Steiner, M., Peer, M., Macdougall, M., & Haskett, R. (2011) "The premenstrual tension syndrome rating scales: an updated version." *Journal of Affective Disorders* 135(1), 82–88.

Stimmel, G. L., Dopheide, J. A., & Stahl, S. M. (1997) "Mirtazapine: an antidepressant with noradrenergic and specific serotonergic effects." *Pharmacotherapy: The Journal of Human Pharmacology and Drug Therapy* 17(1), 10–21.

Thase, M. E., et al. (2015) "Adjunctive brexpiprazole 1 and 3 mg for patients with major depressive disorder following inadequate response to antidepressants: a phase 3, randomized, double-blind study." *The Journal of Clinical Psychiatry* 76(9), 1–478.

Vaidya, V. A., Marek, G. J., Aghajanian, G. K., & Duman, R. S. (1997) "5-HT2A receptor-mediated regulation of brain-derived neurotrophic factor mRNA in the hippocampus and the neocortex." *The Journal of Neuroscience* 17(8), 2785–2795.

Zajecka, J.M., Goldstein, C.N., Siddiqui, U.A., & Schwartz, T.L. (2011) "Using what we have: combining medications to achieve remission." *Clinical Neuropsychiatry* 8(1), 4–27.

Zavodnick, A. D., & Ali, R. (2012) "Lamotrigine in the treatment of unipolar depression with and without comorbidities: a literature review." *Psychiatric Quarterly* 83(3), 371–383.

CHAPTER 6

Insomnia

SECTION 1 Basic Prescribing Practices

Essential Concepts

- The reader should appreciate that insomnia is common as a stand-alone DSM-5 disorder and that insomnia, as a symptom, may be one of the most common to cross the boundaries of multiple DSM-5 disorders.
- Insomnia is the inability to appropriately fall asleep, stay asleep, or perhaps having non-restorative sleep with daytime consequences.
- Insomnia is associated with 4.6% more workplace and non-work-related accidents when compared to patients without insomnia.
- Insomnia is often a residual symptom of major depressive disorder (MDD), anxiety disorder, mania, etc., and should be ameliorated to ensure full remission of the parent psychiatric disorder.
- Insomnia may lead to fatigue and cognitive dysfunction, so treating insomnia may in fact treat multiple psychiatric symptoms.
- Insomnia often leads to substance misuse (alcohol, benzodiazepine).
- Insomnia is considered an acute risk factor for suicide.
- There are many medications approved for treating insomnia (antihistamines, melatonin agonists, orexin antagonists, benzodiazepine receptor agonists).

Phenomenology, Diagnosis, Clinical Interviewing

TIP: Insomnia Specific Complaints

- Difficulty initiating sleep (DIS): 16.4%
- Difficulty maintaining sleep (DMS): 19.9%
- Early morning awakening (EMA): 16.7%
- Non-restorative sleep (NRS): 25%

TIP: Odds Ratio for DSM-5 Insomnia Simultaneous Association with Other Conditions OR Comorbid Condition

2	Adjustment disorder (separation, divorce, widowed)
2.4	Serious medical condition
9.9	Generalized anxiety disorder
15.4	Major depressive disorder

TIP: Prevalence of Psychiatric Comorbidity and Insomnia

- Panic disorder (PD): 7.5%
- Social anxiety disorder (SAD): 16.9%
- Generalized anxiety disorder (GAD): 5.9%
- Post-traumatic stress disorder (PTSD): 9.6%
- Major depressive disorder (MDD): 16.5%
- Persistent depressive disorder (PDD): 4.9%
- Bipolar disorder (BD): 7.8%
- Alcohol use disorder (AUD): 6.7%
- Substance use disorder (SUD): 3.4%

TIP: Insomnia Screening Questions

- How many hours of sleep do you typically get?
- How long does it take you to fall asleep when you go to bed?
- Does lack of sleep ever cause you emotional or work-related problems the next day?

DSM-5 Diagnosis

People with insomnia cannot initiate sleep, maintain sleep, or have non-restorative sleep as their main complaint.

DSM-5 Diagnosis of Insomnia

- Dissatisfaction with sleep quantity or quality with one or more of the following symptoms: difficulty initiating sleep, difficulty maintaining sleep, early morning awakening.

- The sleep disturbance causes significant distress or impairment in social, occupational, educational, academic, behavioral, or other important areas of functioning.
- The sleep difficulty occurs at least three nights per week and is present for at least three months despite having an adequate opportunity for sleep.
- Additionally, insomnia from other psychiatric disorders can be coded separately and treated as an individual comorbidity.

Rating Scales

Regensburg Insomnia Scale (RIS)

- This scale assesses specific insomnia symptoms in a 10-item questionnaire.
- A positive score of 12 or more indicates significant insomnia.
- It takes a few minutes to complete and a few seconds to score.
- This scale is free of charge as it is an open access article and can be found at https://www.ncbi.nlm.nih.gov/pmc/articles/PMC3645970/. Its full citation is Crönlein, T., Langguth, B., Popp, R., Lukesch, H., Pieh, C., Hajak, G., & Geisler, P. (2013). "Regensburg insomnia scale (RIS): a new short rating scale for the assessment of psychological symptoms and sleep in insomnia; study design: development and validation of a new short self-rating scale in a sample of 218 patients suffering from insomnia and 94 healthy controls." *Health and Quality of Life Outcomes* 11(1), 1.

Table 6.1 The Regensburg Insomnia Scale

PLEASE RATE THE FOLLOWING QUESTIONS FOR THE LAST FOUR WEEKS					
0. What time do you usually go to bed? ________				**When do you usually get up? ______**	
1. How many minutes do you need to fall asleep?					
	1–20min	**21–40min**	**41–60min**	**61–90 min**	**91min and more**
	0	1	2	3	4
2. How many hours do you sleep in the night?					
	7h and more	**5–6h**	**4h**	**2–3h**	**0–1h**

HOW OFTEN DO THE FOLLOWING OCCURRENCES HAPPEN?					
	ALWAYS	MOSTLY	SOMETIMES	SELDOM	NEVER
3. My sleep is disturbed.	4	3	2	1	0
4. I wake up too early.	4	3	2	1	0
5. I wake up from the slightest sound.	4	3	2	1	0
6. I feel that I have not slept all night.	4	3	2	1	0
7. I think a lot about my sleep.	4	3	2	1	0
8. I am afraid to go to bed due to my disturbed sleep.	4	3	2	1	0
9. I feel fit during the day.	0	1	2	3	4
10. I take sleeping pills in order to get to sleep.	4	3	2	1	0

Treatment Guidelines

Essential Concepts

- For the novice prescriber attempting to treat an adult with insomnia, it is essential to know the basics of the available guidelines that exist to help provide a high level of care.
- Next, a prescriber must know what psychotropics are specifically approved and the relative side effect profiles of each.
- It is important to disclose to the patient that the approach being used is approved by the FDA (U.S. Food and Drug Administration). A fair amount of off-label prescribing for insomnia occurs and may be warranted (sedating antidepressants, second-generation antipsychotics (SGA), antihypertensives, etc.) at times, especially when treating comorbidities. Sometimes, a non-insomnia medication may simultaneously treat both depression and insomnia.
- Patient education and sleep hygiene approaches are likely warranted prior to prescribing a sleep inducing agent (hypnotic).
- Documenting patient failure or refusal to comply with sleep hygiene should be noted prior to prescribing in most cases.

TIP: Insomnia Approved Medications

- Some agents induce sleepiness as their mechanism and others remove alertness.
- Over-the-counter (OTC) diphenhydramine (Benadryl) and doxylamine succinate (Unisom) are approved for insomnia. These are antihistamines.
- Prescription antihistamines also exist (doxepin [Silenor]) and are approved.
- Melatonin is OTC and stimulates melatonin receptors.
- Ramelteon (Rozerem) is a prescription melatonin receptor agonist.
- Suvorexant (Belsomra) is a prescription orexin receptor antagonist.
- Zolpidem (Ambien), zaleplon (Sonata), and eszopiclone (Lunesta) are benzodiazepine (BZ)-like prescription hypnotics, called benzodiazepine receptor agonists (BZRA).
- True BZ structured hypnotics are less often utilized but still available via prescription (temazepam [Restoril], flurazepam [Dalmane], triazolam [Halcion]).
- See **Prescribing Table** for further details.

TIP: Insomnia Guidelines

- A sleep inventory covering the number of hours slept, time to fall asleep, time of awakening, history of abnormal nighttime movements, use of caffeine or sedatives, etc., should be determined.
- A sleep diary may be kept for several days as well.
- Rating scale use is highly suggested.
- Sleep hygiene and patient education should preceed any use of hypnotic medication. Patients should be made aware that cognitive-behavioral therapy (stimulus control, sleep restriction, relaxation, cognitive restructuring, etc.) also is a side effect–free treatment option.
- If a prescription sleep medication is issued, then short-term use to restore normal circadian function is the primary goal.
- Prior to issuing a prescription, patients should be warned about psychomotor impairment and abnormal nighttime events (sleep walking, driving, eating) even though they are much more common with BZRAs and BZs.

- For mild or infrequent insomnia, OTC antihistamines and melatonin may be used as they are considered to have the best safety profile.
- For more chronic and severe insomnia, use of a prescription hypnotic is warranted and all FDA approved agents can be effective.
- Most are approved over the short term, but can be used longer if the insomnia is more resistant in nature or if the hypnotic is being used to treat insomnia associated with another psychiatric disorder (MDD, GAD, etc.).
- Generally, doses are started at the lowest possible tablet strength and escalated every few days until insomnia is mitigated or side effects mount.
- Maximum allowed doses are warranted prior to determining if the hypnotic has failed clinically.
- It may be warranted to taper off the hypnotic over a few days to avoid rebound insomnia.
- Successive monotherapies are the usual approach. However, rational polypharmacy may be needed for more refractory insomnia.
- Most guidelines suggest starting with BZRA hypnotics (zolpidem [Ambien], zaleplon [Sonata], eszopiclone [Lunesta]) given their high efficacy rate. However, risk of addiction, psychomotor impairment, and abnormal nighttime events may be higher with this approach.
- Alternatives such as doxepin (Silenor), ramelteon (Rozerem), and suvorexant (Belsomra), or off-label approaches such as trazodone (Desyrel) and mirtazapine (Remeron) may have less of these side effects but either have lower effectiveness or less data to support their use.
- When treating insomnia associated with another medical condition, it makes sense to treat that condition first: use central positive airway pressure (CPAP) for obstructive sleep apnea (OSA), use a D2 agonist such as pramipexole (Mirapex) for restless legs syndrome (RLS), or a neuronal calcium channel blocker (gabapentin [Neurontin], pregabalin [Lyrica]) for painful diabetic neuropathy.
- When treating insomnia associated with another psychiatric disorder, the primary disorder should be treated aggressively. A formal hypnotic agent can also be used within the standard of care as needed. Alternatively, a psychotropic indicated for the primary disorder may be chosen based on its proclivity to induce sedation and somnolence, avoiding the use of a formal hypnotic (mirtazapine [Remeron] for depression, quetiapine [Seroquel XR] for mania).
- The specific type of hypnotic chosen may be determined via several different sub-guidelines.
    - If concerned about addiction, psychomotor impairment, or respiratory suppression, then BZRAs, BZs, and orexin antagonists should be avoided.

- If concerned about side effects in general, safer agents should be tried first (ramelteon [Rozerem], doxepin [Silenor]).
- If concerned about initial difficulty falling asleep, then short half-life agents should be selected (zaleplon [Sonata], zolpidem [Ambien]) as these are the shortest acting and theoretically leave the system within 4–5 hours.
- If concerned about maintaining sleep throughout the night, then longer half-life drugs should be chosen (eszopiclone [Lunesta), suvorexant [Belsomra], temazepam [Restoril]), flurazepam [Dalmane]).

TIP: Insomnia Prescribing

- Initiate all hypnotics at the lowest possible dose (even lower than FDA suggested).
- Dosing information is readily available electronically and in print from a myriad of resources. See also the **Prescribing Table** in this chapter.
- Most hypnotics allow for therapeutic effects within a single dose and can be measured over a few days. The dose may be systematically titrated upward every few days.
- Melatonergic drugs may take a few days to become effective and likely should be taken at least an hour beforebed time

SECTION 2 Advanced Prescribing Practices

Introduction

In Section 1, the premise was to convince the reader that they must make an accurate diagnosis and pick an approved agent with well-defined dosing guidelines and expected clinical outcomes. This approach is largely one of pattern recognition: (1) identify the pattern of phenotypic symptoms, (2) choose from a finite list of available, proven effective drugs, (3) start dosing low and escalate through an approved dosing range, (4) assess for effectiveness, and (5) continue medication if effective, and cross-titrate to a new drug if ineffective or not tolerated. This is a methodical, mathematical approach that can improve the standard of care and, ideally, patient outcomes when treated by the novice psychopharmacologist.

Section 2 is designed to provide a greater depth of neuroscience and pharmacodynamic knowledge to the reader and is written for prescribers who are knowledgeable and competent in those skills outlined in Section 1. The section is generally intended for those patients who are felt to be treatment resistant and comorbid with other disorders.

Epidemiology of Insomnia

- 30–48% of the general public will admit to subsyndromal insomnia.
- Severe insomnia with daytime consequences has prevalence between 4% and 15%.
- Up to 60% of patients admit to insomnia lasting greater than two years.
- 57% of patients who present with a chief complaint of insomnia will actually have a different psychiatric disorder.
- 18% of patients who present for insomnia have major depressive disorder (MDD).

Genetics

- Circadian clock genes exist that interact highly with the environment (day/night). These genes create protein products that cycle in concentration according to a 24-hour rhythm.
- These genes are named: Clock; PERIOD 1, 2, and 3; Bmal1; and Timeless.
- Certain sleep disorders have a known gene mutation as a putative cause: most are rare, such as fatal familial insomnia (mutation of prion protein gene PRNP), familial advanced sleep-phase syndrome (mutations in human Period2 (hPER2)), delayed sleep phase syndrome (polymorphism in Per3), and narcolepsy with cataplexy (orexin/hypocretin genes).
- In regard to heritability, 55% of patients with childhood-onset insomnia can identify one family member with sleep difficulties compared to 39% of patients with an onset of insomnia in adulthood.
- According to twin studies, insomnia is felt to be 20–40% heritable.

Neuroanatomy/Physiology of Wakefulness

- The locus coeruleus (LC) promotes norepinephrine (NE) release. The raphe nuclei (RN) promotes serotonin release (SR), and the ventral tegmental area (VTA) promotes dopamine (DA) release. These make up part of the reticular activating system (RAS) and, when firing, promote wakefulness.
- The tuberomammillary nuclei (TMN) promote histamine release, which, when bound to histamine-1 (H1) receptors in the cortex, promote wakefulness.
- Orexins from the hypothalamus also promote wakefulness and are suspected of augmenting the RAS/TMN to maintain their functioning.

- All of these activities promote wakefulness. If they are removed or weakened by psychiatric disorders, diseased process, or psychotropics, then sedation and somnolence may occur.

Neuroanatomy/ Physiology of Sleep

- Via expenditure of cortical energy, ATP is converted to adenosine which ultimately signals the need for sleep.
- The reticular activating system (RAS) lowers its firing at night, likely as a result of a loss of signal from the suprachiasmatic nucleus (SCN), which monitors daylight and helps control the 24-hour circadian clock. Alertness and wakefulness diminish.
- The pineal gland secretes melatonin which also lowers RAS activity.
- The TMN ceases activity and its foil, the ventrolateral preoptic area (VLPO), promotes increased gamma-aminobutyric amino acid (GABA), and galanin activity to promote sleepiness. This also turns off the TMN and lowers histamine (thus diminishing wakefulness propensity).
- Orexin activity diminishes also lowering wakefulness.
- All of these activities remove alertness, wakefulness, or promote somnolence.

TIP: Insomnia Prescribing

Antihistamines: lower histaminergic activity; includes diphenhydramine, doxepin, and eszopiclone.
Melatonin agonists: lower RAS activity; includes melatonin, ramelteon.
BZRAs & BZs: both increase GABA activity; includes *zolpidem and *zaleplon.
Orexin antagonists: lowers orexin activity; includes *Temazepam, *suvorexant, and *Flurazepam.

All of these agents act directly on the neuroanatomic pathways that either remove arousal or increase somnolence.
*These agents have addictive potential.

Neuroscientific Background and Rationale for Medication Use

In treating insomnia, there are five classes of medications frequently used (**see Prescribing Table**) and several off-label pharmacological approaches that may be considered within the standard of care.

1. Antihistamines

MECHANISM OF ACTION

Diphenhydramine (Benadryl), doxylamine (Unisom), doxepin (Silenor)

- The first two agents are available over the counter. The latter is a prescription medication.
- Doxepin is a tricyclic antidepressant, but at lower doses is a pure antihistamine and is not associated with the more severe TCA side effect profiles discussed in other chapters.
- These agents block H-1 histamine receptors in the frontal cortex.
- Histamine promoted by the TMN is not received and arousal is removed, allowing fatigue and somnolence to occur.

2. Melatonin Agonists

MECHANISM OF ACTION

Melatonin, ramelteon (Rozerem), tasimelteon (Hetlioz)

- Melatonin is a naturally occurring chemical secreted by the pineal gland during the evening/overnight hours.
- Ramelteon and tasimelteon are synthetic prescription agents with a high affinity to bind to melatonin receptors.
- When either binds melatonin-1 (MT1) receptors on the RAS, it lowers DA, NE, and SR firing, thus removing cortical arousal and promoting fatigue/somnolence.
- When either binds to MT2 receptors located on the SCN, it entrains the SCN to maintain the usual 24-hour circadian rhythm.

3. Benzodiazepine Receptor Agonists (BZRA)

MECHANISM OF ACTION

Zolpidem (Ambien), zaleplon (Sonata), eszopiclone (Lunesta)

- BZRAs are very similar to the true BZ class of anxiolytics and hypnotics. When GABA-A receptors are bound simultaneously by a GABA transmitter molecule and a BZRA drug, there is an increase in efficiency and opening of chloride neuronal channels, thus decreasing neuronal firing rates.

- BZ2 sub-receptors exist in greater concentrations in the limbic system and activity likely fosters a lowering of anxiety here.
- The BZRA class is very selective for binding the BZ1 sub-receptors, which are much more highly located and concentrated in the sleep inducing center (VLPO).
- Given this, BZRAs are likely less addictive than true BZs, unless they are taken in higher doses than those FDA approved.

4. Benzodiazepines (BZ)

MECHANISM OF ACTION

Temazepam (Restoril), flurazepam (Dalmane), triazolam (Halcion)

- Similar to BZRAs noted above.
- These agents affect the BZ1 and BZ2 equally well and may provide improved sleep onset and duration, as well as anxiolysis and muscle relaxation.
- They likely carry a greater risk for daytime oversedation/psychomotor impairment, addiction, and respiratory suppression.

5. Orexin Receptor Antagonists

MECHANISM OF ACTION

Suvorexant (Belsomra)

- This newer class of hypnotic agents functions by blocking the activity of orexin neurons.
- Orexin-1 and -2 (OX1/OX2) receptors, when stimulated, cause increases in arousal and wakefulness by enhancing the function of the RAS and TMN.
- When OX1 and OX2 are blocked by this agent, cortical arousal is also blocked and fatigue/somnolence ensues.

The following medication options are all considered off-label for insomnia treatment but may be employed in more advanced psychiatric practice.

1. Sedating Antidepressants

MECHANISM OF ACTION

Trazodone (Desyrel), nefazodone (Serzone), mirtazapine (Remeron)

- These three drugs all share a similar side effect in common: antihistamine properties make them sedating in nature. They are sometimes used as hypnotics or anxiolytics. Lowering insomnia and agitation may alleviate two core depressive symptoms. They all may block alpha-1 receptors, also promoting sedation.
- All of these agents antagonize the 5HT-2a and 2c receptor. Mechanistically, this property allows for cortical increases in NE and DA, which are felt to lower depressive symptoms. Blocking 5HT-2a has been shown to promote deeper sleep.
- Trazodone and nefazodone are weaker SSRI agents as well. This property likely becomes more effective at higher doses. These two agents are sometimes termed serotonin antagonist-reuptake inhibitors (SARI). Trazodone may have the highest off-label use for insomnia out of all medications discussed.
- Mirtazapine is different and unique within this class and among all antidepressants, and is sometimes called a norepinephrine antagonist-specific serotonin antagonist (NASSA). In addition to H1, 5HT-2a, and 5HT2c, it also blocks the 5HT-3 receptor, which may stimulate mid-brain release of NE, DA, and SR to the cortex. Additionally, it antagonizes noradrenergic alpha-2 autoreceptors. By inhibiting these autoreceptors, cortical NE neurons are forced to release excess NE, which is also felt to have a strong antidepressant effect.

2. Mood Stabilizers (Anti-epileptic Drugs [AED])

MECHANISM OF ACTION

Divalproex (Depakote), gabapentin (Neurontin), pregabalin (Lyrica), tiagabine (Gabitril)

- AEDs often close down neuronal sodium or calcium channels. Sometimes they lower glutamate activity by blocking glutamate NMDA receptors. Some agents may increase GABA neurotransmitter activity, but this is not accomplished via a GABA-A receptor BZ-like activity.

- Divalproex may increase the synthesis of GABA. Increases in GABA neurotransmission may also have a dampening effect on mania-induced hyperactive limbic structures. It may also lower glutamate neuronal firing by inhibiting NMDA receptors.
- Gabapentin and pregabalin block alpha-2-delta ligand calcium channels. This slows neuronal firing and may lower seizure activity. This mechanism in the periphery also lowers delta pain fiber firing to lower neuropathic pain. There are approvals for this type of prescribing for both gabapentin and pregabalin. Deep sleep may be produced at greater rates.
- Tiagabine is a GABA transporter (called GAT-1) reuptake inhibitor. In some studies it has been shown to promote deeper, more efficient sleep and is mildly sedating. It has largely fallen out of favor due to risk of generating seizures in non-epileptics.
- All of these agents have sedating side effects which may be used therapeutically to improve sleep.
- Similar to the sedating antidepressants above, these agents may be used more often when the patient also has an addiction or medical comorbidity that precludes BZRA use.

3. Antihypertensives

MECHANISM OF ACTION

Clonidine (Catapres), guanfacine (Tenex), prazosin (Minipress)

- Alpha-2 agonists (clonidine and guanfacine) are better known for treating hypertension and were formally discussed in the ADHD and anxiety chapters.
- Their activity centrally lowers noradrenergic tone. Insomnia is hypothesized to begin with elevated NE activity and neuronal firing from the RAS. Theoretically, these agents are poised to directly lower NE firing and potentially improve insomnia.
- There are no approvals and limited evidence base for treating insomnia, though they are used frequently in psychopharmacological practice, perhaps as an alternative to potentially addictive BZs.
- Alpha-1 antagonists are specifically used to treat nightmares associated with PTSD. It is unclear if they can treat insomnia.

4. First- and Second-Generation Antipsychotics (FGA/SGA)

MECHANISM OF ACTION

Chlorpromazine (Thorazine), olanzapine (Zyprexa), quetiapine (Seroquel IR/XR), asenapine (Saphris)

- All approved antipsychotics block D2 receptors to treat psychosis.
- Chlorpromazine was the first approved FGA. The other agents above are SGAs.
- The most commonly prescribed FGAs/SGAs are listed above and in more detail in the Prescribing Table.
- Once 60–65% of D2 receptors are blocked, antipsychotic effects may take effect. If 80% is achieved, then EPS may occur.
- All FGAs/SGAs share this single mechanism of providing efficacy against psychotic symptoms.
- SGAs introduce a second key property: serotonin-2a (5HT-2a) receptor antagonism. These are sometimes called serotonin-dopamine antagonists (SDA).
- This 5HT-2a effect allows for the SGA to selectively and preferentially block DA activity in the mesolimbic DA system, but allows more DA to continue uninterrupted in the nigrostriatal system, which remarkably lowers EPS rates when compared to the low- and high-potency FGAs.
- 5HT-2a antagonism has been shown to promote deeper and more efficient, restorative sleep (see trazodone example above).
- Many of the above FGAs/SGAs have strong antihistamine and anti-alpha-1 properties, also lending to somnolence effects.
- Theoretically, SGAs promote sedation and the ability to attain deeper sleep.

Table 6.2 Prescribing Table for Insomnia

Drugs listed in BOLD are approved agents. Other drugs listed are evidence based and usually second line. Dosing is based upon clinical application. Approved dosing guidelines should be further referenced by the prescriber.						
Brand	Generic	Indication (Bold for FDA Approved)	Drug Mechanism	Dosing Tips	Monitoring Tips	Medicolegal Tips
Antihistamines						
Benadryl	**Diphenhydramine**	• **Insomnia**	• Histamine 1 antagonist	• Usual dose is 25–50mg/day • Take 25–50mg at night for sleep	• Common side effects include sedation, anticholinergic side effects (constipation, dry mouth, blurry vision)	• Generally safe to use • Discourage driving after administration • Avoid in medically sick patients to avoid delirium • Not addicting
Unisom	**Doxylamine**	• **Insomnia**	• Histamine 1 antagonist	• Usual does is 25mg at bed time	• Common side effects include sedation, anticholinergic side effects (constipation, dry mouth, blurry vision)	• Same as above
Silenor	**Doxepin**	• **Insomnia** • **Depression** • Pruritis/itching (topical) • Neuropathic pain	• Selectively blocks histamine 1 receptors at low mg hypnotic doses	• Usual dose for insomnia is 3–6mg/day at night • Usual dose for depression is 75–150mg/day	• Common side effects include sedation, weight gain, anticholinergic side effects, alpha adrenergic side effects (dizziness, orthostasis) • Serious side effects do not include those for TCA that are used at full doses for depression	• Same as above

(*Continued*)

Table 6.2 (Continued)

Brand	Generic	Indication (Bold for FDA Approved)	Drug Mechanism	Dosing Tips	Monitoring Tips	Medicolegal tips
Melatonin Agonists						
	Melatonin	• **Primary insomnia** • **Chronic insomnia** • **Transient insomnia** • **Insomnia associated with shift work, jet lag, or circadian rhythm disturbances**	• Binds to melatonin 1 and 2 receptors to dampen cortical arousal and entrains SCN to maintain the usual circadian rhythm	• Usual dose is 3–10mg at bedtime	• Common side effects include sedation, dizziness, fatigue, headache	• Generally safe to use • Not addicting
Rozerem	**Ramelteon**	• **Insomnia**	• Melatonin 1 and 2 receptor agonist with same effect as above	• Usual dose is 8mg at bedtime	• Same as above	• Generally safe to use • Some reports of daytime fatigue and psychomotor impairment • Not addicting • May temporarily increase prolactin or lower testosterone

Brand	Generic	Indication (Bold for FDA Approved)	Drug Mechanism	Dosing Tips	Monitoring Tips	Medicolegal Tips
Benzodiazepine Receptor Agonists (BZRA)						
Ambien/ Intermezzo	**Zolpidem**	• **Insomnia** • **Insomnia associated with middle of night awakening with difficulty returning to sleep (intermezzo)**	• Selective agonism BZ1 GABA-A subreceptors	• Usual dose is 5–10mg at bedtime for immediate release. 6.25–12.5mg at bedtime for controlled-release. Middle of night dosing using intermezzo is 1.75–3.5 SL • May escalate dose within range after a few nights' use	• Common side effects include sedation, dizziness, ataxia • Other notable side effects: dose-dependent amnesia, paradoxic restlessness/ anxiety, rare psychosis • Serious side effects include respiratory depression when taken with other CNS depressants, sleepwalking events, respiratory suppression, fall risk, addiction	• Clearly explain life-threatening or serious side effects • Discourage driving or operating heavy machinery after administration • Discourage drinking alcohol while taking • Carries risk of dependence (schedule IV) • Carries risk of abnormal night-time events such as sleepwalking, driving, eating, etc.
Sonata	**Zaleplon**	• **Insomnia** • **Insomnia associated with middle of night awakening with difficulty returning to sleep**	• Same as above	• Usual dose is 5–10mg at bedtime • May increase to 20mg at bedtime if needed • May escalate dose within range after a few nights' use	• Same as above	• Same as above

(Continued)

Table 6.2 (Continued)

Lunesta	**Eszopiclone**	• **Insomnia**	• Same as above	• Usual dose is 1–3mg at bedtime • May increase 1mg every few days	• Same as above	• Same as above

Brand	Generic	Indication (Bold for FDA Approved)	Drug Mechanism	Dosing Tips	Monitoring Tips	Medicolegal Tips
Benzodiazepines (BZ)						
Restoril	**Temazepam**	• **Insomnia**	• Agonism BZ1 and BZ2 GABA-A subreceptors	• Dosing is 7.5–30mg at bed time • May increase every few days for effect	• Common side effects include sedation, dizziness, ataxia • Other notable side effects: dose-dependent amnesia, paradoxic restlessness/anxiety • Serious side effects include respiratory depression when taken with other CNS depressants, sleepwalking events, respiratory suppression, fall risk, addiction, poor cognition	• Clearly explain life-threatening or serious side effects • Discourage driving or operating heavy machinery after administration • Discourage drinking alcohol while taking • Carries risk of dependence (schedule IV) • Carries risk of abnormal night time events such as sleepwalking, driving, eating, etc.

Dalmane	**Flurazepam**	• **Insomnia**	• Same as above	• Dosing is 15–30mg at bed time • May increase to full dose range every few days	• Same as above	• Same as above
Halcion	**Triazolam**	• **Insomnia**	• Same as above	• Dosing is 0.125–0.5mg at bed time • May increase to full dose range every few days	• Same as above	• Same as above

Brand	Generic	Indication (Bold for FDA Approved)	Drug Mechanism	Dosing Tips	Monitoring Tips	Medicolegal Tips
Orexin Receptor Antagonists						
Belsomra	**Suvorexant**	• **Insomnia**	• Antagonizes orexin 1+2 receptors which lowers arousal and promotes sleep	• Dosing is 5–20mg at bedtime • May increase 5–10mg every few days	• Common side effects include unpleasant taste, sedation, dizziness, ataxia • Other notable side effects: dose-dependent amnesia, paradoxic restlessness/anxiety, rare psychosis • Serious side effects include respiratory depression when taken with other CNS depressants, memory loss, anxiety, sleep paralysis though this is suspected to be less than the BZ or BZRA. Addiction is possible	• Clearly explain life-threatening or serious side effects • Discourage driving or operating heavy machinery after administration • Discourage drinking alcohol while taking • Carries risk of dependence (schedule IV)

(*Continued*)

Table 6.2 (Continued)

Brand	Generic	Indication (Bold for FDA Approved)	Drug Mechanism	Dosing Tips	Monitoring Tips	Medicolegal Tips
Sedating Antidepressants						
Desyrel	Trazodone	• Insomnia	• SARI (serotonin 2 antagonist/reuptake inhibitor) • H-1 reuptake inhibitor • Alpha-1 antagonist	• Usual dose is 25–300mg at bed time • Increase by 50mg every few days for effect	• Common side effects include dizziness, sedation, hypotension • Serious side effects include priapism, induction of (hypo)mania and suicidal ideation	• In those age <25 there is increased risk of lethality, more frequent monitoring and safety planning is warranted • Warn of psychomotor impairment
Serzone	Nefazodone	• Insomnia	• SARI (serotonin 2 antagonist/reuptake inhibitor) • H-1 reuptake inhibitor	• Usual dose is 50–300mg at bed time • Increase by 50mg every few days for effect	• Same as above except monitor liver functions as rare cases of hepatitis occur • Obtain AST, ALT at baseline, after titration, and annually	• Same as above • Clearly explain life-threatening or serious side effects (e.g., hepatotoxicity)
Remeron	Mirtazapine	• Insomnia	• Serotonin 2 antagonist • H-1 reuptake inhibitor	• Usual dose is 7.5–45mg/day at nighttime • Increase by 7.5–15mg weekly	• Common side effects include dizziness, sedation, hypotension, weight gain • Serious side effects include excessive weight gain and metabolic syndrome, priapism, induction of (hypo)mania, and suicidal ideation • Monitor at baseline and at least annually with, BMP, Lipid Panel. Also conduct more routine weight and vital sign assessment	• Clearly explain life-threatening or serious side effects (e.g., weight gain, metabolic side effects)

Brand	Generic	Indication (Bold for FDA Approved)	Drug Mechanism	Dosing Tips	Monitoring Tips	Medicolegal Tips
Mood Stabilizers (Anti-epileptic Drugs) (AEDs)						
Depakote Depakote ER	Divalproex	• Insomnia	• Increases CNS concentration of GABA via unknown mechanism	• No standard dosing for insomnia exists • 250–1000mg at bed time is theoretical range	• Common initial side effects include sedation, diarrhea, ataxia, tremor • Serious side effects include hepatotoxicity, pancreatitis, thrombocytopenia, polycystic ovarian syndrome, rashes and activation of suicidality • Monitor for LFT, platelets, Amylase/ Lipase at baseline and periodically during treatment	• Clearly explain life-threatening or serious side effects (e.g., hepatotoxicity) as well as risk of weight gain • Should be discontinued before pregnancies (risk category D) due to evidence of increased risk of birth defects (neural tube defects) • Warn of psychomotor impairment
Neurontin	Gabapentin	• Insomnia	• Binds to alpha 2 delta subunit of voltage sensitive calcium channels	• No standard dosing for insomnia exists • 150–600mg at bed time is theoretical range	• Common side effects include sedation, dizziness, sedation, ataxia, tremor, headache	• Warn of psychomotor impairment
Lyrica	Pregabalin	• Insomnia	• Binds to alpha 2 delta subunit of voltage sensitive calcium channels	• No standard dosing for insomnia exists • 25–150mg at bed time is the theoretical range	• Same as above • Serious side effects include mild risk of addiction	• Clearly explain life-threatening or serious side effects (e.g., risk of dependency) • Warn of psychomotor impairment

(*Continued*)

Table 6.2 (Continued)

Gabitril	Tiagabine	• Off-label for sleep disorders and anxiety	• GABA transporter (GAT-1) reuptake inhibitor	• No standard dosing for insomnia exists • Can start at 2mg at night and increase by 2mg every few days to 8–12mg/day	• Same as above • Serious side effects include risk of new-onset seizures in non-epileptics	• Clearly explain life-threatening or serious side effects (e.g., risk of new-onset seizures)

Brand	Generic	Indication (Bold for FDA Approved)	Drug Mechanism	Dosing Tips	Monitoring Tips	Medicolegal Tips
Antihypertensives						
Catapres	Clonidine	• Insomnia	• Stimulates central action of alpha 2A in the prefrontal cortex leading to decreased arousal	• No standard dosing for insomnia exists • 0.1–0.3mg is the theoretical dose range	• Common side effects include dry mouth, dizziness • Serious side effects include sinus bradycardia, AV block, and rare withdrawal hypertensive crisis • Monitor vital signs	• Abrupt discontinuation may lead to rare hypertensive encephalopathy, stroke, and death • Taper over 2–4 days or longer to avoid rebound in blood pressure
Tenex	Guanfacine	• Insomnia	• Same as above	• No standard dosing for insomnia exists • 1–3mg is the theoretical dose range	• Common side effects include sedation and hypotension • Serious side effects include sinus bradycardia and hypotension • Monitor vital signs	• Same as above but less sedating

Minipress	Prazosin	• Insomnia • Nightmares associated with PTSD	• Blocks alpha 1 receptors to reduce noradrenergic tone and decreases arousal	• Usual dose is 1–16mg/day for PTSD nightmares • Theoretical dosing for insomnia may be 1–8mg at bed time	• Common initial side effects include dizziness and lightheadedness due to orthostasis • Serious side effects include syncope • Monitor vital signs	• Clearly explain serious side effects (e.g., orthostasis and syncope, risk of falls)

Brand	Generic	Indication (Bold for FDA Approved)	Drug Mechanism	Dosing Tips	Monitoring Tips	Medicolegal Tips
First- and Second-Generation Antipsychotics (FGA/SGA)						
Thorazine	Chlorpromazine	• Insomnia	• Blocks H1 and alpha 1 receptors removing arousal and promoting sleep	• No standard dosing for insomnia exists • Theoretical dosing is 25–100mg at bed time	• Common initial side effects include dizziness, sedation, dry mouth, blurred vision, constipation • Other notable side effects include risk of all EPS, priapism, weight gain • Serious side effects include risk of TD, NMS, QTc prolongation, urinary retention • Monitor for TD and EPS and metabolics	• Clearly explain life-threatening or serious side effects (e.g., NMS, tardive dyskinesia)

(*Continued*)

Table 6.2 (Continued)

Zyprexa	Olanzapine	• Insomnia	• Blocks serotonin 2A receptors which promotes deeper sleep • Blocks H1 receptors	• No standard dosing for insomnia exists • Theoretical dosing is 2.5-10mg at bed time	• Common initial side effects include dizziness, GI side effects • Other notable side effects include risk of diabetes, dyslipidemia, EPS • Serious side effects include risk of diabetes, increased risk of death in demented elderly, rare NMS and seizures • Monitor for lipids, sugars and vitals at baseline and periodically during therapy	• Clearly explain life-threatening or serious side effects (e.g., NMS, metabolic side effects, tardive dyskinesia) • Weigh and track weight and BMI
Seroquel	Quetiapine	• Insomnia	• Same as above	• No standard dosing for insomnia exists • Theoretical dosing is 25–300mg at bed time	• Same as above	• Same as above
Saphris	Asenapine	• Insomnia	• Same as above	• No standard dosing for insomnia exists • Theoretical dosing is 5–10mg SL at bed time	• Same as above	• Same as above

Practical Applications

TIP: Essential Concepts

- After identifying insomnia, attempt to improve sleep hygiene and refer for cognitive-behavioral therapy (CBT) if available. If not, pharmacologic treatment is fairly linear.
    - If there are no contraindications, short-term use of a low dose BZRA is supported by most guidelines.
    - If longer-term use is required or if there are concerns about addiction, falls, respiratory suppression clinically, then avoid BZRA and BZ agents.
    - If an agent is chosen and appropriately dose-escalated as a monotherapy and it fails, then a second monotherapy from a different hypnotic class should be chosen. Successive monotherapies are appropriate.
- Polypharmacy makes sense in treatment-resistant patients. Combining medications of different mechanisms to improve sleep is possible, for example: combining an antihistamine and a melatonin agonist. This approach makes theoretical sense in a manner similar to that of treating depressive/anxiety disorder.

Good Polypharmacy for Reaching Remission in ***Comorbid*** *Patients*

Insomnia + Major Depressive Disorder (MDD)

- Interestingly, adding BZRA may remarkably lower depression scale scores as insomnia, fatigue, and concentration may improve quickly.
- Use more sedating antidepressants:
    - Trazodone (Desyrel), nefazodone (Serzone), mirtazapine (Remeron).
    - Imipramine (Tofranil), amitriptyline (Elavil), clomipramine (Anafranil) (all are TCAs).

Insomnia + Anxiety Disorder

- The main approvals for anxiety are the SSRI and SNRI classes, which tend to lack remarkable sedation/somnolence qualities.
- Off-label use of the more sedating antidepressants may be warranted as noted above:
    - Trazodone, nefazodone, mirtazapine
    - Imipramine, amitriptyline, clomipramine (TCA)

- If BZs or BZRAs are to be used, then the longer half-life agents may help to improve sleep and linger into the daytime to promote anxiolysis:
  - Eszopiclone (Lunesta), temazepam (Restoril), flurazepam (Dalmane).

Insomnia + Bipolar Disorder

- Use second-generation antipsychotics (SGA) that are sedating, treat mania and possibly depression.
  - Olanzapine (Zyprexa), quetiapine (Seroquel IR/XR), asenapine (Saphris).
- Sometimes, insomnia is the sentinel symptom of a new mania episode, so it is warranted to use a highly efficacious hypnotic that more often guarantees restoration of sleep. BZRAs and BZs are more often reliable in these cases.

Insomnia + Substance Abuse

- Avoiding addictive agents is a priority:
  - Diphenhydramine (Benadryl), doxylamine (Unisom), doxepin (Silenor), and melatonin are examples.
- Non-addictive and more often off-label approaches are used to avoid addiction:
  - Clonidine (Catapres), trazodone (Desyrel), quetiapine (Seroquel), gabapentin (Neurontin), and quetiapine (Seroquel) are examples.

Bibliography

American Psychiatric Association. (2013) *Diagnostic and Statistical Manual of Mental Disorders: DSM-5* (5th ed.). Washington, D.C.: American Psychiatric Association.

Crönlein, T., Langguth, B., Popp, R., Lukesch, H., Pieh, C., Hajak, G., & Geisler, P. (2013) "Regensburg insomnia scale (RIS): a new short rating scale for the assessment of psychological symptoms and sleep in insomnia; study design: development and validation of a new short self-rating scale in a sample of 218 patients suffering from insomnia and 94 healthy controls." *Health and Quality of Life Outcomes* 11(1), 1.

Kessler, R. C., et al. (2012) "Insomnia, comorbidity, and risk of injury among insured Americans: results from the America Insomnia Survey." *SLEEP* 35(6), 825–834.

Luppi, P. H., & Fort, P. (2013) "Neuroanatomy and physiology of sleep." In Eric Nofzinger, Pierre Maquet, and Michael J. Thorpy (eds.), *Neuroimaging of Sleep and Sleep Disorders* (8–14). Cambridge, UK: Cambridge University Press.

McCall, C., & McCall, W. V. (2012) "What is the role of sedating antidepressants, antipsychotics, and anticonvulsants in the management of insomnia?" *Current Psychiatry Reports* 14(5), 494–502.

McCall, W. V., & Black, C. G. (2013) "The link between suicide and insomnia: theoretical mechanisms." *Current Psychiatry Reports* 15(9), 1–9.

Morgenthaler, T., et al. (2006) "Practice parameters for the psychological and behavioral treatment of insomnia: an update." *SLEEP* 29(11), 1415–1419.

Ohayon, M. M. (2002) "Epidemiology of insomnia: what we know and what we still need to learn." *Sleep Medicine Reviews* 6(2), 97–111.

Palagini, L., Biber, K., & Riemann, D. (2014) "The genetics of insomnia–evidence for epigenetic mechanisms?" *Sleep Medicine Reviews* 18(3), 225–235.

Pinto, Jr., L. R., et al. (2010) "New guidelines for diagnosis and treatment of insomnia." *Arquivos de Neuro-Psiquiatria* 68(4), 666–675.

Redfern, P. H., & Lemmer, B. (eds.). (2013) *Physiology and Pharmacology of Biological Rhythms* (Vol. 125). New York: Springer Science & Business Media.

Roth, T., Jaeger, S., Jin, R., Kalsekar, A., Stang, P. E., & Kessler, R. C. (2006) "Sleep problems, comorbid mental disorders, and role functioning in the national comorbidity survey replication." *Biological Psychiatry* 60(12), 1364–1371.

Schutte-Rodin, S., Broch, L., Buysse, D., Dorsey, C., & Sateia, M. (2008) "Clinical guideline for the evaluation and management of chronic insomnia in adults." *Journal of Clinical Sleep Medicine* 4(5), 487–504.

Skaer, T. L., Robison, L. M., Sclar, D. A., & Galin, R. S. (1999) "Psychiatric comorbidity and *pharmacological* treatment patterns among patients presenting with insomnia." *Clinical Drug Investigation* 18(2), 161–167.

Stewart, R., et al. (2006) "Insomnia comorbidity and impact and hypnotic use by age group in a national survey population aged 16 to 74 years." *SLEEP* 29(11), 1391–1397.

Watson, C. J., Baghdoyan, H. A., & Lydic, R. (2012) "Neuropharmacology of sleep and wakefulness: 2012 update." *Sleep Medicine Clinics* 7(3), 469–486.

CHAPTER 7

Neurocognitive Disorders: Delirium, Dementia, and Traumatic Brain Injury

SECTION 1 Basic Prescribing Practices

Essential Concepts

- Patients with delirium often present to the emergency room with confusion and altered mental states.
  - Alternatively, they develop delirium while being treated in a medical-surgical inpatient setting.
  - The onset of confusion is generally abrupt and alarming to the caregivers involved.
  - There are no FDA approved treatments for delirium but the first- and second-generation antipsychotics (FGA and SGA) are the standard of care at times where medical treatment and environmental interventions fail to limit the patient's safety.
- Patients with dementia also will present to the emergency room if there is a crisis resulting from their poor memory, abnormal behaviors, or lapses in judgment.
  - They are typically not disoriented nor have a waxing and waning of consciousness.
  - Given the slow onset and progression of most dementias, caregivers and distant family members often do not notice the deficits or appreciate their depth or severity over time.
  - FDA approvals do exist for slowing the progression of Alzheimer's dementia.
  - There are no medications that reverse the course of illness.
  - Antipsychotics, mood stabilizers, and antidepressants may be used off-label to treat either comorbid psychiatric conditions or behavioral manifestations driven by the dementia process itself.
- Traumatic brain injury (TBI) patients are often treated with psychiatric medications to treat behavioral manifestations driven by their specific injury. All treatments here are off-label.

Phenomenology, Diagnosis, Clinical Interviewing

Similar to previous chapters, the goal here is to teach the clinician to quickly make an accurate diagnosis and choose an approved psychotropic. All of psychiatric prescribing at this beginning level is based on regulatory findings, approvals, and indications that are psychiatric disorder specific. Be warned: much of treating delirium, dementia, and TBI is off-label, with limited evidence base to guide treatment. Similar to treating personality disorder, clinicians are urged to use FDA approvals and the evidence base where possible, but a strategic approach of choosing a specific target symptom to alleviate is warranted. Defining and measuring these symptoms pre- and post-drug titration is critical in avoiding inappropriate polypharmacy.

As seen previously, this chapter will initially teach basic diagnosis and treatment of neurocognitive disorders (NCD), then progress toward more advanced treatment involving comorbid psychiatric states. The DSM-5 recently created the NCD terminology for the disorders in this chapter as well. This chapter assumes the reader is adept and comfortable with descriptive, DSM-5 interviewing and diagnostic assessment.

TIP: Psychiatric Symptoms Associated with NCD

The following target symptoms which may be noticed across the spectrum of NCD are felt to be driven by an underlying medical condition, brain injury, or a neurodegenerative process. As certain brain areas become dysfunctional, psychiatric symptoms may arise. The clinical assumption is that these symptoms may respond to psychopharmacologic interventions just as if these symptoms were due to the separate psychiatric disorder. For example, amotivation in dementia should respond like amotivation in major depressive disorder (MDD), and an antidepressant may be tried on a trial basis for this specific target symptom.

Aggression: verbal or physical resistance, physical aggression
Agitation: pacing, wandering, hyperactivity
Apathy: social withdrawal, anhedonia, amotivation
Affect: irritability, sadness, anxiety
Psychosis: paranoia, illusions/hallucinations
Cognition: distractibility, memory loss, disinhibition/judgement loss

TIP: Delirium Screening Questions

- Unlike ADHD, bipolarity, and anxiety disorders, the typical patient with delirium will likely be unable to answer clinical questions and be a poor historian. They will also likely be unaware that they are suffering from delirium. Similar to mania and other psychotic states, some patients will not recall previous episodes of delirium.

- A possible approach is to ask the non-delirious patient during a psychiatric review of systems (ROS) if they have ever gone through a short bout where they were extremely confused and out of sorts.
- Otherwise, the clinician must ask caregivers about abrupt changes in mental state associated with confusion and waxing of consciousness and arousal.

DSM-5 Diagnosis

People with delirium typically will show an acute (hours to days) change in their mental status and behavior presumed to be directly related to a preceding medical or surgical cause. The formal DSM-5 diagnosis is as follows:

DSM-5 Diagnosis of Delirium

- Disturbance in attention (i.e., reduced ability to direct, focus, sustain, and shift attention) and awareness.
- The disturbance develops over a short period (usually hours to days), representing a clear change from baseline, and tends to fluctuate in severity during the course of the day.
- Additionally, disturbances in cognition are apparent (memory deficit, disorientation, language disturbance, perceptual disturbance).
- These symptoms are not better accounted for by a pre-existing, established, or evolving NCD such as dementia.
- There is evidence from the history, physical examination, or laboratory findings that these symptoms are caused by a direct physiologic consequence of a general medical condition, an intoxicating substance, medication use, or more than one cause.

TIP: Commonly Used Mnemonic for Likely Causes of Delirium

I WATCH DEATH

- Infectious (encephalitis, meningitis, UTI, pneumonia)
    1. Withdrawal (alcohol, barbiturates, benzodiazepines)
    2. Acute metabolic disorder (electrolyte imbalance, hepatic or renal failure)
    3. Trauma (head injury, postoperative)

4. CNS pathology (stroke, hemorrhage, tumor, seizure disorder, Parkinson's)
5. Hypoxia (anemia, cardiac failure, pulmonary embolus)

- Deficiencies (vitamin B12, folic acid, thiamine)
- Endocrinopathies (thyroid, glucose, parathyroid, adrenal)
- Acute vascular (shock, vasculitis, hypertensive encephalopathy)
- Toxins, substance use, medication (alcohol, anesthetics, anticholinergics, narcotics)
- Heavy metals (arsenic, lead, mercury)

Table 7.1 Mnemonic for Differentiating Delirium from Dementia

COCOA PHSS

	Delirium	*Dementia*
Consciousness	Decreased or hyper alert, "clouded"	Alert
Orientation	Disorganized	Disoriented
Course	Fluctuating	Steady slow decline
Onset	Acute or subacute	Chronic
Attention	Impaired	Usually normal
Psychomotor	Agitated or lethargic	Usually normal
Hallucinations	Perceptual disturbances; may have hallucinations	Usually not present
Sleep-wake cycle	Abnormal	Usually normal
Speech	Slow, incoherent	Aphasic, anomic difficulty finding words

Rating Scales

The Delirium Rating Scale (DRS) is a 10-item scale that was one of the original measures utilized at the bedside. It has been revised over time. Unlike previously discussed scales, this one must be completed by the practitioner as the average delirious patient will not have the capacity to provide a good history or complete a checklist. It has a maximum of 32 points and should be completed after the clinician has interviewed the patient a few times over 24 hours or after reviewing nursing and chart notes for a more complete interval history.

A reasonable and faster alternative is the following:

Nursing Delirium Rating Scale (Nu-DESC)

- This scale measures three time intervals that correlate to typical nursing shifts.

- A score of 0, 1, or 2 (most severe) is placed into each eight-hour shift to delineate the severity of each specific delirium symptom. The maximum score is 10.
- A positive total score of 2 or greater indicates the patient likely suffers from delirium.
- This scale is free for clinical use and may be found in the reference section or by visiting http://www.sciencedirect.com/science/article/pii/S0885392405000539 or https://www.researchgate.net/profile/Marc_Andre_Roy2/publication/7879842_Fast_systematic_and_continuous_delirium_assessment_in_hospitalized_patients_The_Nursing_Delirium_Screening_Scale/links/540daad80cf2d8daaacc7785.pdf.

Table 7.2 The Nursing Delirium Rating Scale

Features and Descriptions	Symptoms Rating (0–2)		
Symptom Time Period	Midnight–8 AM	8 AM–4 PM	4 PM–Midnight
I. Disorientation Verbal or behavioral manifestation of not being oriented to time or place or misperceiving the persons in the environment.			
II. Inappropriate behavior Behavior inappropriate to place and/or for the person; e.g., pulling at tubes or dressings, attempting to get out of bed when that is contraindicated, and the like.			
III. Inappropriate communication Communication inappropriate to place and/or for the person; e.g., incoherence, uncommunicativeness, nonsensical or unintelligible speech.			
IV. Seeing or hearing things that are not there; distortions of visual objects.			
V. Psychomotor retardation Delayed responsiveness, few or no spontaneous actions/words; e.g., when the patient is prodded, reaction is deferred and/or the patient is unarousable.			
Total Score			

Dementia

People with dementia typically will show slow and progressive losses in several cognitive and executive functioning areas with the hallmark being that of short-term memory problems. The formal DSM-5 diagnosis, now called neurocognitive disorder (NCD), has been divided into mild versus severe subtypes. Mild NCD suggests there is mild impairment but the patient is capable of safely functioning in society. Major NCD is much more significant and impairing.

TIP: Dementia (NCD) Screening Questions

Screening for common deficits involving memory loss

- Do you find yourself losing things more easily? Are you unable to find the words you want to use? Have you found it difficult to learn new things lately?

Follow up with more intrusive questions about memory

- Have you recently noticed any memory problems?
- Do others point out your lapses in memory?

Mild NCD Diagnosis

The diagnostic criteria for mild NCD include:

1. Evidence of moderate cognitive decline from a previous level of performance in one or more cognitive domains—such as complex attention, executive function, learning, memory, language, perceptual-motor, or social cognition.
   This evidence should consist of:
   - Concern of the individual, a knowledgeable informant (such as a friend or family member), or the clinician that there's been a moderate decline in cognitive function; and
   - A moderate impairment in cognitive performance, preferably documented by standardized neuropsychological testing, or, if neuropsychological testing isn't available, another type of qualified assessment.
2. The cognitive deficits do not interfere with independence in everyday activities (e.g., at a minimum, requiring assistance with complex instrumental activities of daily living, such as paying bills or managing medications).
3. The cognitive deficits don't occur exclusively in context of a delirium, and are not better explained by another mental disorder.

Major NCD Diagnosis

1. Evidence of significant cognitive decline from a previous level of performance in one or more cognitive domains—such as complex attention, executive function, learning, memory, language, perceptual-motor, or social cognition.
   This evidence should consist of:
   - Concern of the individual, a knowledgeable informant (such as a friend or family member), or the clinician that there's been a significant decline in cognitive function; and
   - A substantial impairment in cognitive performance, preferably documented by standardized neuropsychological testing, or, if neuropsychological testing isn't available, another type of qualified assessment.
2. The cognitive deficits interfere with independence in everyday activities (e.g., at a minimum, requiring assistance with complex instrumental activities of daily living, such as paying bills or managing medications).
3. The cognitive deficits don't occur exclusively in context of a delirium and are not better explained by another mental disorder.

TIP: Commonly Used Mnemonics for DSM-5 for Dementia

DEMENTIA (may be used to assess for* reversible *dementia)

D: Drugs
E: Eyes and ears (visual and hearing handicaps may be confused with dementia)
M: Metabolic (hypoglycemia, hyperglycemia, hyponatremia, hypernatremia, hypothyroidism, etc.)
E: Emotional (depression can masquerade as a dementia-pseudodementia)
N: Nutrition (B12 and folic acid deficiency), normal pressure hydrocephalus
T: Tumors, trauma
I: Infections (Lyme disease, syphilis, encephalitis, etc.)
A: Alcoholism, atherosclerosis

C^2I^2: "C-squared-I squared" may be used for diagnosis

C: Cognitive decline
C: Concern of patient or others
I: Impairment measured (severe = major NCD)
I: Interference with daily living

Rating Scales

The Family Questionnaire

- The Family Questionnaire created by the National Chronic Care Consortium and the Alzheimer's Association is free of charge and simple to use by visiting http://www.alz.org/mnnd/documents/Family_Questionnaire.pdf
- It consists of five questions scored 0 to 3 points each. The form is completed by an family member or caregiver with good knowledge of the patient's day-to-day functioning. A score of 3 or more suggests the possibility of an NCD.
- Similar to delirium, patients with NCD may be poor historians, thereby making patient self-rated scales inaccurate as outcome measures, unless family members or caregivers are involved.

Table 7.3 The Family Questionnaire

We are trying to improve the care of older adults. Some older adults develop problems with memory or the ability to think clearly. When this occurs, it may not come to the attention of the physician. Family members or friends of an older person may be aware of problems that should prompt further evaluation by the physician. Please answer the following questions. This information will help us to provide better care for your family member.

In your opinion does ______________________________ have problems with any of the following?
Please circle the answer.

1.	Repeating or asking the same thing over and over?	*Not at all*	*Sometimes*	*Frequently*	*Does not apply*
2.	Remembering appointments, family occasions, holidays?	*Not at all*	*Sometimes*	*Frequently*	*Does not apply*
3.	Writing checks, paying bills, balancing the checkbook?	*Not at all*	*Sometimes*	*Frequently*	*Does not apply*
4.	Deciding what groceries or clothes to buy?	*Not at all*	*Sometimes*	*Frequently*	*Does not apply*
5.	Taking medication according to instructions?	*Not at all*	*Sometimes*	*Frequently*	*Does not apply*

Relationship to patient ______________________________
(spouse, son, daughter, brother, sister, grandchild, friend, etc.)

This information will be given to the patient's primary care provider. If any additional testing is appropriate, he or she will let you know. Thank you for your help.

The Folstein Mini-Mental Status Exam (MMSE)

- If a rating scale is desired for monitoring treatment outcome, there are no reliable patient completed rating scales for treatment monitoring.
- Clinician administered scales do exist and are the standard of care.
- The Folstein Mini-Mental Status Exam (MMSE) has been a standard for many years but now is copyrighted and requires permission to use.
- It is a 30-point scale that tests orientation, immediate memory, recall, concentration, and visuospatial abilities.
- Scores in the mid-20s are suggestive of dementia.

The Montreal Cognitive Assessment (MoCA)

- The clinician must conduct the examination and help the patient complete each step.
- It is conducted similar to the MMSE but covers more functional domains where deficits may be encountered in dementia patients.
- Scores of 18–26 = mild cognitive impairment, 10–17= moderate cognitive impairment, and less than 10 = severe cognitive impairment.
- The Montreal Cognitive Assessment (MoCA) is free to use in the public domain by visiting http://www.mocatest.org/.

Traumatic Brain Injury (TBI)

Diagnosis

Patients with mild TBI may be said to have Postconcussive Syndrome. After a presumed trauma, a heterogeneous and widely varied set of neuropsychiatric symptoms may develop. More severe TBI can present with initial delirium, a full syndromal psychiatric disorder, or develop into a dementia (NCD). TBI is considered an NCD and used to be delineated as a dementia due to an underlying medical condition (brain injury).

TBI Diagnosis

- A TBI is assumed to have occurred if after a blow to the head:
  - It is followed by any period of loss of or a decreased level of consciousness.
  - If any loss of memory for events immediately before or after the injury are noted.
  - If any alteration in mental state at the time of the injury (confusion, disorientation, slowed thinking, etc.) is noted.
  - If any neurological deficits are noted (weakness, loss of balance, change in vision, praxis, paresis/plegia, sensory loss, aphasia, etc.).

Postconcussive Syndrome (PCS) (Mild-TBI) Diagnosis

- PCS presents as three symptom clusters:
  - Mood—depression, anxiety, and irritability.
  - Cognition—decreased attention/concentration and often impaired memory, various degrees of executive dysfunction, and varied levels of conceptual disorganization.
  - Physical—headache, nausea, dizziness, vertigo, diplopia, insomnia, deafness, tinnitus, light and noise sensitivity, fatigue, and problems with coordination.

Rating Scales:

The Quality of Life after Brain Injury (QOLIBRI)

- The QOLIBRI is the first instrument specifically developed to assess health-related quality of life (HRQoL) of individuals after traumatic brain injury and is available in over 20 languages.
- The clinician must conduct the examination and help the patient complete each step.
- It is conducted after a clinical interview with a TBI patient, where the clinician records his/her findings after a typical interview. The approach is similar to the DRS reported above for delirium.
- Scoring is somewhat complex compared to other scales mentioned prior.
  - Responses to the "satisfaction" items (i.e., items on the Cognition, Self, Daily Life & Autonomy, and Social Relationships scales) are coded on a 1 to 5 scale, where 1 = "not at all satisfied" and 5 = "very satisfied." Responses to the "bothered" items (i.e., items on the Emotions and Physical Problems scales) are reverse scored to correspond with the satisfaction items, where 1 = "very bothered" and 5 = "not at all bothered."
  - The responses on each scale are summed to give a total, and then divided by the number of responses to give a scale mean. The scale means have a maximum possible range of 1 to 5. The mean can be computed when there are some missing responses, but should not be calculated if more than one-third of responses on the scale are missing. In a similar manner, the QOLIBRI total score is calculated by summing all the responses and then dividing by the actual number of responses. Again, a total score should not be calculated if more than one-third of responses are missing.
  - The scale means are converted to the 0–100 scale by subtracting 1 from the mean and then multiplying by 25. This produces scale scores which have a lowest possible value of 0 (worst possible quality of life) and a maximum value of 100 (best possible quality of life).
- It can be easily accessed for free at http://www.qolibrinet.com.

NAME :
Education : Date of birth :
Sex : DATE :

MONTREAL COGNITIVE ASSESSMENT (MOCA)
Version 7.1 Original Version

VISUOSPATIAL / EXECUTIVE

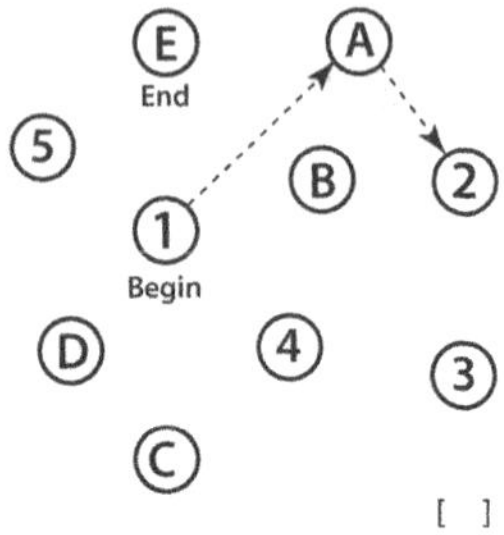

[ ]

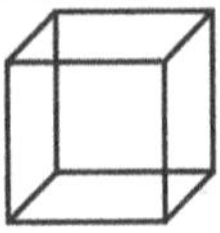

Copy cube

[ ]

Draw CLOCK (Ten past eleven)
(3 points)

[ ] Contour [ ] Numbers [ ] Hands

POINTS __/5

NAMING

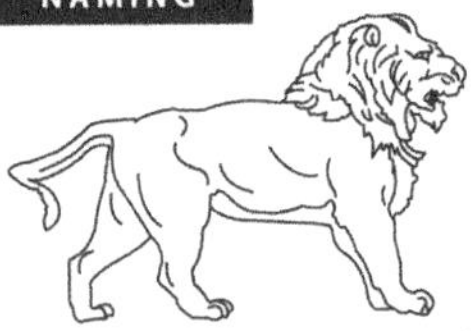

[ ]

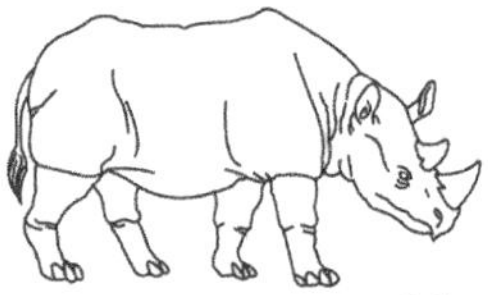

[ ]

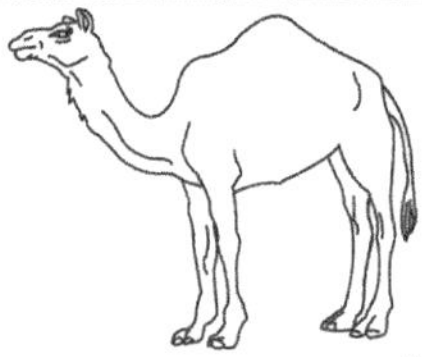

[ ]

__/3

MEMORY Read list of words, subject must repeat them. Do 2 trials, even if 1st trial is successful. Do a recall after 5 minutes.		FACE	VELVET	CHURCH	DAISY	RED	No points
	1st trial						
	2nd trial						

ATTENTION Read list of digits (1 digit/ sec.). Subject has to repeat them in the forward order [ ] 2 1 8 5 4
Subject has to repeat them in the backward order [ ] 7 4 2 __/2

Read list of letters. The subject must tap with his hand at each letter A. No points if ≥ 2 errors
[ ] F B A C M N A A J K L B A F A K D E A A A J A M O F A A B __/1

Serial 7 subtraction starting at 100 [ ] 93 [ ] 86 [ ] 79 [ ] 72 [ ] 65
4 or 5 correct subtractions: **3 pts**, 2 or 3 correct: **2 pts**, 1 correct: **1 pt**, 0 correct: **0 pt** __/3

LANGUAGE Repeat : I only know that John is the one to help today. [ ]
The cat always hid under the couch when dogs were in the room. [ ] __/2

Fluency / Name maximum number of words in one minute that begin with the letter F [ ] ____ (N ≥ 11 words) __/1

ABSTRACTION Similarity between e.g. banana - orange = fruit [ ] train – bicycle [ ] watch - ruler __/2

DELAYED RECALL	Has to recall words **WITH NO CUE**	FACE [ ]	VELVET [ ]	CHURCH [ ]	DAISY [ ]	RED [ ]	Points for UNCUED recall only	__/5
Optional	Category cue							
	Multiple choice cue							

ORIENTATION [ ] Date [ ] Month [ ] Year [ ] Day [ ] Place [ ] City __/6

© Z.Nasreddine MD **www.mocatest.org** Normal ≥ 26 / 30 TOTAL __/30
Administered by: ______ Add 1 point if ≤ 12 yr edu

Figure 7.1 Montreal Cognitive Assessment (MOCA)

The Montreal Cognitive Assessment (Copyright A. Nasreddine MD. Reproduced with permission. Copies are available at www.mocatest.org)

Table 7.4 QOLIBRI—Quality of Life After Brain Injury Scale

In the first part of this questionnaire we would like to know how satisfied you are with different aspects of your life since your brain injury. For each question, please choose the answer which is closest to how you feel now (including the past week) and mark the box with an "X." If you have problems filling out the questionnaire, please ask for help.

PART 1

	A. *These questions are about your thinking abilities now (including the past week).*	**Not at all**	**Slightly**	**Moderately**	**Quite**	**Very**
1.	How satisfied are you with your abilities to concentrate, for example when reading or keeping track of a conversation?					
2.	How satisfied are you with your ability to express yourself and understand others in a conversation?					
3.	How satisfied are you with your ability to remember everyday things; for example, where you have put things?					
4.	How satisfied are you with your ability to plan and work out solutions to everyday practical problems; for example, what to do when you lose your keys?					
5.	How satisfied are you with your ability to make decisions?					
6.	How satisfied are you with your ability to find your way around?					
7.	How satisfied are you with your speed of thinking?					
	B. *These questions are about your emotions and view of yourself now (including the past week).*	**Not at all**	**Slightly**	**Moderately**	**Quite**	**Very**
1.	How satisfied are you with your level of energy?					
2.	How satisfied are you with your level of motivation to do things?					
3.	How satisfied are you with your self-esteem, how valuable you feel?					
4.	How satisfied are you with the way you look?					
5.	How satisfied are you with what you have achieved since your brain injury?					
6.	How satisfied are you with the way you perceive yourself?					
7.	How satisfied are you with the way you see your future?					

(*Continued*)

Table 7.4 (Continued)

	C. These questions are about your independence and how you function in daily life now (including the past week).	**Not at all**	**Slightly**	**Moderately**	**Quite**	**Very**
1.	How satisfied are you with your abilities to concentrate; for example, when reading or keeping track of a conversation?					
2.	How satisfied are you with your ability to express yourself and understand others in a conversation?					
3.	How satisfied are you with your ability to remember everyday things; for example, where you have put things?					
4.	How satisfied are you with your ability to plan and work out solutions to everyday practical problems; for example, what to do when you lose your keys?					
5.	How satisfied are you with your ability to make decisions?					
6.	How satisfied are you with your ability to find your way around?					
7.	How satisfied are you with your speed of thinking?					

	D. These questions are about your social relationships now (including the past week).	**Not at all**	**Slightly**	**Moderately**	**Quite**	**Very**
1.	How satisfied are you with your ability to feel affection toward others; for example, your partner, family, friends?					
2.	How satisfied are you with your relationships with members of your family?					
3.	How satisfied are you with your relationships with your friends?					
4.	How satisfied are you with your relationship with a partner or with not having a partner?					
5.	How satisfied are you with your sex life?					
6.	How satisfied are you with the attitudes of other people towards you?					

PART 2

In the second part, we would like to know how bothered you feel by different problems. For each question please choose the answer which is closest to how you feel now (including the past week) and mark the box with an "X." If you have problems filling out the questionnaire, please ask for help.

E. *These questions are about how bothered you are by your feelings now (including the past week).*		Not at all	Slightly	Moderately	Quite	Very
1.	How bothered are you by feeling lonely, even when you are with other people?					
2.	How bothered are you by feeling bored?					
3.	How bothered are you by feeling anxious?					
4.	How bothered are you by feeling sad or depressed?					
5.	How bothered are you by feeling angry or aggressive?					

F. *These questions are about how bothered you are by physical problems now (including the past week).*		Not at all	Slightly	Moderately	Quite	Very
1.	How bothered are you by slowness and/or clumsiness of movement?					
2.	How bothered are you by effects of any other injuries you sustained at the same time as your brain injury?					
3.	How bothered are you by pain, including headaches?					
4.	How bothered are you by problems with seeing or hearing?					
5.	Overall, how bothered are you by the effects of your brain injury?					

Treatment Guidelines

TIP: Delirium APA GUIDELINES

- The APA guideline suggests the first-generation antipsychotic (FGA) haloperidol is the drug of choice if the delirious patient is agitated, combative, thought disordered, or is experiencing delusions or hallucinations.
- Second-generation antipsychotics (SGA) are being used more often for treating delirium but may be fraught with akathisia and sedation depending upon which SGA is chosen. There is mounting evidence for the ability of these SGAs to clear delirium symptoms comparably to haloperidol. Of the SGAs, risperidone (Risperdal), olanzapine (Zyprexa), and quetiapine (Seroquel) have the most data.
- Generally, pharmacological management is provided along with environmental and social support, all while the underlying medical cause is being treated.
- FGA/SGA use is generally limited to low doses over several days as delirium tends to resolve as the underlying medical condition is being concomitantly treated.
- A few days after delirium symptoms have resolved, the FGA/SGA should be stopped.
- Use of antipsychotics may lower incidence of injury to the patient or hospital staff, lessen the need for physical restraint, improve medical outcomes, and lead to a shorter hospital stay.
- Benzodiazepines (BZs) are generally not used for elderly patients who may become disinhibited, over-sedated, respiratory suppressed, or suffer from falls.
- BZs are the treatment of choice if the delirium is caused by BZ withdrawal or alcohol withdrawal. Lorazepam (Ativan) is most often used as it is available in PO, IM, and IV preparations and is easily metabolized outside of the hepatic P450 enzyme system. Doses are increased until withdrawal symptoms dissipate, and dosing may be higher than those used when treating anxiety.

TIP: Delirium Prescribing—Haloperidol

- Haloperidol (Haldol) is generally started at 0.25–2mg (PO or IM) every 2–4 hours as needed until delirium symptoms are controlled.
- IM doses have twice the bioavailability as oral doses and likely should be lower at initiation.
- Direct IV pushes are contraindicated due to risk of fatal ventricular arrhythmia. Sometimes, slow soluset drips may be utilized but greater cardiac monitoring is warranted.

- After 24 hours of dosing, the cumulative dose may be divided and administered daily until the delirium fully clears.
- It should be continued a few days after remission then discontinued.
- Haloperidol is a high-potency FGA and, as such, is very specific for blocking the dopamine D-2 receptor.
- It does not block histamine, cholinergic, or adrenergic receptors and thus is not sedating and likely will not complicate the patient's mental state further.
- There is little risk of tardive dyskinesia (TD) as patients are generally treated for less than two weeks.
- Akathisia may be the only extrapyramidal syndrome (EPS) noted.
- The only monitoring required may be that of an EKG to observe for QTc prolongation.

TIP: Delirium Prescribing—SGAs

- SGAs are being used more often for treating delirium as they are felt to have less extrapyramidal symptoms (EPS).
- Given the short-term use of these drugs in delirium, TD and Parkinsonism are rare but there is likely an increase in akathisia, dystonia, and neuroleptic malignant syndrome (NMS) when haloperidol or other FGAs are used.
- SGAs will have less risk of EPS overall. Unfortunately, when EPS develops in a delirious patient it is often seen as agitation and combativeness and assumed to be a worsening delirium. This often requires greater dosing and more medical risk with greater testing and procedures. Use of SGAs may alleviate some of these clinical dilemmas.
- SGAs, unfortunately, carry more risk of sedation, somnolence, and hypotension. This may cloud the delirious patient's sensorium or, frankly, sedate them. These side effects may also be confused for the waxing and waning symptoms of delirium.
- SGAs mostly have PO routes of administration, making them less versatile than haloperidol. However, olanzapine (Zyprexa) has an IM version that could be utilized, again at lower doses given higher IM bioavailability.
- Risperidone (Risperdal), olanzapine (Zyprexa), and quetiapine (Seroquel) have the greatest evidence base for use in delirium.
- Average oral doses of 1.4mg/day, 4.6mg/day, and 73mg/day, respectively, are utilized (compared to an average daily dose of 4.6mg of haloperidol).
- Starting at the lowest tablet strength and use of divided dosing is warranted.
- Obtaining an EKG at baseline and periodically during treatment may be warranted similar to that of haloperidol use.

TIP: Delirium Prescribing—BZs

- Benzodiazepines (BZs) are generally not used for elderly patients who may become disinhibited, over-sedated, respiratory suppressed, or suffer from falls.
- Regardless of age, BZs may cause sedation and alter the patient's mental status and level of consciousness, thus making it difficult to assess if the delirium is clearing.
- BZs are used primarily if the withdrawal is medically due to alcohol, BZ, or barbiturate withdrawal. Sometimes, BZs are incorporated into the treatment of non-alcohol delirium sparingly and if a few doses of a FGA/SGA have failed to lower combativeness.
- A typical protocol for moderate alcohol withdrawal is outlined in the next table.

TIP: Alcohol Withdrawal/Delirium BZ Prescribing

- All alcohol withdrawal patients should receive 100mg of thiamine to prevent permanent brain damage and memory problems. Folate and thiamine are generally added.
- The Clinical Institute Withdrawal Assessment for Alcohol-Revised (CIWA-Ar) symptom scale may be used to assess the level of withdrawal and to determine improvement. CIWA-Ar scores of ≤8 are suggestive of mild withdrawal symptoms, while those ≥15 confer an increased risk for confusion and seizures.
- Lorazepam (Ativan) may be given from 2–4mg every six hours for four doses to control symptoms and lower CIWA-Ar scores for mild cases.
- CIWA-Ar score ≥15 likely requires inpatient detoxification.
- Of note, carbamazepine (Tegretol) and divalproex (Depakote) also have some evidence to support their use in alcohol withdrawal.

TIP: Neurocognitive Disorder (NCD) Guidelines

- Readers should note that the only approvals for NCD are to slow the progression of Alzheimer's dementia. There are no current preventatives, reversing, or curative agents.
- Psychotropics are often used to treat the behavioral complications of NCD (agitation, combativeness, delirium or other psychoses, etc.)

- Anticholinesterase inhibitors (donepezil [Aricept], galantamine [Razadyne], rivastigmine [Exelon]) may be used as early as possible in the course of mild to moderate NCD due to Alzheimer's to preserve function and delay the need for nursing home care.
- Memantine (Namenda) is a glutamate dampening agent approved for use in moderate NCD.
- The current evidence also supports combining memantine and an anticholinesterase together.
- The above medications are used long term.
- SGAs may be warranted for psychosis due to NCD. They may be considered for use in agitation and combativeness in the absence of psychosis if potentially treatable causes of these symptoms are first addressed.
    - SGAs are used only after social and behavioral options have been tried.
    - After a few weeks, if patient has responded to an SGA, it should be removed to avoid long-term side effects (TD, EPS, increased cardio/cerebrovascular mortality). If behavioral symptoms return, it can be started and used over longer terms.
- SSRIs have shown limited effectiveness in NCD for agitation.
- Epilepsy mood stabilizers (AED) have generally failed to prove effectiveness in this area.
- Small studies indicate that NCD apathy may respond to low dose stimulant therapy.
- BZ sedatives are generally avoided as they may worsen memory and psychomotor functioning.

TIP: TBI Guidelines

- TBI causes a wide variety of psychiatric disturbances that are associated with functional impairments and a lower quality of life. These disturbances include disorders of mood, behavior, cognition, and changes in personality.
- Not only is TBI associated with higher rates of psychiatric disorders, but psychiatric illness is also a risk factor for TBI.
- Dementia is a progressive and lengthy degenerative process, and depending upon which brain area is involved in this process, different symptoms may emerge. TBI causes direct and immediate tissue damage, and depending upon which brain area is injured and becomes poorly functional, different psychiatric symptoms may emerge, comparable to a dementia.
- There are no FDA approved treatments for the behavioral disturbances associated with TBI. Similar to the off-label treatment of these symptoms

in delirium and NCD, clinicians should clearly target, describe, and measure baseline neuropsychiatric symptoms that they wish to treat.

- Ideally, doses should be started and escalated slowly, as TBI patients are presumed to have more severe CNS side effects or greater idiosyncratic, paradoxical effects.
- If there is a clear reduction in these symptoms, then the prescribing should continue. If not, then another treatment option should be pursued.
- The approach to prescribing is very similar to those taught regarding NCD.

TIP: TBI Prescribing

- Post-TBI depressive/anxious symptoms should be treated with entry-level antidepressants, such as SSRIs, and there is a limited but positive evidence base to support this approach.
- Post-TBI depression with remarkable cognitive symptoms may respond to stimulant (ex. methylphenidate [Ritalin]) augmentation.
- ECT has been shown to be effective in a small sample of patients as well.
- Post-TBI induced manic episodes have been successfully treated per the literature with divalproex (Depakote), lithium, or ECT.
- Post-TBI psychosis should be treated with SGAs instead of FGAs, as there is a presumptive increased risk of TD and EPS in patients with pre-existing CNS neuronal compromise
- Small trials support the use of melatonin, amitriptyline (Elavil), lorazepam (Ativan), and eszopiclone (Lunesta) for the treatment of post-TBI insomnia. Ideally, use of less psychomotor/cognitive impairing (non-BZ) hypnotic agents is warranted. Off-label use of melatonin, ramelteon (Rozerem), doxepin (Silenor), trazodone (Desyrel) makes clinical sense.
- Finally, as many TBI patients will develop symptoms of impulsivity, affective lability/dyscontrol, anxiety, and depression that may resemble those of borderline personality disorder (BPD) patients, see that chapter for help in off-label prescribing of mood stabilizers (AEDs) and SGAs.

SECTION 2 Advanced Prescribing Practices

Introduction

In Section 1, the premise is to convince the reader that they must make an accurate diagnosis and pick an approved agent with well-defined dosing guidelines and expected clinical outcomes. This approach is largely one of pattern recognition: (1) identify the pattern of phenotypic symptoms, (2) choose from a finite list of available, proven effective drugs, (3) start dosing low and escalate through an approved dosing range, (4) assess for effectiveness, and (5) continue medication if effective and cross-titrate to a new drug if ineffective or not tolerated. This methodical and mathematical approach can improve the standard of care and, ideally, patient outcomes when treated by the novice psychopharmacologist.

Section 2 is designed to provide a greater depth of neuroscience and pharmacodynamic knowledge to the reader and is written for prescribers who are knowledgeable and competent in those skills outlined in Section 1. The section is generally intended for those patients who are felt to be treatment-resistant and comorbid with other disorders.

To start, this chapter will briefly cover three distinct treatment entities instead of exhaustively discussing one single disorder.

Neurocognitive disorder (NCD) encompasses what was known in the DSM-IVTR as dementia. It is also broader in categorizing a disorder of variable etiologies that may yield deficits in attention, concentration, executive function, learning and memory, language, perceptual and motor function, and social cognition. These disorders may be reversible and short in duration (delirium) or may be progressive and permanent (Alzheimer's dementia, vascular dementia, frontotemporal dementia, traumatic brain injury, etc.). TBI is a type of NCD and will be discussed in short. Delirium is an acute condition that causes cognitive symptoms which will also be compared and contrasted to other NCD.

Epidemiology of Delirium

- Delirium is often called an acute confusional state or encephalopathy.
- Generally, there is a medical cause that acutely changes global brain function. Diffuse global slowing is often seen on electroencephalograms (EEG). Patients will wax and wane into and out of consciousness, and become disoriented and cognitively impaired.
- Once the medical condition is diagnosed and treated, often delirium resolves without any permanent cognitive deficits.
- At any given time, medically hospitalized patients may be suffering from delirium. The prevalence is approximately 20%.

Epidemiology of Dementia

- Dementia is now called neurocognitive disorder (NCD) in the DSM-5.
- Generally, these are chronic and progressive disorders where there is gradually a loss of cognitive function. Faster onset conditions do exist (prion disease, trauma, embolic shower strokes, etc.) as do some reversible conditions (vitamin B12 deficiency, hypothyroidism, normal pressure hydrocephalus, etc.).

- The most common conditions are Alzheimer's disease, Lewy Body disease, vascular disease, frontotemporal lobar degeneration, and traumatic brain injury.
- The prevalence of dementia in those below age 70 is about 1.5% and may reach as high as 20% for nonagenarians.

Epidemiology of TBI

- Currently, approximately 5.3 million Americans suffer from a TBI.
- An average of 1.4 million TBIs occur each year, including 1.1 million emergency department visits, 235,000 hospitalizations, and 50,000 deaths.
- The leading causes of TBI are falls, motor vehicle crashes, struck by or against objects, and assaults.
- 1.6 million–3.8 million sports-related TBIs occur each year, as many are unreported.
- Work productivity loss attributed to TBI is 14 times that associated with spinal cord injury.
- The costs of TBIs in the United States, including medical costs and lost productivity, total an estimated $60 billion annually.

Genetics of Delirium

- For delirium, candidate risk genes often include those responsible for mediating inflammatory processes (cytokines such as the interleukins) or dopamine neurocircuitry (dopamine receptors and metabolic enzymes). The latter are implicated as delirious patients may become thought disordered, delusional, or may experience hallucinations.
- There are minimal genetic studies to discuss. Two have shown an association between the APOE4 gene and longer, complicated delirium episodes. This gene is often implicated in Alzheimer's and has links to lowered acetylcholine (Ach) activity in the CNS, which harms short-term memory. Only one study has confirmed that within the dopamine system DRD2 dopamine-2 receptor gene mutations may convey risk for delirium.

Genetics of Dementia

- Given the variety of specific dementia types, the amount of research dollars supporting dementia research, and the marketability for current and future drug treatments in this area, there is much in the way of risk-gene data. It is beyond this chapter to cover much of this, but key findings are quickly detailed below.
- One finding does include the APOE e4 mutation noted for delirium above. The heritability of Alzheimer's may be upwards of 70%, where that of vascular dementia is 20% based upon twin studies.
- There are well-known causative genes for Alzheimer's disease: *APP*, *PSEN1*, and *PSEN2* all are implicated in the creation of amyloid plaques and neurofibrillary tangles. Three risk genes may explain a majority of frontotemporal dementia risk: *MAPT*, *GRN*, and *C9ORF72*, which may cause abnormalities in TAU or ubiquitin proteins.
- There is a 40% family history in those suffering from Alzheimer's dementia.
- Results from genetic association studies in vascular dementia suggest the following risk genes: *APOE*, renin–angiotensin, *TRIM65* and *TRIM47*, as well as the Notch3 signaling pathway genes.
- The APOEe4 allele is also associated with poor outcome in adults who have suffered a traumatic brain injury (TBI).

Neuroanatomy of Delirium

- Again, the available research for delirium when compared to that of dementia is quite limited. For delirium, neuroanatomic findings suggest that ischemic or hypoxia-based lesions are often noted in the hippocampus, pons, and striatum.
- Neuroanatomic findings suggest abnormal connectivity between the dorsolateral prefrontal cortex (DLPFC) where alertness and executive function dominate and the posterior cingulates.
- In fact, during a delirium the connectivity and direction of neural information flow may be reversed. These findings are somewhat similar to those found in ADHD and during sedative intoxication. Interestingly, these fMRI findings may be noted several days after a delirium clinically remits. Typical guidelines suggest treating a delirium with antipsychotics for a few days after symptom remission, as such.

- Although not an imaging technique, EEGs may be helpful in the diagnosis of delirium. In a two-electrode model, relative delta power can delineate delirious from non-delirious patients with a 1–2 minute limited EEG protocol. Formal, full electrode EEG will show diffuse global background activity slowing as an alternative option. These findings are not typically found in schizophrenia or dementia.

Neuroanatomy of Dementia

- For dementia, we will briefly review the neuroanatomic findings for a few dementia subtypes.
- Loss of hippocampal volume is noted across many dementia types (Alzheimer's, Parkinson's, Lewy body, and vascular).
- Temperal lobe atrophy seems most common in Alzheimer's dementia.
- White matter lesions (strokes) may be seen across dementia types but are clearly more common and predictive of vascular dementia and its severity and progression. These are most often seen in the deep white matter.
- Even though there are differential areas of brain atrophy across dementias, total brain volume loss may be comparable across different dementia types (Alzheimer's, Lewy body, vascular).
- Generally, functional neuroimaging studies will show differences in activity depending on the dementia type and its level of progression. Overall, there appears to be an inability to activate full brain areas responsible for task completion in these paradigms. The dementia brain seems to lack the normal capacity to use and activate key brain areas to complete tasks (facial recognition, short-term memory, visuospatial, etc.).
- In TBI patients, there may be clear evidence of swelling and bruising of brain tissue related to the area of the brain that was injured. There is often diffuse axonal injury that also is not easy to detect. Functional imaging, especially for working memory, is often abnormal early in the healing process, but over several months can be seen to improve. The most implicated area of dysfunction is around the right corticofrontal region.
- Unlike other dementias, TBI dementias do not seem to have hippocampal atrophy and loss of cholinergic tone. An alternative hypothesis suggests that brain damage itself may impair neuronal functioning, but dopamine- and norepinephrine-based neuronal tone and connectivity is more likely lost post-trauma.

- In conclusion, genetic risk and environmental insult appear to lead to brain tissue loss and brain functional abnormalities. These, in turn, lead to phenotypic symptoms that may be detected upon a clinical interview.

Neuroscientific Background and Rationale for Medication Use

In treating NCD, there are three classes of frequently used medications. (**See Prescribing Table.**)

1) Anticholinesterase Inhibitors for Dementia

MECHANISM OF ACTION

Donepezil (Aricept), galantamine (Razadyne), rivastigmine (Exelon)

- The mechanism of slowing dementia symptom progression is likely due to the increase, or at least preservation of, acetylcholine (ACh) in the CNS and preservation of hippocampal function.
- This class of medication inhibits the enzyme acetylcholine esterase. This enzyme's purpose is to degrade and lower ACh concentrations in the synapse. By blocking this enzymatic activity, ACh concentrations elevate enhancing cholinergic tone throughout the CNS.
- This is likely very important in hippocampal structures, where short-term memory is thought to be temporarily stored and ultimately begins the process of long-term memory encoding.
- Elevating or preserving ACh here may preserve or maintain what short-term memory function is left in the brain that is undergoing neurodegeneration from a dementia process.

2) NMDA Antagonists for Dementia

MECHANISM OF ACTION

Memantine (Namenda)

- Glutamate is the main excitatory transmitter in the CNS. Theoretically, hyperactivity of glutamate neurons may lead to excess glutamate in synapses which can cause neuronal cell death (excitotoxicity).

- The NMDA glutamate receptor may be blocked, thus lowering glutamate activity and neuronal depolarization. This may slow the rate of neuronal cell death.
- This may preserve brain tissue and function as long as possible, again, slowing the progression and course of Alzheimer's dementia.
- To improve medication compliance, there exists a combination pill that includes memantine plus the anticholinesterase inhibitor donepezil.

3) First- and Second-Generation Antipsychotics for Delirium

MECHANISM OF ACTION

FGAs/SGAs

- The reader is referred to the bipolar and schizophrenia chapters for further discussion regarding this class of medication.
- This class of medication may be utilized to treat psychosis from any disorder but is specifically indicated for the treatment of schizophrenia.
- Of the 11 available SGA agents in this class, all are approved for schizophrenia. Some SGAs are approved for autism aggression, mania, bipolar depression, and/or major depressive disorder (MDD) as well. These drugs are complicated, as they manipulate many different monoamine receptors and neuronal transporters giving each a unique profile.
- All of these agents block the D-2 dopamine receptor and, in the limbic system, this should restore a lower, more normal activity, thus alleviating mood swings, hostility, aggression, and psychosis even if associated with a medical delirium.
- All SGAs, therefore, may help treat the cognitive-perceptual symptoms of delirium or dementia in an off-label manner.
- In delirium, this may lower confusion, agitation, hallucinations, or delusions.
- In dementia (except for Lewy body disease where symptoms may escalate), this may lower agitation, hallucinations, and delusions as well.

Table 7.5 Prescribing Table for Neurocognitive Disorders

Drugs listed in BOLD are approved agents. Dosing is based upon clinical application. Approved dosing guidelines should be further referenced by the prescriber.
Alzheimer's Dementia Medications

Brand	Generic	Indication (Bold for FDA Approved)	Drug Mechanism	Dosing Tips	Monitoring Tips	Medicolegal Tips
Anticholinesterase Inhibitors						
Aricept	**Donepezil**	• **Alzheimer's disease (mild, moderate, severe)** • Memory impairments in other types of dementia • Mild cognitive impairment	• Reversible inhibition of centrally acting acetylcholinesterase (AChE), making more acetylcholine available for degenerating cholinergic neurons	• Usual dose is 5–23mg at night • Start 5mg/day and increase to 10mg/day after 4–6 weeks. May increase to 23mg/day after 90 days if needed (ER preparation)	• Common initial side effects include nausea, vomiting, diarrhea, weight loss, sleep disturbances	• Generally free of serious side effects
Exelon/ Exelon Patch	**Rivastigmine**	• **Alzheimer's disease (mild to moderate)** • **Parkinson's disease dementia (mild to moderate)** • Memory impairments in other types of dementia • Mild cognitive impairment	• Same as above	• Usual dose is 1.5–6mg twice daily • Start 1.5mg twice a day and increase by 3mg every 2 weeks • Transdermal usual dose is 4.6mg/24 hrs to 13.3mg/24 hrs increasing after 4 weeks if needed	• Same as above	• Same as above

(*Continued*)

Table 7.5 (Continued)

Drugs listed in BOLD are approved agents. Dosing is based upon clinical application. Approved dosing guidelines should be further referenced by the prescriber.

Alzheimer's Dementia Medications

Brand	Generic	Indication (Bold for FDA Approved)	Drug Mechanism	Dosing Tips	Monitoring Tips	Medicolegal Tips
Razadyne/ER	**Galantamine**	• **Alzheimer's disease (mild to moderate)** • Memory impairments in other types of dementia • Mild cognitive impairment	• Same as above and may modulate nicotinic receptors that enhances actions of acetylcholine	• Usual dosing 4mg–12mg twice daily • May increase by 4mg every 4 weeks • Usual ER dose is 8–24mg/day. Increase by 8mg/day every 4 weeks if needed	• Same as above	• Same as above
NMDA Antagonist						
Namenda/ER	**Memantine**	• **Alzheimer's disease (moderate to severe)** • Memory impairments in other types of dementia • Mild cognitive impairment	• NMDA receptor antagonist which interferes with excessive glutamatergic transmission	• Usual dose is 5–20mg/day • Starting dose is 5mg daily and after several days may increase to 5mg twice daily • For ER: start at 7mg/day and increase by 7mg every week. Maximum daily dose is 28mg	• Common initial side effects include dizziness, headache, and constipation.	• Generally free of serious side effects

Delirium Treatment Medications

First-Generation Antipsychotics						
Haldol	Haloperidol	• Delirium • Behavioral disturbances in dementias	• Blocks dopamine 2 receptors which reduces psychosis, confusion, agitation, and combativeness	• Usual dose is 1–2mg/day if elderly and 4–5mg/day if younger • Start at 0.25–0.5mg for medically frail patients and repeat every few hours until symptoms are controlled • Half the dose for IM use • After 24 hrs of as-needed (PRN) dosing, a total daily dose can be tabulated and, starting the next day, the daily dose can be divided into 4 doses and used routinely throughout the day until the delirium clears • Stop a few days after symptom remission	• Common initial side effects include mild sedation • Other notable side effects include akathisia. Other EPS, TD, galactorrhea, amenorrhea. Though these latter are not expected with short-term use • Serious side effects include rare neuroleptic malignant syndrome, QTc prolongation • Monitoring includes baseline and follow-up EKG	• Clearly explain life-threatening or serious side effects (e.g., NMS, dystonia, akathisia) • Higher doses and IV administration may be associated with increased risk of QT prolongation and torsades de pointes • Never administer via IV push • Risk of akathisia is high

(*Continued*)

Table 7.5 (Continued)

Brand	Generic	Indication (Bold for FDA Approved)	Drug Mechanism	Dosing Tips	Monitoring Tips	Medicolegal Tips
Second-Generation Antipsychotics						
Risperdal	Risperidone	• Delirium • Behavioral disturbances in dementias	• Blocks dopamine 2 receptors reducing psychosis and stabilizing affective symptoms • Blocks serotonin 2A receptors which promotes less pronounced EPS	• A similar dosing protocol may be used as that described for haloperidol • Start at 0.25–0.5mg for medically frail patients and repeat every few hours until symptoms are controlled • There is no IM formulation • After 24 hrs of as-needed (PRN) dosing, a total daily dose can be tabulated and, starting the next day, the daily dose can be divided into 4 equal doses and be given routinely throughout the day until the delirium clears • Stop a few days after symptom remission	• Common initial side effects include mild sedation, dizziness, GI side effects • Other notable side effects include risk of diabetes, dyslipidemia, EPS, hyperprolactinemia, and gynecomastia, though these are not expected over short-term use • Monitoring for metabolics may not be needed given short-term use, but serial EKG may be warranted	• Clearly explain life-threatening or serious side effects (e.g., EPS, QTc prolongation) • Risk of EPS akathisia is moderate

Zyprexa Zydis	Olanzapine	• Delirium • Behavioral disturbances in dementias	• Same as above	• A similar dosing protocol may be used as that described for haloperidol • Start at 2.5–5mg for medically frail patients and repeat every few hours until symptoms are controlled • Zydis is a dissolving preparation that can be used for patients with swallowing difficulty • Olanzapine does have an IM preparation but it has very little data for use in delirium. It is dosed at 5–10mg and may be repeated at 2 hrs and 4 hrs as needed • After 24 hrs of as-needed (PRN) dosing, a total daily dose can be tabulated and, starting the next day, the daily dose can be divided into 4 smaller equal doses and be given routinely as a standing order • Stop a few days after symptom remission	• Common initial side effects include moderate sedation, dizziness, dry mouth, blurred vision, GI side effects • Other notable side effects include risk of diabetes, dyslipidemia, EPS, hyperprolactinemia, and gynecomastia, though these are not expected over short-term use • Serious side effects include risk of diabetes, increased risk of death in demented elderly, rare NMS, and seizures • Monitoring for metabolics may not be needed given short-term use, but serial EKG may be warranted	• Same as above

(*Continued*)

Table 7.5 (Continued)

Brand	Generic	Indication (Bold for FDA Approved)	Drug Mechanism	Dosing Tips	Monitoring Tips	Medicolegal Tips
Seroquel Seroquel XR	Quetiapine	• Delirium • Behavioral disturbances in dementias	• Same as above	• A similar dosing protocol may be used as that described for haloperidol • Start at 25–50mg for medically frail patients and repeat every few hours until symptoms are controlled • There is no IM formulation • The XR preparation starts at 50mg and given its slow release may have less sedating side effects	• Common initial side effects include severe sedation, dizziness, GI side effects • Other notable side effects include risk of diabetes, dyslipidemia, EPS, though these are not expected over short-term use • Serious side effects include risk of diabetes, increased risk of death in demented elderly, rare NMS, and seizures • Monitoring for metabolics may not be needed given short-term use, but serial EKG may be warranted	• Same as above though EPS akathisia risks are lowest in this class and sedation may be highest

Practical Applications

TIP: Essential Concepts

- Unlike the previous disorders, there are not many second- or third-line treatments. There is not much rational polypharmacy for delirium where a monotherapy is almost always warranted with an FGA or an SGA.
- For delirium, if the first few doses of FGA/SGA fail to lower agitation and combativeness, then a low dose of a BZ may be administered as a secondary option. A typical protocol may include three successive doses of haloperidol, and, if little effect, then a low dose benzodiazepine may be issued.
- Polypharmacy of the NCD of Alzheimer's dementia occurs generally as the disease progresses. The anticholinesterase inhibitors are utilized in the early phases with NMDA-blocking memantine added for more moderate decline. Some practitioners are starting both agents as a combination (memantine + donepezil) earlier in treatment, though this is not as established in the literature. Namzaric is the combination preparation currently available.
- Polypharmacy of dementia often relates to the treatment of the secondary symptoms of dementia (psychosis, combativeness, depression, apathy, impulsivity, etc.).

Good Polypharmacy to Be Used

DO

- Start low dose to minimize side effects.
- Dosing escalations of NCD/dementia medications are often done every month instead of every few to every several days as noted in previous chapters for other psychiatric disorders.
- Escalate dosing within full range for optimal effectiveness.
- Monitor for EPS and EKG changes when using an FGA/SGA.
- Add drugs from different pharmacologic classes for treatment resistant cases where progression into further dementia symptoms is apparent.
  - Anticholinesterase inhibitors + NMDA Receptor Antagonists.
- Add antidepressants, stimulants, SGAs as needed to anti-dementia medications to treat behavioral manifestations of depression, anxiety, apathy, psychosis, agitation, or combativeness.
  - Use low doses and escalate gingerly.
  - Particularly for FGAs/SGAs, if successful, after several weeks attempt to lower dose and/or remove medication. Re-start as needed if target symptoms re-emerge.

DON'T

- Add two anticholinesterase inhibitors together.
- Increase monotherapy dosing too rapidly.
- Avoid BZs in delirium and other NCD.

Final Advanced Prescribing Thoughts

Patients with NCD typically are poor historians, so prescribers must enlist family and other caregivers to obtain up-to-date information about ongoing symptoms and side effects. Like personality disorder treatment, ideally clinicians should identify a clear target symptom to address (ex. memory loss, combativeness, apathy, etc.) and succinctly monitor over time. As these patients tend to be more frail and more side effect prone, agents should be prescribed carefully and closely monitored. If there is no clear effect, they should be removed to avoid further risk and inappropriate polypharmacy.

Bibliography

American Psychiatric Association. (1997) "Practice guideline for the treatment of patients with Alzheimer's disease and other dementias of late life." *The American Journal of Psychiatry* 154(5), 1–39.

American Psychiatric Association. (2006) *American Psychiatric Association Practice Guidelines for the Treatment of Psychiatric Disorders: Compendium 2006*. Arlington, VA: American Psychiatric Association.

American Psychiatric Association. (2013) *Diagnostic and Statistical Manual of Mental Disorders: DSM-5* (5th ed.). Washington, D.C.: American Psychiatric Association.

Asplund, C. A., Aaronson, J. W., & Aaronson, H. E. (2004) "3 regimens for alcohol withdrawal and detoxification." *Journal of Family Practice* 53(7), 545–554.

Barr, J., et al. (2013) "Clinical practice guidelines for the management of pain, agitation, and delirium in adult patients in the intensive care unit." *Critical Care Medicine* 41(1), 263–306.

Choi, S. H., Lee, H., Chung, T. S., Park, K. M., Jung, Y. C., Kim, S. I., & Kim, J. J. (2012) "Neural network functional connectivity during and after an episode of delirium." *American Journal of Psychiatry* 169(5), 498–507.

Folstein, M. F., Robins, L. N., & Helzer, J. E. (1983) "The mini-mental state examination." *Archives of General Psychiatry* 40(7), 812.

Gaudreau, J. D., Gagnon, P., Harel, F., Tremblay, A., & Roy, M. A. (2005) "Fast, systematic, and continuous delirium assessment in hospitalized patients: the nursing delirium screening scale." *Journal of Pain and Symptom Management* 29(4), 368–375.

Kurowski, B., Martin, L. J., & Wade, S. L. (2012) "Genetics and outcomes after traumatic brain injury (TBI): what do we know about pediatric TBI?" *Journal of Pediatric Rehabilitation Medicine* 5(3), 217.

Langlois, J. A., Rutland-Brown, W., & Wald, M. M. (2006) "The epidemiology and impact of traumatic brain injury: a brief overview." *The Journal of Head Trauma Rehabilitation* 21(5), 375–378.

Loy, C. T., Schofield, P. R., Turner, A. M., & Kwok, J. B. (2014) "Genetics of dementia." *The Lancet* 383(9919), 828–840.

McAllister, T. W., Flashman, L. A., McDonald, B. C., & Saykin, A. J. (2006) "Mechanisms of working memory dysfunction after mild and moderate TBI: evidence from functional MRI and neurogenetics." *Journal of Neurotrauma* 23(10), 1450–1467.

Meagher, D. J., McLoughlin, L., Leonard, M., Hannon, N., Dunne, C., & O'Regan, N. (2013) "What do we really know about the treatment of delirium with antipsychotics? Ten key issues for delirium pharmacotherapy." *The American Journal of Geriatric Psychiatry* 21(12), 1223–1238.

O'Brien, J. T., et al. (2001) "Progressive brain atrophy on serial MRI in dementia with Lewy bodies, AD, and vascular dementia." *Neurology* 56(10), 1386–1388.

Qiu, C., De Ronchi, D., & Fratiglioni, L. (2007) "The epidemiology of the dementias: an update." *Current Opinion in Psychiatry* 20(4), 380–385.

Reus, V. I., et al. (2016) "The American Psychiatric Association Practice Guideline on the use of antipsychotics to treat agitation or psychosis in patients with dementia." *American Journal of Psychiatry* 173(5), 543–546.

Rombouts, S. A., Damoiseaux, J. S., Goekoop, R., Barkhof, F., Scheltens, P., Smith, S. M., & Beckmann, C. F. (2009) "Model-free group analysis shows altered BOLD FMRI networks in dementia." *Human Brain Mapping* 30(1), 256–266.

Sanchez-Carrion, R., et al. (2008) "A longitudinal fMRI study of working memory in severe TBI patients with diffuse axonal injury." *Neuroimage* 43(3), 421–429.

Schwartz, T. L., & Masand, P. S. (2002) "The role of atypical antipsychotics in the treatment of delirium." *Psychosomatics* 43(3), 171–174.

Simpson, J. R. (2014) "DSM-5 and neurocognitive disorders." *Journal of the American Academy of Psychiatry and the Law Online* 42(2), 159–164.

Trzepacz, P. T. (1999) "The Delirium Rating Scale: its use in consultation-liaison research." *Psychosomatics* 40(3), 193–204.

Trzepacz, P. T., Baker, R. W., & Greenhouse, J. (1988) "A symptom rating scale for delirium." *Psychiatry Research* 23(1), 89–97.

van der Kooi, A. W., Zaal, I. J., Klijn, F. A., Koek, H. L., Meijer, R. C., Leijten, F. S., & Slooter, A. J. (2015) "Delirium detection using EEG: what and how to measure." *CHEST Journal* 147(1), 94–101.

van Munster, B. C., De Rooij, S. E., & Korevaar, J. C. (2009) "The role of genetics in delirium in the elderly patient." *Dementia and Geriatric Cognitive Disorders* 28(3), 187–195.

von Steinbuechel, N., Petersen, C., Bullinger, M., & QOLIBRI group. (2005) "Assessment of health-related quality of life in persons after traumatic brain injury—development of the Qolibri, a specific measure." In Klaus von Wild (ed.) *Re-Engineering of the Damaged Brain and Spinal Cord* (43–49). Vienna: Springer.

CHAPTER 8

Schizophrenia Spectrum Disorders

SECTION 1 Basic Prescribing Practices

Essential Concepts

- Typically, hallucinations and delusions are noted as hallmarks of psychosis in schizophrenia (SP), but other forms of psychosis may include disorganized thought processes (loose associations) or behaviors (catatonia).
- Many times the patient presents with negative symptoms where they can appear withdrawn or isolated, with depressed, flat, or blunted affect. Misdiagnosis as major depressive disorder (MDD) may occur. Other, patients are agitated, restless, and may be diagnosed with an anxiety disorder.
- In the absence of positive symptoms, clinicians must be perceptive so as to detect and establish the longer, more gradual onset of prodromal negative symptoms, depressive and anxiety symptoms, and milder forms of thought disorder.
- Psychotic disorders exist along a spectrum based upon the type and duration of symptoms experienced.
- Antipsychotics will be able to treat psychotic symptoms regardless of the assigned DSM-5 diagnosis (schizophrenia [SP], schizophreniform disorder, brief psychotic disorder, delusional disorder, schizoaffective disorder).
- Psychosis due to mania, depression, or delirium may also be treated by antipsychotics.
- Psychosis is felt to be due to excessive dopamine (DA) neuronal firing in the CNS limbic system. All antipsychotics tend to correct this abnormal hyperactivity.

Phenomenology, Diagnosis, Clinical Interviewing

For any new practitioner in any field, the goal is to be able to make an accurate diagnosis. All of psychiatric prescribing at this beginning level is based on regulatory findings, approvals, and indications that are psychiatric disorder specific.

Psychotropics will only deliver the outcomes promised if the patient at hand actually has been accurately identified as having SP or a spectrum disorder. Diagnosis may be difficult as patients often are poor historians with little insight into their disorder. However, some patients do retain insight and also fear repercussion if they discuss their psychosis. They may be guarded and unwilling to elaborate on their more obvious positive (delusions, hallucinations) symptoms. Sometimes, patients may be seen talking when no one is around, or looking or reacting to their hallucinations (responding to internal stimuli). More subtly, they experience these symptoms but do not exhibit them for clinicians to witness. Commonly, SP in adults is confounded by other psychiatric disorders, such as a formal anxiety, substance use, or depressive disorders.

TIP: Comorbidity with SP

Patients with SP may also present with the following high prevalence comorbidities:

- 15% panic disorder (PD)
- 29% posttraumatic stress disorder (PTSD)
- 23% obsessive-compulsive disorder (OCD)
- 50% major depressive disorder (MDD)
- 47% substance use disorder (SUD)

Similar to previous chapters, this book will initially teach diagnosis and treatment of SP in a simplified, single-disorder state and then progress toward more advanced treatment of comorbid psychiatric states. This chapter will teach and then assume the reader is adept and comfortable with descriptive, DSM-5 interviewing and diagnostic assessment. Furthermore, in the absence of DSM-5 mastery, patient administered rating scales should become the standard of care.

TIP: Diagnostic Concepts Regarding the Schizophrenia Spectrum

- Brief psychotic disorder—lasts a month or less and has no negative SP symptoms.
- Schizophreniform disorder—lasts 1–6 months with full SP symptoms.
- Schizophrenia—lasts greater than six months with full SP symptoms.
- Delusional disorder—only has delusions but never has hallucinations, thought disorder, or negative symptoms.

- Schizoaffective disorder—meets full SP criteria while predominantly experiencing MDD or bipolar disorder (BD) as well.
- The key to diagnosis of schizophrenia is to confirm the *sustained* nature of the course of illness.
- Typically, patients with SP proceed with normal psychosocial milestones until the schizophrenia develops, most often in the late teens or early 20s.
- Sometimes, patients who present as depressed or anxious may admit during the Psychiatric Review of Systems interview that they have had psychotic experiences. At other times, paranoid or bizarre stories may emerge when discussing their developmental and social history.

TIP: Schizophrenia Screening Questions

Screening for perceptual disturbances

- In your life, have you ever had hallucinations? Perhaps saw or heard things that did not make sense or seem part of reality? Do you see or hear things that others cannot?
    - Note that hallucinations of taste, touch, and smell are not typical of SP and may herald an organic (brain tumor, epilepsy, drug induced) cause.

Screening for delusions

- Have you ever been paranoid and felt people were out to get you, trying to harm you, or following you around?
- When you watch TV or listen to music, do you detect hidden messages or feel these are speaking specifically to or about you?

DSM-5 Diagnosis

People with SP often will show an initial several months of a prodrome prior to meeting full DSM-5 criteria. Often, patients become socially isolated, appear to lose abstract thought, and operate in a more concrete pattern of thought. They may experience lapses in grooming and hygiene. They may appear depressed or as if strung out on drugs. Many SP patients are erroneously treated for MDD in this timeframe. Once full SP symptoms are established, there should be an absence of full MDD or mania symptoms as well. The following pages describe the multiple diagnoses within the SP spectrum.

DSM-5 Diagnosis of Brief Psychotic Disorder

- Presence of one (or more) of the following symptoms:
  - delusions
  - hallucinations
  - disorganized speech (e.g., frequent derailment or incoherence)
  - grossly disorganized or catatonic behavior
- Duration of an episode of the disturbance is at least one day but less than one month, with eventual full return to premorbid level of functioning.

DSM-5 Diagnosis of Schizophreniform Disorder

- Two (or more) of the following, each present for a significant portion of time during a one-month period (or less if successfully treated). At least one of these must be (1), (2), or (3):
  1. delusions
  2. hallucinations
  3. disorganized speech (e.g., frequent derailment or incoherence)
  4. grossly disorganized or catatonic behavior
  5. negative symptoms (i.e., diminished emotional expression or avolition)
- An episode of the disorder lasts at least one month but less than six months.

DSM-5 Diagnosis of Schizophrenia

- Two (or more) of the following, each present for a significant portion of time during a one-month period (or less if successfully treated). At least one of these must be (1), (2), or (3):
  1. delusions
  2. hallucinations
  3. disorganized speech (e.g., frequent derailment or incoherence)
  4. grossly disorganized or catatonic behavior
  5. negative symptoms (i.e., diminished emotional expression or avolition)
- For a significant portion of the time since the onset of the disturbance, level of functioning in one or more major areas, such as work, interpersonal relations, or self-care, is markedly below the level achieved prior to the onset.
- Continuous signs of the disturbance persist for at least six months.

TIP: Mnemonic for SP Criteria

- DHSBN or "dustbin" = **D**elusions **H**erald **S**chizophrenic **B**ad **N**ews
- **D**elusions, **H**allucinations, **S**peech disorganization, **B**ehavior disorganization, **N**egative symptoms

Rating Scales

Interestingly and unlike every other chapter in this book, there is not a widely used or accepted rating scale that patients self-complete in order to detect or measure schizophrenia symptoms. Almost all that are discussed in the literature are conducted and completed by a clinician. The approach may resemble that used in neurocognitive disorders (NCD) such as delirium or dementia.

Community Assessment of Psychic Experiences (CAPE-42)

- The CAPE is not validated as yet and uses Likert Scale items for positive, negative, and distress symptoms. It takes several minutes to complete as it is 42-items long.
- Scoring is more difficult as it uses an algorithm, but it is an easy way to track a variety of symptoms associated with psychotic symptoms over time.
- It is free in the public domain and can be obtained at cape42.homestead.com.

Table 8.1 The Community Assessment of Psychic Experiences

CAPE-42

1. Do you ever feel sad?
(please tick)
Never Sometimes Often Nearly always

If you ticked never, please go to Question 2.
If you ticked sometimes, often, or nearly always, please indicate how distressed you are by this experience:

(please tick)
Not distressed A bit distressed Quite distressed Very distressed

2. Do you ever feel as if people seem to drop hints about you or say things with a double meaning?
(please tick)
Never Sometimes Often Nearly always

If you ticked never, please go to Question 3.
If you ticked sometimes, often, or nearly always, please indicate how distressed you are by this experience:

(please tick)
Not distressed A bit distressed Quite distressed Very distressed

3. Do you ever feel that you are not a very animated person?
(please tick)
Never Sometimes Often Nearly always

If you ticked never, please go to Question 4.
If you ticked sometimes, often, or nearly always, please indicate how distressed you are by this experience:

(please tick)
Not distressed A bit distressed Quite distressed Very distressed

4. Do you ever feel that you are not much of a talker when you are conversing with other people?
(please tick)
Never Sometimes Often Nearly always

If you ticked never, please go to Question 5.
If you ticked sometimes, often, or nearly always, please indicate how distressed you are by this experience:

(please tick)
Not distressed A bit distressed Quite distressed Very distressed

5. Do you ever feel as if things in magazines or on TV were written especially for you?
(please tick)
Never Sometimes Often Nearly always

If you ticked never, please go to Question 6.
If you ticked sometimes, often, or nearly always, please indicate how distressed you are by this experience:

(please tick)
Not distressed A bit distressed Quite distressed Very distressed

6. Do you ever feel as if some people are not what they seem to be?
(please tick)
Never Sometimes Often Nearly always

If you ticked never, please go to Question 7.
If you ticked sometimes, often, or nearly always, please indicate how distressed you are by this experience:

(please tick)
Not distressed A bit distressed Quite distressed Very distressed

7. Do you ever feel as if you are being persecuted in some way?
(please tick)
Never Sometimes Often Nearly always

If you ticked never, please go to Question 8.
If you ticked sometimes, often, or nearly always, please indicate how distressed you are by this experience:

(please tick)
Not distressed A bit distressed Quite distressed Very distressed

(*Continued*)

8. Do you ever feel that you experience few or no emotions at important events?
(please tick)
Never Sometimes Often Nearly always

If you ticked never, please go to Question 9.
If you ticked sometimes, often, or nearly always, please indicate how distressed you are by this experience:

(please tick)
Not distressed A bit distressed Quite distressed Very distressed

9. Do you ever feel pessimistic about everything?
(please tick)
Never Sometimes Often Nearly always

If you ticked never, please go to Question 10.
If you ticked sometimes, often, or nearly always, please indicate how distressed you are by this experience:

(please tick)
Not distressed A bit distressed Quite distressed Very distressed

10. Do you ever feel as if there is a conspiracy against you?
(please tick)
Never Sometimes Often Nearly always

If you ticked never, please go to Question 11.
If you ticked sometimes, often, or nearly always, please indicate how distressed you are by this experience:

(please tick)
Not distressed A bit distressed Quite distressed Very distressed

11. Do you ever feel as if you are destined to be someone very important?
(please tick)
Never Sometimes Often Nearly always

If you ticked never, please go to Question 12.
If you ticked sometimes, often, or nearly always, please indicate how distressed you are by this experience:

(please tick)
Not distressed A bit distressed Quite distressed Very distressed

12. Do you ever feel as if there is no future for you?
(please tick)
Never Sometimes Often Nearly always

If you ticked never, please go to Question 13.
If you ticked sometimes, often, or nearly always, please indicate how distressed you are by this experience:

(please tick)
Not distressed A bit distressed Quite distressed Very distressed

13. Do you ever feel that you are a very special or unusual person?
(please tick)
Never Sometimes Often Nearly always

If you ticked never, please go to Question 14.
If you ticked sometimes, often, or nearly always, please indicate how distressed you are by this experience:

(please tick)
Not distressed A bit distressed Quite distressed Very distressed

14. Do you ever feel as if you do not want to live anymore?
(please tick)
Never Sometimes Often Nearly always

If you ticked never, please go to Question 15.
If you ticked sometimes, often, or nearly always, please indicate how distressed you are by this experience:

(please tick)
Not distressed A bit distressed Quite distressed Very distressed

15. Do you ever think that people can communicate telepathically?
(please tick)
Never Sometimes Often Nearly always

If you ticked never, please go to Question 16.
If you ticked sometimes, often, or nearly always, please indicate how distressed you are by this experience:

(please tick)
Not distressed A bit distressed Quite distressed Very distressed

16. Do you ever feel that you have no interest to be with other people?
(please tick)
Never Sometimes Often Nearly always

If you ticked never, please go to Question 17.
If you ticked sometimes, often, or nearly always, please indicate how distressed you are by this experience:

(please tick)
Not distressed A bit distressed Quite distressed Very distressed

17. Do you ever feel as if electrical devices such as computers can influence the way you think?
(please tick)
Never Sometimes Often Nearly always

If you ticked never, please go to Question 18.
If you ticked sometimes, often, or nearly always, please indicate how distressed you are by this experience:

(please tick)
Not distressed A bit distressed Quite distressed Very distressed

(*Continued*)

18. Do you ever feel that you are lacking in motivation to do things?
(please tick)
Never Sometimes Often Nearly always

If you ticked never, please go to Question 19.
If you ticked sometimes, often, or nearly always, please indicate how distressed you are by this experience:

(please tick)
Not distressed A bit distressed Quite distressed Very distressed

19. Do you ever cry about nothing?
(please tick)
Never Sometimes Often Nearly always

If you ticked never, please go to Question 20.
If you ticked sometimes, often, or nearly always, please indicate how distressed you are by this experience:

(please tick)
Not distressed A bit distressed Quite distressed Very distressed

20. Do you believe in the power of witchcraft, voodoo, or the occult?
(please tick)
Never Sometimes Often Nearly always

If you ticked never, please go to Question 21.
If you ticked sometimes, often, or nearly always, please indicate how distressed you are by this experience:

(please tick)
Not distressed A bit distressed Quite distressed Very distressed

21. Do you ever feel that you are lacking in energy?
(please tick)
Never Sometimes Often Nearly always

If you ticked never, please go to Question 22.
If you ticked sometimes, often, or nearly always, please indicate how distressed you are by this experience:

(please tick)
Not distressed A bit distressed Quite distressed Very distressed

22. Do you ever feel that people look at you oddly because of your appearance?
(please tick)
Never Sometimes Often Nearly always

If you ticked never, please go to Question 23.
If you ticked sometimes, often, or nearly always, please indicate how distressed you are by this experience:

(please tick)
Not distressed A bit distressed Quite distressed Very distressed

23. Do you ever feel that your mind is empty?
(please tick)
Never Sometimes Often Nearly always

If you ticked never, please go to Question 24.
If you ticked sometimes, often, or nearly always, please indicate how distressed you are by this experience:

(please tick)
Not distressed A bit distressed Quite distressed Very distressed

24. Do you ever feel as if the thoughts in your head are being taken away from you?
(please tick)
Never Sometimes Often Nearly always

If you ticked never, please go to Question 25.
If you ticked sometimes, often, or nearly always, please indicate how distressed you are by this experience:

(please tick)
Not distressed A bit distressed Quite distressed Very distressed

25. Do you ever feel that you are spending all your days doing nothing?
(please tick)
Never Sometimes Often Nearly always

If you ticked never, please go to Question 26.
If you ticked sometimes, often, or nearly always, please indicate how distressed you are by this experience:

(please tick)
Not distressed A bit distressed Quite distressed Very distressed

26. Do you ever feel as if the thoughts in your head are not your own?
(please tick)
Never Sometimes Often Nearly always

If you ticked never, please go to Question 27.
If you ticked sometimes, often, or nearly always, please indicate how distressed you are by this experience:

(please tick)
Not distressed A bit distressed Quite distressed Very distressed

27. Do you ever feel that your feelings are lacking in intensity?
(please tick)
Never Sometimes Often Nearly always

If you ticked never, please go to Question 28.
If you ticked sometimes, often, or nearly always, please indicate how distressed you are by this experience:

(please tick)
Not distressed A bit distressed Quite distressed Very distressed

(*Continued*)

28. Have your thoughts ever been so vivid that you were worried other people would hear them?
(please tick)
Never Sometimes Often Nearly always

If you ticked never, please go to Question 29.
If you ticked sometimes, often, or nearly always, please indicate how distressed you are by this experience:

(please tick)
Not distressed A bit distressed Quite distressed Very distressed

29. Do you ever feel that you are lacking in spontaneity?
(please tick)
Never Sometimes Often Nearly always

If you ticked never, please go to Question 30.
If you ticked sometimes, often, or nearly always, please indicate how distressed you are by this experience:

(please tick)
Not distressed A bit distressed Quite distressed Very distressed

30. Do you ever hear your own thoughts being echoed back to you?
(please tick)
Never Sometimes Often Nearly always

If you ticked never, please go to Question 31.
If you ticked sometimes, often, or nearly always, please indicate how distressed you are by this experience:

(please tick)
Not distressed A bit distressed Quite distressed Very distressed

31. Do you ever feel as if you are under the control of some force or power other than yourself?
(please tick)
Never Sometimes Often Nearly always

If you ticked never, please go to Question 32.
If you ticked sometimes, often, or nearly always, please indicate how distressed you are by this experience:

(please tick)
Not distressed A bit distressed Quite distressed Very distressed

32. Do you ever feel that your emotions are blunted?
(please tick)
Never Sometimes Often Nearly always

If you ticked never, please go to Question 33.
If you ticked sometimes, often, or nearly always, please indicate how distressed you are by this experience:

(please tick)
Not distressed A bit distressed Quite distressed Very distressed

33. Do you ever hear voices when you are alone?
(please tick)
Never Sometimes Often Nearly always

If you ticked never, please go to Question 34.
If you ticked sometimes, often, or nearly always, please indicate how distressed you are by this experience:

(please tick)
Not distressed A bit distressed Quite distressed Very distressed

34. Do you ever hear voices talking to each other when you are alone?
(please tick)
Never Sometimes Often Nearly always

If you ticked never, please go to Question 35.
If you ticked sometimes, often, or nearly always, please indicate how distressed you are by this experience:

(please tick)
Not distressed A bit distressed Quite distressed Very distressed

35. Do you ever feel that you are neglecting your appearance or personal hygiene?
(please tick)
Never Sometimes Often Nearly always

If you ticked never, please go to Question 36.
If you ticked sometimes, often, or nearly always, please indicate how distressed you are by this experience:

(please tick)
Not distressed A bit distressed Quite distressed Very distressed

36. Do you ever feel that you can never get things done?
(please tick)
Never Sometimes Often Nearly always

If you ticked never, please go to Question 37.
If you ticked sometimes, often, or nearly always, please indicate how distressed you are by this experience:

(please tick)
Not distressed A bit distressed Quite distressed Very distressed

37. Do you ever feel that you have only a few hobbies or interests?
(please tick)
Never Sometimes Often Nearly always

If you ticked never, please go to Question 38.
If you ticked sometimes, often, or nearly always, please indicate how distressed you are by this experience:

(please tick)
Not distressed A bit distressed Quite distressed Very distressed

(*Continued*)

38. Do you ever feel guilty?
(please tick)
Never Sometimes Often Nearly always

If you ticked never, please go to Question 39.
If you ticked sometimes, often, or nearly always, please indicate how distressed you are by this experience:

(please tick)
Not distressed A bit distressed Quite distressed Very distressed

39. Do you ever feel like a failure?
(please tick)
Never Sometimes Often Nearly always

If you ticked never, please go to Question 40.
If you ticked sometimes, often, or nearly always, please indicate how distressed you are by this experience:

(please tick)
Not distressed A bit distressed Quite distressed Very distressed

40. Do you ever feel tense?
(please tick)
Never Sometimes Often Nearly always

If you ticked never, please go to Question 41.
If you ticked sometimes, often, or nearly always, please indicate how distressed you are by this experience:

(please tick)
Not distressed A bit distressed Quite distressed Very distressed

41. Do you ever feel as if a double has taken the place of a family member, friend, or acquaintance?
(please tick)
Never Sometimes Often Nearly always

If you ticked never, please go to Question 42.
If you ticked sometimes, often, or nearly always, please indicate how distressed you are by this experience:

(please tick)
Not distressed A bit distressed Quite distressed Very distressed

42. Do you ever see objects, people, or animals that other people cannot see?
(please tick)
Never Sometimes Often Nearly always

If you ticked sometimes, often, or nearly always, please indicate how distressed you are by this experience:

(please tick)
Not distressed A bit distressed Quite distressed Very distressed

Treatment Guidelines

Essential Concepts

- The use of an antipsychotic is essentially mandated as no other class of pharmacologic agent has been determined to alleviate psychotic symptoms.
- Generally, it is best to use a medication that can safely treat SP over a longer duration, as SP is most often considered a chronic, life-long disorder.
- Treatment begins with education of the patient and, when possible, significant others can be involved.
- Pharmacotherapy is the only treatment option when a patient suffers from psychotic symptoms.
- Certain psychotherapies may lower relapse risk (family therapy) and may improve executive functioning (CBT) to some degree.
- Both first- and second-generation antipsychotics (FGAs/SGAs) carry significant risks (tardive dyskinesia [TD], extrapyramidal syndromes [EPS], metabolic syndrome, cardiac QTc prolongation, agranulocytosis, etc.) and, despite having limited capacity, SP patients must understand and be offered informed consent about their treatment.

TIP: Meta-Guidelines

- Stephen Stahl (2014) published one of the most recent guidelines, and it is considered a "meta-guideline," as it combines material from other national SP guidelines into one document.
- The clinician must take a history and make an accurate diagnosis based upon lifetime history and associated impairments.
- DSM-5 criteria should be utilized.
- Comorbidities should be ruled out.
- Family history of SP may be found.
- Many SP patients may experience their first symptoms in their late teens to early 20s, so a longitudinal history must be taken.
- Treatment begins with education of the patient and, if necessary, significant others can be involved. As schizophrenia patients tend to lose insight and may be poor historians at times given their psychotic symptoms, it is often important to involve family or friends in the process

of education and informed consent, and to help with visit and medication compliance. SP patients often legitimately forget their psychotic episodes, making ongoing treatment difficult.

- Pharmacotherapy should be started after reasonable informed consent.
- Family therapy to lower expressed emotion within the household and certain forms of executive functioning training have been shown to lower psychotic relapse and improve daily functioning.
- The front-line treatment is an SGA. These have been approved since the mid-1990s and have largely replaced the use of the older, first-generation FGAs.
    - SGAs generally have much less risk of EPS (akathisia, parkinsonism, dystonia, and neuroleptic malignant syndrome [NMS]).
    - SGAs have less risk over the long term of developing the permanent movement disorder tardive dyskinesia (TD).
    - Despite these advantages, SGAs may have a greater risk for the development of metabolic syndrome (hyperlipidemia, hypertension, hyperglucosemia, increased abdominal girth/weight gain).
    - Both of these significant side effects must be discussed in the informed consent process and monitored throughout the course of patient care.
    - Typically, a full dose range is needed and the minimal therapeutic dose must be achieved and used to lower psychotic symptoms. Some patients will require higher doses that may be above the FDA approved norm.
- Some SGAs are being termed "third-generation antipsychotics" (TGA) as they are partial agonists (this means they become net antagonists in the synapse), whereas FGAs/SGAs are complete and full antagonists or dopamine-2 (D2) receptor blockers.
- FGAs may be used, but generally are reserved for those patients who have failed to respond to a few SGA trials first.
- Clozapine is an antipsychotic that predates the formal class of SGA, but itself is the most atypical and is relatively devoid of TD/EPS risks. It has great propensity for creating metabolic disorder and may cause agranulocytosis. It is technically an SGA and has clear data suggesting it may be the most effective in class.
- For SP, the SGA is generally used long term to indefinitely, but determining the optimal lowest dose is ideal over time.
- Patients must be monitored for TD, EPS, metabolic disorder, and agranulocytosis routinely.
- Polypharmacy using multiple SGAs is considered to be less clinically sanctioned versus aggressive monotherapy use (sometimes off-label higher doses are required).

TIP: Psychopharmacology

- SGAs may be divided into three distinct families and may be delineated by their common chemical structures: —DONEs, PINEs, RIP/PIPs. See the **Prescribing Table** for further details.
  - DONEs: risperi*done* (Risperdal), paliperi*done* (Invega), ziprasi*done* (Geodon), iloperi*done* (Fanapt), lurasi*done* (Latuda).
  - PINEs: olanza*pine* (Zyprexa), quetia*pine* (Seroquel XR), asena*pine* (Saphris), cloza*pine* (Clozaril).
  - RIP/PIPs (the TGAs): ari*pip*razole (Abilify), brex*pip*razole (Rexulti), ca*rip*razine (Vraylar).
- The DONEs tend to have higher EPS rates and the PINEs tend to have more sedation, hypotension, and metabolic disorder. There are certainly exceptions, as risperidone/paliperidone have higher metabolic rates and asenapine has higher akathisia rates. The PIP/RIPs share a blend of side effects with mild to moderate risks for metabolic syndrome and elevated akathisia rates.
- FGAs may be divided into two distinct families, called high- and low-potency agents. Typically, high-potency FGAs have high affinities for D2 receptor antagonism, require lower dosing, and have higher EPS rates. The low-potency FGAs tend to have greater rates of sedation, hypotension, weight gain, and anticholinergic effects (blurred vision, dry mouth, constipation, urinary retention, memory problems, etc.). Moderate-potency FGAs share both characteristics, albeit at lower levels of each.
  - Low potency: chlorpromazine (Thorazine), thioridazine (Mellaril).
  - Moderate potency: loxapine (Loxitane), perphenazine (Trilafon).
  - High potency: haloperidol (Haldol), fluphenazine (Prolixin), thiothixene (Navane).

TIP: SP Prescribing

- Choose initially any of the SGAs/TGAs outside of clozapine initially for treating psychosis, as they all treat psychosis equally well at therapeutic doses.
- Titrate for effect. Either side effects will mount to an intolerable level or psychosis will dissipate over several days. Must use full FDA approved dosing range!
- A typical course of an aggressive monotherapy should occur over several days for hospitalized patients and several weeks for outpatients.
- Dosing parameters are shown in the Prescribing Table.

- Most often, clinicians will choose a drug based upon side effects to be avoided or where side effects might be used to become therapeutic effects.
  - Some SGAs are more *Parkinsonism and EPS* prone (risperidone, olanzapine) and others are fairly safe in this regard (quetiapine, iloperidone).
  - Some SGAs are more *sedating* than others (olanzapine, quetiapine, asenapine). Notice that SGAs that end in PINE are more sedating.
  - Some SGAs create more *akathisia* in certain patients (risperidone, olanzapine, ziprasidone, aripiprazole, cariprazine, brexpiprazole).
  - Some SGAs create more *weight gain and metabolic issues* (risperidone, olanzapine, quetiapine, clozapine) and some are much safer (ziprasidone, aripiprazole, lurasidone).
  - Some increase cardiac QTc (ziprasidone, iloperidone).
- A variety of formulations exist to improve compliance:
  - Some drugs are used once daily.
  - Other patients like to take smaller doses spread throughout the day to lower peak plasma side effects, like sedation.
  - Certain SGAs have slow release formulas which can be helpful (quetiapine XR).
  - Some SGAs come in long-acting injectables so that oral tablets may not be needed at all (risperidone, paliperidone, aripiprazole).
- Finally, successive, aggressive monotherapies are the guideline-based approach of choice.
  - It may make sense to switch from one SGA family to another if there are therapeutic failures (ex. If a patient has failed taking a DONE, then a trial of a PINE or a RIP/PIP may be warranted.)

SECTION 2 Advanced Prescribing Practices

Introduction

In Section 1, the premise was to convince the reader that they must make an accurate diagnosis and pick an approved agent with well-defined dosing guidelines and expected clinical outcomes. This approach is largely one of pattern recognition: (1) identify the pattern of phenotypic symptoms, (2) choose from a finite list of available, proven effective drugs, (3) start dosing low and escalate through an approved dosing range, (4) assess for effectiveness, and (5) continue medication if effective or cross-titrate to a new drug if ineffective or not tolerated. This methodical, mathematical approach that can improve the standard of care and, ideally, patient outcomes when treated by the novice psychopharmacologist.

Section 2 is designed to provide a greater depth of neuroscience and pharmacodynamic knowledge to the reader and is written for prescribers who are knowledgeable and competent in those skills outlined in Section 1. The section is generally intended for those patients who are felt to be treatment-resistant and comorbid with other disorders.

Epidemiology

- Schizophrenia is believed to affect 1 out of 100 individuals.
- Over the long term, it appears to affect men and women equally, but more recent data suggests men are affected more, at a ratio of 1.4:1.
- Additionally, data suggests that migrant groups and city dwellers have increased rates of schizophrenia.
- Despite being a 1% illness, schizophrenia may account for the largest expense upon governmental healthcare agencies among any of the psychiatric disorders. It is estimated that the annual cost may be $20,000–$30,000 per patient, with the highest expense being that of inpatient hospitalization.

Genetics

- Depending on the methodology, the heritability of schizophrenia may range from 24–55%.
- At the highest end, in more localized populations, heritability may top 80%. This may be comparable to findings associated with bipolar disorder/ADHD, but perhaps less heritable than depressive or anxiety disorders.
- Genetic research in schizophrenia reveals several replicated linkages, including implicating chromosome arms 1q, 5q, 6p, 6q, 8p, 10p, 13q, 15q, and 22q. However, none of these linkage findings has led to cloning of clearly causative genes for schizophrenia.
- Consortium-findings suggest that there may be 128 statistically independent genes associated with the risk of developing schizophrenia, implicating a minimum of 108 better defined mutations from this group. Twenty-five mutations have been identified and replicated in multiple studies. These are believed to be rare but highly penetrant mutations.
    - Key mutations may include those involved in glutamate neurotransmission (i.e., GRM3, GRIN2A, GRIA1, and SLC38A7), neuronal calcium signaling (CACNA1C, CACNB2, CAMKK2, CACNA1I, NRGN, and RIMS1), or dopamine neurotransmission (DRD2).

Neuroanatomy

- Over time, the SP brain may develop tissue atrophy and ventriculomegaly, appearing as if a dementia process has occurred.
- Neurodevelopmentally, patients with SP may not obtain the correct normal asymmetry associated with normal development.
- There are several key functional neuroanatomic findings that suggest where in the brain SP symptoms develop.
- Patients who experience hallucinations may activate subcortical nuclei (thalamic, striatal), limbic structures (especially hippocampus), and paralimbic regions (parahippocampal and cingulate gyri, as well as orbito-frontal cortex).
- Furthermore, negative emotional symptoms of SP seem more related to the functioning of the ventrolateral prefrontal cortex (vmPFC) and ventral striatum. Negative cognitive symptoms may involve hypofunctioning of the dorsolateral prefrontal cortex (DLPFC).
- Positive symptoms, particularly persecutory ideation, tend to be related to hyperfunctioning of the medial prefrontal cortex, amygdala, and hippocampus/parahippocampal region.
- Disorganization/thought disorder symptoms, although less frequently evaluated, appear mostly related to poor functioning of the dorsolateral prefrontal cortex (DLPFC).
- Many SP patients suffer from cognitive decline and executive dysfunction, implicating hypofunctioning of the DLPFC, also known as hypofrontality.
- Similarly, SP patients may show lower activation in ventrolateral areas of the frontal cortex. The VMPFC has also been shown to be relatively underactive when patients are tasked with deciphering emotional states of others. This may account for a certain amount of negative symptom development (social isolation, etc.).
- For deeper cortical structures, amygdala and hippocampus firing rates may also be increased when patients are asked to observe a variety of neutral to more threatening stimuli.
- However, when presented with faces showing anger or fear, amygdala activations become lower and more abnormal.
- The ventral striatum may be less active when SP patients are asked to complete rewarding tasks.
    - This may represent the cause of negative symptom of amotivation or abulia.

Neuroscientific Background and Rationale for Medication Use

In treating schizophrenia, there are two distinct classes of frequently used medications. Antipsychotics are commonly divided into first-generation antipsychotics (FGA), often called typical antipsychotics, which were approved from the 1950s through the 1980s. Second-generation antipsychotics (SGA), which include TGAs, essentially were approved from the 1990s through present day. As mentioned in Section 1, SGAs/TGAs can actually be divided into the DONEs, PINEs, and PIPs/RIPs. Section 2 will discuss each individual SGA as a stand-alone, novel product in a more thorough manner.

1) FGAs

MECHANISM OF ACTION

Chlorpromazine (Thorazine), thioridazine (Mellaril), loxapine (Loxitane), perphenazine (Trilafon), haloperidol (Haldol), fluphenazine (Prolixin), thiothixene (Navane)

- All approved antipsychotics fully block (antagonize) D2 receptors to treat psychosis.
- Chlorpromazine was the first approved FGA.
- The most commonly prescribed FGAs are listed above, in Section 1, and in greater detail in the Prescribing Table.
- Once 60–65% of D2 receptors are blocked, antipsychotic effects may take effect. If 80% is achieved, then EPS may occur.
- All FGAs share this single mechanism of providing efficacy against psychotic symptoms.
- FGAs may be categorized based on potency:
    - Low-potency (affinity) FGAs are a sub-group within this class of FGA medications. These agents are a bit weaker at providing D2 antagonism, so must be used at higher oral doses. They also are more likely to create side effects outside of EPS. For example, many of these agents have a high affinity for histamine-1 (H1) receptor blockade and create excessive sedation and weight gain. Also, many are aggressive at anticholinergic muscarinic (AchM) blockade which creates constipation, blurred vision, dry mouth, etc. Finally, many of these agents antagonize alpha-1 (a-1) noradrenergic receptors, adding a greater risk of dizziness and hypotension.

- High-potency FGAs are the other sub-class, and these are fairly selective for the D2 receptor. They have minimal impact upon the side effects reported above for low-potency agents. Therefore, the high-potency SGAs provide for greater EPS side effects but less sedation, weight gain, hypotension, dry mouth, blurred vision, etc.

Table 8.2 Extrapyramidal Symptoms and Management

Reaction	*Onset*	*Features*	*Treatment*
Acute dystonia	Hours–days	Spasm usually around neck but may affect tongue, eyes, neck, jaw, trunk	Anticholinergics (benztropine, trihexyphenidyl or diphenhydramine)
Parkinsonism	Days–weeks	Rest tremor, shuffling gait, cogwheel rigidity, bradykinesia, postural instability	Anticholinergics (benztropine, trihexyphenidyl or diphenhydramine)
Akathisia	Days–weeks	Psychomotor agitation, pacing, foot tapping, restlessness	Benzodiazepines (alprazolam, clonazepam), Beta blockers (propranolol, atenolol), Anticholinergics (benztropine, trihexyphenidyl or diphenhydramine)
Neuroleptic Malignant Syndrome (NMS)	Days–years	Most often occurs after dose increase, dehydration, or increased environmental temperature. Hyperthermia, autonomic instability, leadpipe rigidity, elevated liver functions, and CPK values	Discontinue the FGA/SGA. Start IV fluids and support vitals. Consider reversal with dantrolene, bromocriptine, amantadine, or apomorphine
Tardive Dyskinesia (TD)	Months–years	Choreic or athetotic movements that are not tic/spasm related often involve lips/tongue and perioral movements, may involve trunk and extremities	Discontinue or reduce dose of antipsychotics. Consider changing antipsychotic to quetiapine or clozapine Consider tetrabenazine, branched chain amino acid therapy, ginko biloba, dextromethorphan off-label antidotes to lower TD or hasten recovery. One-third of cases are permanent. Valbenazine (Ingrezza) was just FDA approved

1) SGAs

MECHANISM OF ACTION

Risperidone (Rispderal), paliperidone (Invega), olanzapine (Zyprexa), quetiapine (Seroquel XR), ziprasidone (Geodon), aripiprazole (Abilify), asenapine (Saphris), iloperidone (Fanapt), lurasidone (Latuda), brexpiprazole (Rexulti), cariprazine (Vraylar)

- SGAs capitalize on the same D2 receptor blockade to lower psychotic symptoms but introduce a second key property, serotonin-2a (5HT-2a) receptor antagonism. These are sometimes called serotonin-dopamine antagonists (SDA).
- Three third-generation antipsychotics (TGAs) exist whose mechanism is D2 receptor partial agonism with a net effect to partially antagonize D2 in areas of high dopamine (DA) activity. Partial agonists act as antagonists in the face of high transmitter concentrations.
- The 5HT-2a antagonism effect allows for the SGA to selectively and preferentially block DA activity in the mesolimbic DA system, but allows more DA to continue uninterrupted in the nigrostriatal system, which remarkably lowers EPS rates when compared to low- and high-potency FGAs.

TIP: Pharmacodynamic Receptor Effects of SGAs

- SGAs/TGAs are very complex drugs that manipulate many receptors, and each appears to have a unique profile in this regard:
  - D2 antagonism—improves psychosis, mania, and causes EPS/TD.
  - D2 partial agonism—improves drive, motivation, reward in areas of low DA for depression and lowers DA activity similar to above in areas of high DA activity. Sometimes referred to as DA stabilization.
  - D3 partial agonism—improves alertness, wakefulness, and is associated with the TGA.
  - 5HT-1a partial agonism—improves anxiety and depression.
  - 5HT-2a antagonism—lowers EPS, and improves depression and deep sleep.
  - 5HT-2c antagonism—improves depression, worsens weight gain.
  - 5-HT3 antagonism—improves depression and GI distress.
  - 5-HT7 antagonism—improves cognition and circadian function.
  - H1 antagonism – improves anxiety/insomnia, worsens fatigue and weight gain.
  - ACHm antagonism—worsens dry mouth, blurred vision, constipation.
  - a1 antagonism—improves nightmares, worsens lightheadedness, hypotension, and fatigue

Table 8.3 Prescribing Table for Schizophrenia

Brand	Generic	Indication (Bold for FDA Approved)	Drug Mechanism	Dosing Tips	Monitoring Tips	Medicolegal Tips
Drugs listed in BOLD are approved agents. Dosing is based upon clinical application. Approved dosing guidelines should be further referenced by the prescriber.						
First-Generation Antipsychotics (FGAs)						
Haldol	**Haloperidol**	• **Psychotic disorders, esp. schizophrenia** • Bipolar mania • Delirium	• Blocks dopamine 2 receptors reducing positive symptoms of psychosis • High potency	• Usual dose is 1–100mg/day • Starting dose usually 5–10mg and increased 5–10mg as tolerated every few days • For 1 month decanoate injection 50–100mg/4wk • For acute injection for combativeness 5–10mg every 1–2 hours • Do not use via IV push	• Common initial side effects include mild sedation, insomnia • Other notable side effects include higher risk of all EPS • Serious side effects include risk of TD, NMS, QTc prolongation, prolactinemia • Monitor for TD and EPS	• Clearly explain life-threatening or serious side effects (e.g., NMS, TD) • Greater risk for TD/EPS

Thorazine	**Chlorpromazine**	• Same as above	• Blocks dopamine 2 receptors reducing positive symptoms of psychosis • Low potency	• Usual dose is 25–250mg 4 times daily • Increase 25–50mg every few days	• Common initial side effects include dizziness, sedation, dry mouth, blurred vision, constipation • Other notable side effects include risk of all EPS, priapism, weight gain, hypotension • Serious side effects include risk of TD, NMS, QTc prolongation, urinary retention • Monitor for TD and EPS and metabolics	• Same as above
Trilafon	**Perphenazine**	• Same as above	• Blocks dopamine 2 receptors reducing positive symptoms of psychosis • Moderate potency • Has mild 5HT-2a blocking properties	• Usual dose is 4–16mg, 2–4 times daily • Increase 4mg every few days • For acute injection for combativeness 5–10mg every 1–2 hours	• Same as above	• Same as above

(*Continued*)

Table 8.3 (Continued)

Brand	Generic	Indication (Bold for FDA Approved)	Drug Mechanism	Dosing Tips	Monitoring Tips	Medicolegal Tips
Prolixin	**Fluphenazine**	• Same as above	• Blocks dopamine 2 receptors reducing positive symptoms of psychosis • High potency	• Usual dose is 5–40mg/day • Increase 5mg every few days • Long-acting injections are 12.5–100mg every 2–3 weeks • For acute injection for combativeness, 5–10mg every 1–2 hours	• Common initial side effects include mild sedation, insomnia • Other notable side effects include higher risk of all EPS • Serious side effects include risk of TD, NMS, QTc prolongation, prolactinemia • Monitor for TD and EPS	• Same as above • Greater risk for TD/EPS
Mellaril	**Thioridazine**	• Same as above	• Blocks dopamine 2 receptors reducing positive symptoms of psychosis • Low potency	• Usual dose is 25–200 mg 4 times daily • Increase 50 mg every few days	• Common initial side effects include dizziness, sedation, dry mouth, blurred vision, constipation • Other notable side effects include risk of all EPS, priapism, weight gain, hypotension • Serious side effects include risk of TD, NMS, QTc prolongation, urinary retention • Monitor for TD and EPS and metabolics	• Clearly explain life-threatening or serious side effects (e.g., NMS, tardive dyskinesia, QTc increase) • This drug increases QTc 90msec

Loxitane	**Loxapine**	• **Same as above**	• Blocks dopamine 2 receptors reducing positive symptoms of psychosis • Moderate potency • Has mild 5HT-2a blocking properties	• Usual dose is 10–125mg twice daily • Increase 25mg every few days	• Same as above	• Clearly explain life-threatening or serious side effects (e.g., NMS, tardive dyskinesia)
Navane	**Thiothixene**	• **Same as above**	• Blocks dopamine 2 receptors reducing positive symptoms of psychosis • High potency	• Usual dose is 2–30mg twice daily • Increase 5mg every few days	• Common initial side effects include mild sedation, insomnia • Other notable side effects include higher risk of all EPS • Serious side effects include risk TD, NMS, QTc prolongation, prolactinemia • Monitor for TD and EPS	• Clearly explain life-threatening or serious side effects (e.g., NMS, tardive dyskinesia) • Greater risk for TD/EPS

(*Continued*)

Table 8.3 (Continued)

Brand	Generic	Indication (Bold for FDA Approved)	Drug Mechanism	Dosing Tips	Monitoring Tips	Medicolegal Tips
Second-Generation Antipsychotics (SGAs): -dones						
Risperdal	**Risperidone**	• **Schizophrenia** • Other psychotic disorders • **Acute mania/mixed mania** • **Bipolar maintenance** • Bipolar depression • Depression augmentation • Behavioral disturbances in dementia • Impulse control disorders	• Blocks dopamine 2 receptors reducing psychosis and stabilizing affective symptoms • Blocks serotonin 2A receptors lowering EPS/TD risks	• Usual dosing is 2–16mg/day • Usual dose for depot injection is 25–50mg every 2 weeks • Start at 1mg/day and increase daily by 1mg/day to therapeutic dose • Slower titration is acceptable and lowers akathisia	• Common initial side effects include dizziness, GI side effects, fatigue • Other notable side effects include risk of diabetes, dyslipidemia, EPS, hyperprolactinemia, and gynecomastia • Serious side effects include risk of metabolic syndrome, TD/EPS, increased risk of death in demented elderly, rare NMS, and seizures • Monitor at baseline, after titration, and then semi-annually to annually for VS, BMI, BMP, Lipids, and for TD/EPS	• Clearly explain life-threatening or serious side effects (e.g., NMS, metabolic side effects, tardive dyskinesia) • Should be discontinued before pregnancies (risk category C) • Weigh and track weight and BMI • This drug is a higher risk for EPS and metabolic disorder

Invega	**Paliperidone**	• **Schizophrenia** • **Schizoaffective disorder** • Acute mania/mixed mania • Bipolar maintenance • Other psychotic disorders • Behavioral disturbances in dementia • Impulse control disorders	• Same as above	• Usual dose is 3– 12mg/day for oral formulation and 39–234mg/month for injections • May increase by 3mg/day every 5 days	• Same as above	• Clearly explain life-threatening or serious side effects (e.g., NMS, metabolic side effects, tardive dyskinesia) • This drug is renally metabolized and safer for hepatic impairment patients
Geodon	**Ziprasidone**	• **Schizophrenia** • **Acute agitation in schizophrenia** • **Acute mania/mixed mania** • **Bipolar maintenance** • Bipolar depression • Depression augmentation • Other psychotic disorders • Behavioral disturbances in dementia • Impulse control disorders	• Same as above • May have SNRI properties	• Usual dose is 20–80mg twice daily • Increase every 2 days by 40mg • For injection for agitation control, 10mg IM every 2 hr with max 40mg/d • Must take with food	• Same as above but carries warning of 20msec QTc prolongation and less prolactinemia	• Same as above • This drug is known for either increased sedation or increased activation/akathisia and initial reaction may be unpredictable • This SGA has one of the safest profiles against the development of metabolic side effects

(*Continued*)

Table 8.3 (Continued)

Brand	Generic	Indication (Bold for FDA Approved)	Drug Mechanism	Dosing Tips	Monitoring Tips	Medicolegal Tips
Fanapt	**Iloperidone**	• **Schizophrenia** • Acute mania/mixed mania • Bipolar maintenance • Other psychotic disorders • Behavioral disturbances in dementia • Impulse control disorders	• Same as above • May have one of the highest alpha-1 receptor antagonism	• Usual dose is 1–12mg twice daily and must be titrated slowly to avoid orthostasis • Start at 2mg in 2 divided doses on day 1 and increase to 4mg on day 2, 8mg on day 3, 12 mg on day 4, 16mg on day 5, 20mg on day 6, and 24mg on day 7, all on divided doses	• Same as above but carries higher risk of hypotension and orthostasis	• Same as above • This drug has one of the lowest rates of EPS
Latuda	**Lurasidone**	• **Schizophrenia** • **Bipolar depression** • Acute mania/mixed mania • Bipolar maintenance • Depression augmentation • Other psychotic disorders • Behavioral disturbances in dementia • Impulse control disorders	• Same as above • May have high level of 5-HT7 antagonism allowing antidepressant and possibly pro-cognitive and pro-circadian symptoms reduction	• Usual dose is 20–160mg/day for schizophrenia • Start at 40–80mg/day once daily • Must take with food or 50% of dose is lost via poor absorption	• Same as above	• Same as above • This SGA has one of the safest profiles against the development of metabolic side effects

Second-Generation Antipsychotics (SGAs): -pines						
Seroquel XR	**Quetiapine**	• **Schizophrenia, acute and maintenance** • **Acute mania** • **Bipolar maintenance** • **Bipolar depression** • **Depression Augmentation** • Generalized anxiety • Other psychotic disorders • Behavioral disturbances in dementia • Impulse control disorders	• Same as above • Has potent NRI antidepressant mechanism	• Dosing is 150-800mg/day in a single dose for XR preparation or twice daily for IR • Schizophrenia: start 300mg/day in the evening, increase by 300mg/day in divided doses, increase by up to 100mg/day as tolerated to therapeutic dose	• Common initial side effects include dizziness, fatigue, somnolence • Other notable side effects include risk of diabetes, dyslipidemia • Serious side effects include risk of metabolic syndrome, TD/EPS, increased risk of death in demented elderly, rare NMS, and seizures • Monitor at baseline, after titration and then semi-annually to annually for VS, BMI, BMP, Lipids, and for TD/EPS	• Clearly explain life-threatening or serious side effects (e.g., NMS, metabolic side effects, tardive dyskinesia) • This drug has likely the lowest risk of EPS/TD • This SGA has a higher risk of metabolic disorder • This SGA carries the warning to observe for cataracts

(*Continued*)

Table 8.3 (Continued)

Brand	Generic	Indication (Bold for FDA Approved)	Drug Mechanism	Dosing Tips	Monitoring Tips	Medicolegal Tips
Zyprexa	**Olanzapine**	• **Schizophrenia, acute and maintenance** • **Acute agitation associated with schizophrenia and bipolar disorder** • **Bipolar disorder, acute and maintenance** • **Bipolar depression (in combination with fluoxetine)** • **Treatment-resistant depression (in combination with fluoxetine)** • Other psychotic disorders • Behavioral disturbances in dementia • Impulse control disorders	• Blocks dopamine 2 receptors reducing psychosis and stabilizing affective symptoms • Blocks serotonin 2A receptors • May have the most anticholinergic potential in the SGA class	• Usual dose is 5–20mg/day • Start at 5–10mg once daily and increase by 5mg/day once a week	• Same as above	• Same as above except EPS/TD risks are moderate to higher and metabolic disorder may be highest in class only behind clozapine
Saphris	**Asenapine**	• **Schizophrenia, acute and maintenance** • **Acute mania/mixed mania** • Other psychotic disorders • Behavioral disturbances in dementia • Impulse control disorders	• Same as above • May antagonize alpha-2 receptors similar to antidepressant mirtazapine	• Usual dose is 5–10mg twice daily • Start at 10mg/day and increase to 20mg/day if needed after several days • Drug must be taken sublingually or it may not be absorbed or be	• Same as above	• Same as above but with less severe risk of metabolic disorder compared to olanzapine • EPS rates are lower except for akathisia

Clozaril	**Clozapine**	• **Treatment-resistant schizophrenia** • **Reduction of suicidal behaviors in schizophrenia** `	• Same as above • May also antagonize D1 and D4 receptors and NMDA glutamate receptors	• Usual dose is 12.5–450mg twice daily • May increase by 25–50mg/day every day until target efficacy; maintenance dose is 300–450mg/day • This drug requires visiting the REMS website and blood monitoring. ANC should be done before treatment, weekly for first 6 months of treatment, every 2 weeks for months 6–12, and every month after 12 months. For details, refer to clozapine REMS	• Same as above but has highest agranulocytosis risk in class • Marked sedation and orthostasis have been noted • Avoid combining with sedatives • Sialorrhea often reported	• Same as above but note agranulocytosis risk • Lowest in class for EPS and TD risk • Highest in class for metabolic disorder induction

(*Continued*)

Table 8.3 (Continued)

Brand	Generic	Indication (Bold for FDA Approved)	Drug Mechanism	Dosing Tips	Monitoring Tips	Medicolegal Tips
Second-Generation Antipsychotics (SGAs): -rips/-pips (Sometimes Referred to as TGAs)						
Abilify	**Aripiprazole**	• **Schizophrenia, acute and maintenance** • **Acute mania/mixed mania** • **Bipolar maintenance** • **Depression augmentation** • **Acute agitation associated with schizophrenia or bipolar disorder** • Other psychotic disorders • Behavioral disturbances in dementia • Impulse control disorders	• Blocks dopamine 2 receptors reducing psychosis via partial agonism and stabilizing affective symptoms • Also agonizes D3 receptors partially • Blocks serotonin 2A receptors without marked EPS	• Usual dose is 5–30mg/day • Start 5–10mg/day. Increase every 2 weeks by same amounts • 15mg/day generally required for psychosis	• Common initial side effects include dizziness, sedation, GI side effects • Other notable side effects include risk of diabetes, dyslipidemia, EPS, TD • Serious side effects include risk of death in demented elderly, rare NMS, and seizures • Monitor at baseline, after titration, and then semi-annually to annually for VS, BMI, BMP, Lipids, and for TD/EPS	• Clearly explain life-threatening or serious side effects (e.g., NMS, metabolic side effects, tardive dyskinesia) • This drug is a substrate of p4502D6 and should be halved when in use with a major 2D6 inhibitor • This SGA has higher akathisia rates • This SGA has low to moderate metabolic risks • This drug has a long half-life, and side effects may accumulate or dissipate more slowly upon cessation

Rexulti	Brexpiprazole	• Depression augmentation • Acute mania/mixed mania • Schizophrenia • Bipolar maintenance • Depression augmentation • Acute agitation associated with schizophrenia or bipolar disorder • Other psychotic disorders	• Same as above	• Usual dose is 0.25–4mg/day • May increase 0.5–1mg every few days to reach 3–4mg/day as effective dose	• Same as above	• Same as above • Akathisia rates may be half that of aripiprazole above
Vraylar	**Cariprazine**	• **Schizophrenia** • **Acute mania/mixed mania** • Bipolar maintenance • Depression augmentation • Bipolar depression • Agitation	• Same as above	• Usual dose is 1.5–6mg/day • May increase to 3mg on day 2 to reach therapeutic level for schizophrenia	• Same as above	• Same as above • Akathisia rates are moderate to higher

(Continued)

Table 8.3 (Continued)

Brand	Generic	Indication (Bold for FDA Approved)	Frequency	Dosing Tips	Administration
Long-Acting Injectable (LAI) Antipsychotics					
Haldol Decanoate	**Haloperidol**	• Schizophrenia	• Every 4 weeks	• Usual dose is 10–20 times the previous daily dose of oral antipsychotic • Demonstrate tolerability with PO haloperidol prior • Initial dose is 10–15 times the previous oral dose for patients maintained on up to 10mg/day of PO haldol (10mg PO is equivalent to 100mg of decanoate) • For doses higher than 10mg/day PO haloperidol, initial dose may be as high as 20 times	• Intramuscular • Time to Tmax is about 1 week which means the patient may require additional oral medication for at least a week • PO dosing is sometimes continued for first few injections • Monitor similar to PO
Prolixin Decanoate	**Fluphenazine**	• Psychotic disorders	• Every 2 weeks	• Usual dose is 12.5– 25mg/mL • Demonstrate tolerability with PO fluphenazine prior • Initial dose is 12.5–25mg. May increase dose by 12.5mg increments up to 100mg (12.5mg is equivalent to 10mg of PO fluphenazine)	• Intramuscular • Onset of antipsychotic action within 48–96 hours • EPS is also most common in the first 48 hours; thus anticholinergic medications may be given for 48 hours and then discontinued if there are no EPS • PO dosing is sometimes continued for first few injections • Monitor similar to PO

Risperdal Consta	**Risperidone**	• **Schizophrenia**	• Every 2 weeks	• Usual dose is 25–50mg injection every 2 weeks • Demonstrate tolerability with PO risperidone • Initial dose is 25mg (equivalent to 2–3mg/day of oral risperidone). May increase dose to 50mg after 2 weeks	• Intramuscular • Onset of antipsychotic action delayed for 2 weeks while microspheres are being absorbed • For antipsychotic coverage during initiation phase, continue oral treatment for 3–4 weeks • PO dosing is sometimes continued for first few injections • Monitor per PO
Invega Sustenna	**Paliperidone**	• **Schizophrenia**	• Every 4 weeks	• Usual dose is 39–234mg injection every month • Demonstrate tolerability with PO risperidone or paliperidone (paliperidone is an active metabolite of risperidone), though not required • Initiation phase: initial 234mg on day 1; 156mg one week later • Maintenance phase: give 117mg every 4 weeks; range 39–234mg/month (3mg oral equivalent to 39–78mg injection; 6 mg oral to 117mg injection; 12mg oral to 234mg injection)	• Intramuscular (deltoid) • No oral supplementation required given rapid onset of antipsychotic action • Monitor per PO • Loading strategy may not require concurrent oral use initially

(*Continued*)

Table 8.3 (Continued)

Brand	Generic	Indication (Bold for FDA Approved)	Frequency	Dosing Tips	Administration
Relprevv	**Olanzapine**	• **Schizophrenia**	• Every 2 weeks	• Usual dose is 210–405mg every 2–4 weeks depending on dose • Demonstrate tolerability with PO olanzapine • If stabilized on 10mg/day of PO olanzapine, then give 210mg LAI every 2 weeks or 405mg LAI every 4 weeks, then 150mg LAI every 2 weeks or 300mg LAI every 4 weeks • If stabilized on 15mg/day then 300mg LAI every 2 weeks for the first 8 weeks, then 210mg LAI every 2 weeks or 405mg LAI every 4 weeks • If stabilized on oral 20mg/day, then 300mg LAI every 2 weeks	• Intramuscular • No oral supplementation required given rapid onset of antipsychotic action • 3-hour post-injection monitoring required due to FDA blackbox warning of PDSS (post-injection delirium/sedation syndrome) • Monitor per PO
Abilify Maintena	**Aripiprazole**	• **Schizophrenia**	• Every 4 weeks	• Usual dose is 300–400mg every 4 weeks • Demonstrate tolerability with PO aripiprazole • Initial and maintenance doses are both 400mg/month; can decrease to 300mg/month if needed	• Intramuscular • Need 14-day oral supplementation overlap • Monitor per PO

Practical Applications

Good Polypharmacy for Reaching Remission in Resistant Patients

DO

- Start low dose to minimize side effects.
- May use a higher dosing strategy/higher dose at initiation strategy for severe psychosis.
- May use lower doses for elderly, frail, medically compromised, or those prone to neuromuscular side effects.
- Escalate dosing within full range for optimal effectiveness.
- Some patients may need doses higher than approved norms. This data exists in the literature to support this practice.
- Aggressive, higher-dosed monotherapies are favored over polypharmacy trials.
- Monitor for weight gain, hypertension, abnormal movements, metabolic lab values (glucose, lipids), agranulocytosis, and perhaps QTc prolongation.
- Consider adding an FGA to a failing SGA to make it better at dampening DA activity. This is called *making an atypical look typical.*
- Consider adding a low-dose SGA to an FGA to make it have less EPS. This is called *making a typical look atypical.* This can also be accomplished by adding a sedating antidepressant (nefazodone, trazodone, mirtazapine) in certain cases due to 5HT2A blockade.
- Augmenting an FGA or SGA with lithium, a benzodiazepine (BZ), or divalproex sometimes may help lower schizophrenia symptoms in more refractory cases.
- Consider switching to a long-acting injectable (LAI) for patients who are non-compliant taking their medications or require frequent admissions.
- Consider clozapine for patients with remarkable suicidality or those who do not respond to the first few SGA trials as the key is to lower psychosis and prevent relapses to improve long-term outcomes.

DON'T

- Add two SGAs together for psychosis.
- Wait several years and several FGA/SGA trials before considering a clozapine trial, as it is the most effective antipsychotic.

Good Polypharmacy for Reaching Remission in Comorbid Patients

Schizophrenia + ADHD

- **Use of NDRI:** bupropion (Wellbutrin XL).
- **Use of NRI:** atomoxetine (Strattera).
- **Use alpha-2 agonists:** guanfacine (Tenex), clonidine (Catapres).
- **Use second-generation antipsychotics (SGA)** with D2/D3 partial agonism (RIPS/PIPS): aripiprazole (Abilify), brexpiprazole (Rexulti), cariprazine (Vraylar).
- **Do not use stimulant medication** (risk increasing psychosis). Consider modafinil/armodafinil (Provigil/Nuvigil) as less risky alternative.

Schizophrenia + Anxiety Disorder

- **Use of SSRI:** fluoxetine (Prozac), sertraline (Zoloft), paroxetine (Paxil), citalopram (Celexa), escitalopram (Lexapro).
- **Use of BZ:** alprazolam (Xanax XR), clonazepam (Klonopin). Some literature suggests that BZs are effective at treating free-floating anxiety, ambivalence, and other forms of schizophrenia-induced anxiety and agitation.
- **Use alpha-2 agonists:** guanfacine (Tenex), clonidine (Catapres).
- **Use of antihistamine (H1 receptor antagonist):** the SGA–PINEs may provide anxiolysis or treatment for insomnia given their greater risk of sedation.

Schizophrenia + Bipolar (Schizoaffective) Disorder

- **Use of second-generation antipsychotic (SGA)** monotherapy should help treat both conditions.
- **If remaining affective symptoms,** may utilize strategies listed in the bipolar chapter (addition of lithium, lamotrigine [Lamictal], divalproex [Depakote], etc.).

Bibliography

American Psychiatric Association. (2013). *Diagnostic and Statistical Manual of Mental Disorders: DSM-5* (5th ed.). Washington, D.C.: American Psychiatric Association.

Buckley, P. F., Miller, B. J., Lehrer, D. S., & Castle, D. J. (2009) "Psychiatric comorbidities and schizophrenia." *Schizophrenia Bulletin* 35(2), 383–402.

Cannon, T. D., Kaprio, J., Lönnqvist, J., Huttunen, M., & Koskenvuo, M. (1998) "The genetic epidemiology of schizophrenia in a Finnish twin cohort: a population-based modeling study." *Archives of General Psychiatry* 55(1), 67–74.

Goghari, V. M., Sponheim, S. R., & MacDonald, A. W. (2010) "The functional neuroanatomy of symptom dimensions in schizophrenia: a qualitative and quantitative review of a persistent question." *Neuroscience & Biobehavioral Reviews* 34(3), 468–486.

McGrath, J. J. (2007) "The surprisingly rich contours of schizophrenia epidemiology." *Archives of General Psychiatry* 64(1), 14–16.

Mossaheb, N., Becker, J., Schaefer, M. R., Klier, C. M., Schloegelhofer, M., Papageorgiou, K., & Amminger, G. P. (2012) "The Community Assessment of Psychic Experience (CAPE) questionnaire as a screening-instrument in the detection of individuals at ultra-high risk for psychosis." *Schizophrenia Research* 141(2), 210–214.

Schwartz, T. L., & Stahl, S. M. (2011) "Treatment strategies for dosing the second generation antipsychotics." *CNS Neuroscience & Therapeutics* 17(2), 110–117.

Stahl, S. M., et al. (2013) "'Meta-guidelines' for the management of patients with schizophrenia." *CNS Spectrums* 18(03), 150–162.

Tansey, K. E., Owen, M. J., & O'Donovan, M. C. (2015) "Schizophrenia genetics: building the foundations of the future." *Schizophrenia Bulletin* 41(1), 15–19.

CHAPTER 9

Substance Related and Addictive Disorders: Nicotine, Alcohol, Opiates, and Food

SECTION 1 Basic Prescribing Practices

Essential Concepts

- Hallmark of addiction is loss of control over the use of substances that ultimately leads to distress or dysfunction (psychological, social, legal, financial, medical, etc.).
- Substance use disorder (SUD) in adults is commonly confounded by other psychiatric disorders, such as anxiety, depression, bipolarity, and personality disorder.
- Currently, there are only approved pharmacological treatments for alcohol use disorder (AUD), nicotine use disorder (NUD), and opioid use disorder (OUD).

Phenomenology, Diagnosis, Clinical Interviewing

For any new practitioner in any field, the goal is to be able to make an accurate diagnosis. All of psychiatric prescribing at this beginning level is based on regulatory findings, approvals, and indications that are psychiatric disorder specific. Psychotropics will only deliver the outcomes promised if the patient at hand actually has been accurately identified as having a substance use disorder. Currently, there are only approved treatments for AUD, OUD, and NUD. In regard to obesity and weight gain as a clinical entity (not an addiction), there are also several approved medications. Obesity is not an addiction, per se, but is covered in this chapter to ensure these pharmacological interventions are included in this book.

As this chapter progresses to discuss intermediate and advanced psychopharmacologic prescribing, the use of off-label approaches and the need to appreciate that certain psychiatric symptoms can cross the barriers of categorical diagnostic and regulatory processes is addressed. Understanding and appreciating this concept is often needed to treat the more treatment-resistant or comorbidly afflicted patient.

Commonly, an addiction develops when patients find the need to spend more time and resources obtaining and using the substance in question. Patients appear to lose control over their use and ultimately get into more psychosocial distress with time. This progression likely mirrors functional brain findings where the addictive drive centers of the brain become hyperactive while the behavior dampening cortical centers become hypoactive and unable to curtail the addictive behavior. Later in this section, there will be a formal discussion about DSM-5 diagnosis and use of rating scales, but, regardless of these constructs, a common definition might include excessive use of a drug or engagement in a behavior where the patient experiences an inability to contain and control the deleterious conduct, specifically resulting in distress or dysfunction (psychological, social, legal, financial, medical, etc.).

Substance use disorder (SUD) in adults is more often than not confounded by other psychiatric disorders, such as anxiety, depression, bipolarity, and personality disorder. Comorbidity with AUD is listed in the table below. Interestingly, personality disorders (antisocial, schizotypal, borderline) seem to predict ongoing and treatment-resistant substance misuse more so than depression, anxiety, etc.

TIP: Addiction and Psychiatric Comorbidity

% of AUD patients suffering from psychiatric comorbidity

- 15.6%: Major depression
- 2.2%: Persistent depressive disorder
- 5.1%: Bipolar disorder
- 5.5%: Social anxiety disorder
- 5.8%: Panic disorder or agoraphobia
- 7.1%: Generalized anxiety disorder
- 10.6%: Specific phobia
- 10.8%: Posttraumatic stress disorder
- 9.6%: Antisocial personality

In this book, each chapter will initially address the pure, non-comorbid condition in advising the novice psychopharmacologist. This chapter assumes the reader is adept and comfortable with descriptive, DSM-5 interviewing and diagnostic assessment. Furthermore, in the absence of DSM-5 mastery, patient-administered rating scales should become more the standard of care. Outside of aiding in diagnosis, routine use of validated scales likely will aid in obtaining outcomes found in regulatory trials used as evidence-based medicine. These trials utilize these scales to drive treatment and can alert and motivate the prescriber to address residual symptoms, much like how abnormal lab values prompt responses from primary care clinicians when monitoring and treating relevant medical conditions (hypertension, hyperglycemia, etc.).

Regarding this chapter that focuses on substance use disorder (SUD), the authors will use alcohol use disorder (AUD) as the hallmark condition for teaching about diagnosis. Nicotine use disorder (NUD) and opioid use disorder (OUD) also are diagnosed with the same DSM-5 construct. Beyond the scope of this chapter is the delineation of substance specific intoxication and withdrawal states. The goal of this chapter is to teach the overall diagnosis of a SUD rather than the nuances of each possible addictive substance or behavior. Finally, abnormal weight gain, or obesity, will also be discussed as prescription weight loss agents are more readily available for prescription by psychopharmacologists.

DSM-5 Diagnosis of Alcohol Use Disorder (AUD)

- People with AUD show a problematic pattern of use leading to clinically significant impairment or distress, manifested by two or more of the following within a 12-month period:
  - Alcohol is often taken in larger amounts or over a longer period than was intended.
  - There is a persistent desire or unsuccessful efforts to cut down or control alcohol use.
  - A great deal of time is spent in activities necessary to obtain alcohol, use alcohol, or recover from its effects.
  - Craving or a strong desire or urge to use alcohol.
  - Recurrent alcohol use resulting in a failure to fulfill major role obligations at work, school, or home.
  - Continued alcohol use despite having persistent or recurrent social or interpersonal problems caused or exacerbated by the effects of alcohol.
  - Important social, occupational, or recreational activities are given up or reduced because of alcohol use.
  - Recurrent alcohol use in situations in which it is physically hazardous.
  - Alcohol use is continued despite knowledge of having a persistent or recurrent physical or psychological problem that is likely to have been caused or exacerbated by alcohol.
  - Tolerance, as defined by either of the following: (a) a need for markedly increased amounts of alcohol to achieve intoxication or desired effect, or (b) a markedly diminished effect with continued use of the same amount of alcohol.
  - Withdrawal, as manifested by either of the following: (a) the characteristic withdrawal syndrome for alcohol, or (b) alcohol is taken to relieve or avoid withdrawal symptoms.
- The presence of two to three symptoms suggests mild AUD and six or more is severe.
- This list of 11 DSM-5 symptoms reflects a merging of the old DSM-IVTR system of delineating substance *abuse* versus substance *dependence*.

The key to diagnosis is confirming that the substance is in fact taken. Patient self-reports may be biased by the use of denial or minimization. If patients fear legal or occupational repercussion, they may be hesitant to self-disclose at all.

Urine or blood screening is readily available for definitive testing for many drugs. However, drugs with short half-lives or synthetically modified drugs are increasingly hard to detect. Use of a sober-support person to gather collateral information to corroborate the extent of the disorder may be the most reliable approach.

The use of the DSM-5 model may seem effortful in regard to memorization and implementation of a rigorous black and white, symptom-based approach to the SUD diagnosis. This may be true, but it does promote a very sensitive and specific validated way to make the diagnosis and apply accurate and efficacious treatments. Following this approach should allow the prescriber and patient to obtain the pharmacological outcomes that are reported in the literature. Use of rating scales will be discussed later and allows the clinician to rely less on the DSM-5 clinical interview and more on patient driven self-report and repeated measures. Ideally, both approaches will be used.

In regard to screening approaches, adult practitioners usually see adult patients presenting with comorbidities such as anxiety or depression. A patient will typically present with a non-SUD complaint, such as sadness or suicidality. After the clinician clearly delineates the presenting problem, the screening for SUD often then occurs in the Psychiatric Review of Systems or Social History component of obtaining a full psychiatric history. Patients may state they "do not drink much," or that they "drink socially." If there is ever a positive admission to any use of caffeine products, nicotine products, alcohol, cannabis, etc., then the clinician must proceed to delineate the pattern of use. It is important to know the last time used, the number of days used in a row, the quantity used, etc. It may be important to trace backwards from the last day used and delineate the pattern of use for each previous day. This may detect a pattern of loss of control, missed social obligations, legal ramification, and clearly reveal if there is tolerance or withdrawal.

If the patient presents in a depressed or anxious state, it may be important to interview for these syndromes in two phases. The clinician may need to ask about these DSM-5 diagnoses presently while the patient is using drugs or alcohol in excess and assess retrospectively if the other psychiatric conditions existed when the patient was relatively sober. In the past, getting the patient sober was a priority prior to treating the other known psychiatric conditions in order to prove in some ways that the depression or anxiety wasn't just alcohol induced. More commonly now, if the condition was present while sober at all, it generally makes clinical sense to treat the addiction and the comorbid psychiatric condition simultaneously.

Screening Questions

TIP: Substance Use Screening Questions

3-Step Screen:

- Do you drink coffee or caffeinated beverages?
- Do you smoke cigarettes or drink alcohol?
- Do you smoke pot, do other drugs?

Screen for Substance History and Loss of Control

- Do you drink or use drugs at all? Ever?
- Have you ever gotten in trouble legally, in relationships, or at work because you lost control over the amount you used?

This approach askes three short questions, starting from innocuous, non-threatening legal drugs of common use and then progresses toward more serious, controlled drug use. This progression tends to make the patient comfortable answering addiction questions as the less invasive questions are asked first.

Rating Scales

Alcohol Use Disorders Identification Test (AUDIT)

- Is a 10-item scale with a wider variety of self-report answers than the DAST.
- A score of 8+ on the AUDIT generally indicates harmful or hazardous drinking. Questions 1–8 are scored as 0, 1, 2, 3, or 4 points. Questions 9 and 10 are scored 0, 2, or 4 only.
- This scale is copyrighted but does not require permission to use and is property of the World Health Organization: https://www.drugabuse.gov/sites/default/files/files/AUDIT.pdf.

Drug Abuse Screening Test (DAST-10)

- Is a 10-item scale that is usually completed by the interviewer asking the patient a series of questions. It takes only a few minutes to take and score.
- Each of the 10 questions is worth one point. A score of 6+ suggests that an intensive clinical investigation should continue as addiction is likely present.
- This scale is copyrighted but does not require permission to use and is property of the World Health Organization: www.drugabuse.gov/sites/default/files/files/DAST-10.pdf.

World Health Organization Tobacco Questions

- These are a subset of questions from the Global Adult Tobacco Survey (GATS) and are free to use in clinical interviewing.
- There is no scoring key but these outcomes can identify the severity of misuse and outcomes over time by tabulating answers.
- These are available at: www.who.int/tobacco/surveillance/en_tfi_tqs.pdf.

Treatment Guidelines

For the novice prescriber who attempts to treat an adult with a SUD, it is essential to know the basics of the available guidelines that exist to help provide a high level of care. Next, a prescriber must know what psychotropics are specifically approved for these patients. The following subsections will be devoted to alcohol cessation, opioid cessation/maintenance, smoking cessation, and obesity management, as this is where regulatory approvals and indications exist.

Nicotine Cessation

- The NICE Guidelines for Stop Smoking Services are succinct and suggest the following pharmacotherapy approaches. It is generally assumed that patients will be evaluated, offered opportunistic advice, and, ideally, given some bona-fide education about behavioral approaches to nicotine cessation.
- Pharmacotherapy may always be considered unless there is a medical or psychiatric contraindication. Clinicians may recommend and prescribe nicotine replacement therapy (NRT), varenicline, or bupropion, as these are all approved.
- Some patients may obtain NRT on their own over the counter (OTC), ordered from state or county run Quit Smoking agencies, or have it prescribed. This is often a frontline approach given a minimum of side effects and ease of access.
- Bupropion SR (Wellbutrin SR) is an antidepressant that was found to aid in smoking cessation. It is generally well tolerated and also an effective choice. It is discussed in further detail in the depression chapter.
- Finally, varenicline (Chantix) may have the greatest effectiveness (especially when combined with NRT for more resistant cases) but has carried a controversial warning that it may induce suicidality or worsen psychiatric conditions in those who use it to quit smoking. Most recent reviews and meta-analyses suggest these events are minimal and may not reach significance versus placebo. A recent study also suggested no exacerbation of bipolar or schizophrenia symptoms.
- It has also been unclear if these drugs increase life span if cessation successfully occurs. Most recent studies have not shown any increase in cardiovascular events, and some safety trials exist for patients who have suffered a cardiac arrest and desire to quit.
- In smoking cessation approaches, it is generally necessary for the patient to set a clear quit date. They are asked to reduce as much cigarette use as possible, and for NRT they start a full dose on their quit date. For oral medications, generally the patient is started on a low dose one week prior to quitting and then a full dose is taken on the quit date when complete cessation of cigarette use is expected.

Alcohol Sobriety Maintenance

- Similar to smoking cessation, patients with AUD should similarly be approached at opportunistic times to suggest quitting. Abstinence, harm reduction, and the use of motivational interviewing approaches may be helpful. Working with any SUD patient to lower daily intake may also be helpful in achieving sobriety.
- Generally, alcohol cessation and sobriety maintenance medications are applied after the patient has become sober from alcohol. This may require inpatient or outpatient formal detoxification prior to starting acamprosate (Campral), naltrexone (ReVia), or disulfiram (Antabuse).
- This chapter does not cover acute alcohol detoxification procedures, and it is assumed that the patient has become safely sober prior to using one of these three medications.
- Guidelines for use of these medication-assisted treatment approaches are available at the U.S. Substance Abuse and Mental Health Services Association (http://store.samhsa.gov/shin/content//SMA15-4907/SMA15-4907.pdf). All have been shown to be effective.
- Most recently, acamprosate (Campral) has been shown to have higher effect sizes overall compared to naltrexone (ReVia), except in those patients with much higher days of heavy drinking noted at treatment onset. These two drugs seem to lower the craving or drive to drink as their mechanism.
- Disulfiram (Antabuse) is different in that it acts as a deterrent. If a patient drinks while taking this medication, they become remarkably ill with profuse nausea and vomiting.
- Generally, the least side effect-prone agent, acamprosate, is used first, then naltrexone, and finally disulfiram.

Opioid Sobriety Maintenance

- SAMHSA also offers treatment guidelines for maintaining sobriety for those patients with OUD (http://store.samhsa.gov/shin/content//SMA12-4214/SMA12-4214.pdf).
- Currently, available options include the use of methadone to replace the misused opioid. Buprenorphine (Buprenex, Subutex, Suboxone) is an alternative. The latter brand name agent also is a combination product where naloxone is combined with buprenorphine.
- The use of these agents is generally governed by state agencies as these controlled medications are routinely issued to those who are highly addicted to opioids. This is a harm reduction model where a less addictive drug is given to patients to lower their risks from using the more harmful, illegal opioid agents.

- Ideally, patients are tapered off of these maintenance medications over time. Given their longer half-lives and the need to see clinicians routinely to obtain limited supplies, addictive use is better controlled and detoxification may proceed over months to years. Some patients may need to stay on the drugs for a substantial part of their lifetime.

Obesity and Weight Gain Management

- Overeating is not truly an addiction either. The author felt that the average psychopharmacologist tends to underutilize weight loss medications in a similar way to underutilizing anti-addiction medications. Hence, given this pattern, anti-obesity medications have landed in this particular chapter.
- The U.S. Endocrine Society has published a comprehensive guideline regarding the pharmacotherapy for treating obesity.
- Similar to the use of psychotropics to help with SUD, it is expected that prescription of weight loss agents generally be accompanied by education and behavioral therapeutic approaches. Further education about diet and exercise counseling is assumed.
- Harm reduction and motivational interviewing approaches have been found to be helpful and to aid pharmacological outcomes. Use of drug treatment can be escalated earlier in the guideline approach if the patient is unable to diet or exercise.
- Many psychiatric patients take medications known to increase weight and, given their symptomatology (amotivation, executive dysfunction, etc.), may not be able to readily comply with lifestyle change suggestions as easy as non-psychiatric patients.
- An intense area of ongoing research is antipsychotic associated weight gain (AAWG), as the newer second-generation antipsychotics (SGA) have a tendency to promote weight gain and metabolic disorder. The anti-obesity medications are poorly studied in this specific population, but in clinical practice are reasonable for the psychopharmacologist to consider.
- If patients have gained weight and have developed comorbidities (diabetes, hypertension, hyperglucosemia, arthritis, etc.), again, use of prescription weight loss agents may be considered earlier per most guidelines and insurance panels.
- Use of medication is considered successful if 5% of baseline weight is lost within 90 days. Medications that fail to help should be stopped. Successive, aggressive monotherapies are warranted to obtain optimal weight loss. Sometimes, polypharmacy is warranted.
- Phentermine (Adipex), phentermine-topiramate combination (Qsymia), lorcaserin (Belviq), orlistat (Xenical), naltrexone-bupropion combination (Contrave) are all currently approved for weight loss.
- Once an accurate DSM-5 diagnosis is established for a SUD (or obesity), the prescriber should choose from one of the FDA approved and

indicated medications outlined above and in tables below. Generally, safer products are chosen as front line, especially in the absence of any clear efficacy superiority.

- Monotherapies that use the full dose range of each drug are recommended. If sobriety is not maintained, or weight gain diminished, a cross titration to a new monotherapy is warranted.

NUD Prescribing

TIP: Nicotine Replacement Therapy (NRT) (Nicotrol)

- NRTs are considered low level, stimulating medications.
- They allow for therapeutic effects within a single dose.
- Transdermal patches, lozenges, chewing gum, and other preparations are available for use.
- The dose started depends upon the number of cigarettes that the patient smokes daily. The package directions should be consulted for each delivery product.
- Generally, longer use and greater amounts of cigarettes will increase the chance of nictotine withdrawal, onset of cravings, and relapse back into NUD. Therefore, higher doses are generally started first and tapered down in a detoxification protocol.
- There are no clear end-organ or permanent side effect risks. At one time, controversy existed where it was suggested that patients who use NRT and begin smoking again were at increased risk of cardiac complications. This, more recently, has not been found to be a clear risk.
- Common side effects include headache, palpitations, nausea, and insomnia. Use of transdermal patches may cause skin irritation.

TIP: Bupropion (Zyban)

- This is an antidepressant (Wellbutrin SR) used for treatment of major depressive and seasonal depressive disorder.
- It is approved for smoking cessation. It likely has a greater side effect burden than NRT.
- There are no clear end-organ or permanent side effect risks outside of the chance of inducing generalized seizures in patients with a history of epilepsy or eating disorder.
- Dry mouth, nausea, anxiety, agitation, insomnia, and diaphoresis may be noted. Subtle blood pressure and heart rate increases may occur.

TIP: Varenicline (Chantix)

- This agent may have the greatest efficacy for treatment in smoking cessation patients. It also may carry a greater overall risk given some of its warnings.
- As noted above, this drug had warnings that it may increase psychosis, and create depression, hostility, or suicidality, but the FDA has now decreased severity of the warnings.
- Nausea, vomiting, headache, and abnormal dreams may be the most common side effects.

AUD Prescribing

TIP: Acamprosate (Campral)

- Acamprosate may have the least amount of side effects and best tolerability in this class. It is often a frontline agent given this fact.
- There are no severe, end-organ side effects.
- Diarrhea, insomnia, and anxiety are the most common side effects.

TIP: Naltrexone (oral ReVia, injected Vivitrol)

- Naltrexone has slightly more side effects but is generally considered equally effective.
- Initially, it was felt to have a greater impact upon those who binge drink instead of having daily drinking patterns.
- There is a warning for liver toxicity. When used with patients who are actively drinking or have known pre-existing liver disease, liver function monitoring is suggested at baseline and at certain follow-up points.
- Nausea, vomiting, insomnia, anxiety, headache, and abdominal pain may be the most common side effects.

TIP: Disulfiram (Antabuse)

- Disulfiram is an effective drug, but it works as an aversive conditioning agent.
- Patients must take it daily, sometimes under observation. If it is not taken, it will not deter drinking.
- It does not mechanistically lower alcohol cravings as the previous drugs may, but is used to keep the patient sober due to the fear of flushing and vomiting when alcohol is taken in the presence of disulfiram.

- Rare cases of liver toxicity, peripheral neuropathy, and optic neuritis have been reported. Baseline and follow-up liver functions are suggested.
- Nausea, vomiting, and diaphoresis occur if combined with alcohol. Otherwise, rash, sedation, headaches, metallic tastes, and acne are reported as being more common.

OUD Medications

TIP: Methadone (Dolophine)

- Methadone is a controlled medication with addictive potential.
- Given its slower absorption and longer half-life it likely is not as addictive as shorter acting opioids of abuse.
- It is taken daily often under observation and may be used for maintenance or in detoxification protocols. It has been the standard of care for opioid addiction for the longest period of time.
- Addiction, respiratory suppression, and QTc prolongation are notable.
- Fatigue, hypotension, dizziness, constipation, nausea, and psychomotor impairment are often reported.

TIP: Buprenorphine (Subutex), buprenorphine-naloxone combination (Suboxone)

- Buprenorphine agents are controlled substances and generally require additional training and licensing for clinicians to administer in an addiction treatment program setting.
- Similar to methadone replacement, one addictive drug is replaced with a safer, better-monitored drug in a clinical setting.
- Reports of elevated liver functions and hepatotoxicity are rare.
- Fatigue, headache, insomnia, rhinitis, and dizziness are often reported.

Obesity Medications

TIP: Orlistat (Xenical)

- This agent has been studied for acute and long-term weight loss.
- It inhibits lipase enzymes causing fatty foods to be poorly absorbed.
- This is not an addictive agent and does not work through appetite suppression.

- Liver toxicity, nephrotoxicity and drug-induced vitamin deficiency have been reported and monitoring is suggested.
- Gastrointestinal distress, diarrhea, and fecal incontinence are common and drug quit-rates are quite high as a result.

TIP: Lorcaserin (Belviq)

- This agent has been studied for acute weight loss. It promotes serotonergic receptor activity, which tends to improve metabolism by lessening fat storage.
- There are no end-organ damage concerns and this is not an addictive agent.
- Headaches, dizziness, nausea, vomiting, and diarrhea are often reported.

TIP: Phentermine (Adipex)

- This agent has been studied for acute weight loss. It has mild stimulant/addictive properties and curbs appetite.
- Addictive potential is possible but mild.
- May cause hypertension.
- Palpitation, arrhythmia, agitation, insomnia, tremors, and headaches are often reported.

TIP: Phentermine-topiramate combination (Qsymia)

- This agent has been studied for acute weight loss.
- It has mild stimulant/addictive properties and curbs appetite by combining two medications. It may also improve carbohydrate metabolism.
- The same risks apply as discussed above for phentermine. The addition of lower-dose topiramate adds warning for inducing metabolic acidosis, acute glaucoma, oligohydrosis, and psychomotor impairment.
- Palpitations, agitation, insomnia, tremors, and headaches are often reported with phentermine. Additionally, patients may report paresthesias, xerostomia, constipation, sedation, or cognitive dulling.

TIP: Naltrexone-bupropion combination (Contrave)

- This agent has been studied for acute weight loss. It combines a known antidepressant with a weight loss side effect profile and an opioid blocking agent to curb appetitive reward.
- Bupropion, when used for depression management, carries warnings for inducing suicidality in young adults. It is contraindicated for patients with known history of seizures or eating disorder. This drug may promote acute opioid withdrawal if the patient is taking other opioids. There are some reports of hepatotoxicity with naltrexone.
- Nausea, vomiting, dizziness, insomnia, agitation, xerostomia, and diarrhea are often reported.

Practical Application

For smoking cessation, patients should be educated about behavioral approaches to cessation as medications are often used in studies in conjunction with support and education protocols. Generally, starting with NRT is warranted, as this may have the lowest side effect burden. If two to three attempts to quit smoking with NRT fail, then it makes sense to escalate to a prescription approach. Considering that bupropion SR and varenicline are generally well tolerated on a day-to-day basis, either could be considered next. Bupropion is a bit more activating and may be less well tolerated by anxious patients or those that suffer from insomnia. It is a good choice for smokers who are overweight or are worried about post-smoking weight gain effects. It may treat those who suffer depression or ADHD as a comorbid condition. Varenicline had a more ominous warning about inducing new psychiatric syndromes but this again is controversial. It is generally associated with worsening sleep by inducing dreams or nightmares. It makes sense to try successive monotherapies of each type of agent. Polypharmacy may be considered by adding two or all three agents together for patients who fail all monotherapies and are at greater risk for smoking-related complications.

For alcohol maintenance or sobriety, acamprosate has minimal side effects and is likely the best tolerated. After a few days of sobriety it can be started at a full dose. With all of these agents, if the patient relapses, the drug can be stopped. A new alcohol quit date can be chosen and the drug restarted. Naltrexone is also a reasonable choice but has a slightly higher side effect burden. Naltrexone comes in a monthly injection, which may help those patients with a history of medication noncompliance. For more resistant cases, polypharmacy may be considered. In regard to disulfiram, the approach is different. This drug does not promote abstinence by decreasing cravings but creates an aversive behavioral paradigm where the patient chooses not to drink to avoid a toxicity reaction of severe nausea and vomiting. This approach requires definitive sobriety and adequate education about substances outside of beer, liquor, and wine that contain alcohol (ex. perfume, mouthwash, etc.). This drug only works if taken, so it may make sense for the drug to be started initially in the office setting under observation or have a sober support person administer it daily. Given the level of informed consent, it makes sense to have a handout for the patient to read, take home, and, ideally, share with a support person as well. It used to be common practice to induce an alcohol reaction in the office setting to prove to the patient the penalty for drinking but this practice has fallen out of favor.

For opioid addiction management, enrollment into a licensed methadone or buprenorphine maintenance program may be warranted. This is the treatment gold standard. A patient is titrated to a dose ideally equivalent to the other opioids that were being misused and they are maintained initially on this equivalent dose. Over time, the patient may be detoxed from the medication. Use of buprenorphine products have rapidly escalated to frontline use. The ability to control withdrawal, avoid intoxication, and detox away from opioids more readily make this approach easier. There also is no requirement for daily observation of dosing.

For weight loss, patients should have routine vital signs and BMI monitored. Ideally an analysis of eating habits will identify a bona-fide eating disorder or not. If bulimia nervosa (BN) or binge eating disorder (BED) are confirmed, than appropriate treatments should be initiated. If the patient engages in stress eating or maladaptive eating behaviors, these can be addressed via education and psychotherapy. If the patient suffers from obesity that is drug-induced (antipsychotic associated weight gain (AAWG)), then education about diet (portion control) and exercise should follow. Assuming these interventions have failed or the patient cannot comply, then a medication intervention is warranted. Generally, a behavioral approach plus medication use will yield the greatest long-term results. Usually these agents are used as successive monotherapies. A reasonable trial is three months per drug. If the patient does not lose a substantial amount of weight, then the trial is considered a failure and the next drug may be considered. Theoretically, some agents curb appetite and caloric intake, others lower fat absorption, and some improve carbohydrate metabolism. Clinicians might attempt to determine if the patient overeats fats, carbohydrates, or both and select the agent that may more directly address the dietary issue.

Another option is to select the drug with the least systemic side effects. In this group, orlistat is not systemically absorbed and could be chosen. However, the quit-rate due to excessive diarrhea is quite high. Patients with addiction or hypertension should not take phentermine products. Patients treated with opioids should not take naltrexone products.

SECTION 2 Advanced Prescribing Practices

Introduction

In Section 1, the premise was to convince the reader that they must make an accurate diagnosis and pick an approved agent with well-defined dosing guidelines and expected clinical outcomes. This approach is largely one of pattern recognition: (1) identify the pattern of phenotypic symptoms, (2) choose from a finite list of available, proven effective drugs, (3) start dosing low and escalate through an approved dosing range, (4) assess for effectiveness, and (5) continue medication if effective, cross-titrate to a new drug if ineffective or not tolerated. This methodical, mathematical approach can improve the standard of care and, ideally, patient outcomes when treated by the novice psychopharmacologist.

Section 2 is designed to provide a greater depth of neuroscience and pharmacodynamic knowledge to the reader. It is written for prescribers who are knowledgeable and competent in those skills outlined in Section 1. It is also written for those clinicians who treat patients who fail to respond to first-level treatments. The section is generally intended for those patients who are felt to be treatment resistant. This means that the adult addicted or overweight patient has failed to respond to the frontline treatments outlined in Section 1.

Epidemiology

- Recently, the DSM-5 converted from the more traditional terms of alcohol abuse and dependence to the term alcohol use disorder (AUD). This also holds true in describing other substances that are used in an addictive manner. The prevalence of AUD likely is a combination of the prevalences of abuse and dependence, and could be as high as 8.46% based on catchment study protocols in the U.S. using DSM-5 definitions. More recent data suggest lifetime AUD rates as high as 29.1% using DSM-5 terminology.
- Opioid use disorder (OUD) prevalence may be as high as 2.2% in those who use prescription opioids for non-medical/addictive purposes. Heroin use may account for an additional 0.2%.
- Cigarette induced nicotine use disorder (NUD) is prevalent and may be as high as 27% in certain populations. NUD may be decreasing in employed populations and increasing in those where unemployment rates are higher. The overall rate in the U.S. is 16%.
- Addiction to eating or food is controversial. This concept is covered in this chapter to make the reader aware of the pharmacological treatments that are available to treat obesity and weight gain rather than that of food addiction. As weight gain is often promulgated via psychotropic prescribing as a side effect, prescribers should be able to monitor for abnormal weight gain and treat it as necessary.
- The prevalence of excessive food or addictive style intake is felt to be from 8–25% with the caveat that some of the patients may in fact suffer from a formal eating disorder like BN or BED.

Genetics

- AUD shows a heritability of 60% based upon twin studies.
- Certain gene mutations have been implicated for contributing risk for developing AUD and also for predicting treatment outcomes. Mutations in certain opioid receptors (OPRM1, OPRD1, and OPRK1) are implicated, but evidence here is equivocal. The opioids and their receptors clearly modulate the limbic system in regard to its drive pathways which are felt to be governed

mostly by dopamine facilitation. Certain opioid receptors may disinhibit DA neuronal firing by impairing GABA inhibitory interneurons. Mutations along glutamatergic pathways suggest that metabotropic glutamate receptor alterations may predispose to drinking excess alcohol or drinking more frequently. These genes may include *GRM1, GRM5, HOMER1, HOMER2, EEF2K, MTOR, EIF4E, EEF2, CAMK2A, ARC, GRIA1,* and *GRIA4.*

- OUD twin studies suggest a heritability of 9.5% and suggest findings of genetic vulnerability in both the inhibitory GABA and stimulatory glutamate neurocircuitry. These mutations generally involve GABA-A (GAD1, GABRB3) or NMDA receptor (GRIN2A) mutation. Finally, mu-opioid receptor genes (OPRM1) have been implicated and may interact with the hypothalamic-pituitary (HPA) axis and the stress response system in human models.
- NUD is associated with mutations in cholinergic nicotinic receptors (*CHRNA5, CHRNA3* and *CHRNB4, CHRNA6* and *CHRNB3) and DRD2/DBH* dopaminergic genes are also implicated. Genetic heritability for development of severe NUD may be as high as 51–75%.
- Abnormal weight gain and obesity may have a heritability from 40–80% depending upon risk genes being studied. The FTO (fat mass and obesity-associated) gene has been implicated. Birthweight itself may be 40% heritable. The melanocortin-4 receptor gene (MC4R) has several mutations that may contribute to abnormal weight gain and was one of the first recognized to cause obesity and dysregulation of blood sugar. MC4R, TMEM18, GNPDA2, BDNF, NEGR1, SH2B1, ETV5, MTCH2, and KCTD15 are also implicated as weight gain risk genes. Interestingly, mutations in the serotonin-2c gene have shown to create risk for excessive weight gain and leptin insensitivity as well. This may have direct implications for antipsychotic associated weight gain (AAWG) side effects and metabolic disorder.

Neuroanatomy

- For addiction in general, animal and human models have shown increased dopamine (DA) neuronal activations at their origin in the brain stem, called the ventral tegmental area (VTA). Secondary activations are noted in the striatum.
- Limbic reward structures appear to be hyperactive in addicted animals and humans. Frontal cortex structures may become hypoactive (dorsolateral prefrontal cortex (DLPFC), orbitofrontal cortex (OFC)), which allows even greater abnormal limbic activity and perpetuation of self-destructive addictive behavior. Patients seem not to be able to calculate the psychosocial consequences of their behavior, nor cease their activity (poor response prevention or delay in gratification).
- Internet, gambling, eating, and pornography addiction findings have not necessarily been replicated in similar models as that for drug

addiction. Sometimes these non-drug habits are not considered to be "addictive in a neuroanatomical sense," but clinically may be observed and treated in a similar manner.

Neuroscientific Background and Rationale for Medication Use

In treating NUD, there are three types of medications that are often utilized:

1) Nicotine Replacement Therapy (NRT)

MECHANISM OF ACTION

Nicoderm, Nicorette, etc.

- Cigarette smoking allows nicotine to be inhaled and enter the blood stream and then the CNS. Here, nicotinic cholinergic receptors are bound and the limbic dopamine pathways are excited and rewarded for this behavior, thus creating an addictive state.
- Endogenous nicotine is a 100% agonist, as is inhaled nicotine. Inhaled nicotine activates normal reward pathways to excess using a full agonist mechanism. Cigarettes are fast-acting and quickly metabolized. Generally, faster onset and offset of a drug's clinical efficacy creates more addictive potential.
- NRT patches, gums, lozenges, etc., provide slower absorption and a longer half-life situation where nicotine still enters the system as a 100% agonist but the process is slowed down. This may be similar to a detox protocol where a slower pharmacokinetic agent replaces an addictive agent to prevent withdrawal symptoms (diazepam for alcohol, methadone for heroin) and helps cessation be more successful. This harm-reduction approach replaces harmful inhaled nicotine with oral or transdermal nicotine.

2) Norepinephrine Reuptake Inhibitors (NDRIs)

MECHANISM OF ACTION

Bupropion SR (Zyban/Wellbutrin XL)

- This class of drug has been discussed in prior chapters for use in treating ADHD off-label or MDD as indicated. This drug is a norepinephrine transporter (NET) inhibitor and likely a dopamine transporter (DAT) inhibitor. This drug blocks the reuptake of norepinephrine (NE) and dopamine (DA) creating excesses of NE and DA in neuronal synapses and thus increases neuronal firing.

- Bupropion products are believed to act predominantly in the cortex, thus avoiding limbic activation and addiction. Theoretically, when patients quit smoking they lose DA tone throughout the CNS, which may trigger addictive cravings, fatigue, cognitive dulling, etc. Some elevations in DA may alleviate addictive cravings, but likely the DAT and NET inhibition is allowing for more CNS activation where the patient can still feel alert and energetic despite the loss of nicotine. Indirectly, they still may get a stimulating effect despite quitting cigarettes. Appetite may be curbed, allowing for less post-cigarette cessation weight gain.
- NDRIs are not NRT and do not prevent nicotine withdrawal symptoms.

3) The Nicotine Receptor Partial Agonists

MECHANISM OF ACTION

Varenicline (Chantix)

- This medication has the most recent approval and may have the best efficacy data. As mentioned before, NRT is a 100% full nicotine agonist. Varenicline is a partial agonist at the alpha-4-beta-2 nicotinic receptor subunit. It will bind to nicotinic receptors even when cigarette-based nicotine is gone and it will partially activate the receptor. This allows for some activity but not to an addictive level.
- This drug will also bind the receptor longer to avoid cravings when short-acting nicotine is absent. Patients may feel some nicotine-like effects, so that being off cigarette nicotine is not as difficult an experience.

In treating NUD, there are other types of medications that may be utilized in an off-label manner as there is an evidence base to support their use. Nortriptyline (Pamelor) is likely the best example. It is a tricyclic antidepressant (TCA) that is largely an NRI and provides for excellent NRI activity. It likely acts similar to the bupropion SR product noted above. As this is a TCA, it has far more side effects and is harder to tolerate. The reader is referred to the depression chapter for further details.

In treating OUD, there are two types of medications that are often utilized:

4) Opioid Agonist or Partial Agonist Substitution and Maintenance

MECHANISM OF ACTION

Methadone (Dolophine), buprenorphine (Subutex), buprenorphine-naloxone combination (Suboxone)

- Using illegal or prescription opioids allows the drug to be ingested, inhaled, or injected entering the blood stream and then the CNS. Here, these agents bind to the mu-opioid receptors.

- Endogenous endorphins are agonists. When activated, they provide relief from stress and pain and may produce a euphoria and activate reward pathways. Opioid misuse activates normal reward pathways to excess using a full mu-agonist mechanism. Many abused opioids have a high affinity for mu receptors and are quickly absorbed and distributed. Generally, faster onset and offset of a drug's clinical efficacy creates more addictive potential.
- Methadone is a full agonist and the latter drugs are partial agonists at mu receptors. They provide slower absorption and longer half-life, so opioids still enter the system as a 100% agonist down to a partial agonist, but the process is slowed down. This may replace missed opioid doses and helps cessation be more successful. OUD patients may stay on these permanently or become slowly detoxed.
- The partial agonists are more difficult to abuse as they cannot produce a full drug high or euphoria. Naloxone is further added to block euphoric effects in some patients.

In treating OUD, there are other types of medications that may be utilized in an off-label manner as there is an evidence base to support their use. Clonidine (Catapres) is an antihypertensive that has utility in treating ADHD by indication, and anxiety and insomnia states in an off-label manner. It is often used to help patients deal with the agitation and distress during opiate detoxification and withdrawal. Alpha-2 agonist activity and inhibition may mimic what is lost to mu-opioid receptors and may provide symptomatic relief. The risks are generally sedation, dizziness, and hypotension. Clonidine is further referenced in the ADHD and anxiety chapters. Clonidine can be used alone or more often in conjunction with an initial but abbreviated (sometimes single day) use of a buprenorphine product in some innovative outpatient settings.

In treating AUD, there are three types of medications that are often utilized:

1) Glutamate Receptor Antagonists

MECHANISM OF ACTION

Acamprosate (Campral)

- This drug likely antagonizes the NMDA, mGluR1, and mGluR5, though these findings are controversial.
- Chronic use of alcohol increases and enhances inhibitory GABAergic tone. The brain attempts to calm this inhibition by promoting an excess of excitatory glutamate (GLU) activity to maintain homeostasis.
- Upon alcohol abrupt cessation, GABA activity plummets while GLU activity remains or even accelerates. This relative GLU excess may cause

insomnia or agitation and may ultimately lead to full alcohol withdrawal. Even a hint of this may cause an AUD patient to start drinking again to avoid these symptoms.

- Acamprosate, by dampening GLU partially, may decrease mild withdrawal symptoms and triggers and urges to drink again, thus possibly helping to gain better sobriety or less severity in heavy drinking.

2) Opioid Mu, Kappa Antagonists

MECHANISM OF ACTION

Naltrexone (ReVia/Vivitrol)

- This drug serves to block endogenous opioid receptors and to dampen euphoria and reward-driving responses to alcohol use.
- Some patients (binge) drink to feel happy or calm or find an intrinsic reward to drinking (social lubrication or disinhibition), where these positive rewards drive future drinking to excess. Naltrexone dampens these endogenous positive rewards, theoretically lowering the behavioral drive to drink more.

3) Acetaldehyde Dehydrogenase Inhibitors

MECHANISM OF ACTION

Disulfiram (Antabuse)

- When alcohol is ingested, it is usually converted to less toxic metabolites by the enzyme acetaldehyde dehydrogenase.
- When this enzyme is inhibited or blocked by disulfiram (or by genetic mutation), AUD patients cannot efficiently detoxify themselves from alcohol, and acetaldehyde accumulates systemically.
- This toxicity causes acute diaphoresis, flushing, nausea, and vomiting episodes that are very unpleasant.
- AUD patients learn via a punishment-reinforcing paradigm that if they drink, they will have an extremely difficult few hours. In this behavioral model, AUD patients start to gain an ability to choose not to drink.

In treating AUD, there are other types of medications that may be utilized in an off-label manner, as there is an evidence base to support their use. Topiramate (Topamax) is likely the best example. It is an anti-epileptic drug (AED) that may lower neuronal firing by blocking sodium influx channels and may also dampen GLU receptors and enhance GABA activity. All of these may lower alcohol withdrawal hyperarousal and decrease the drive to drink while trying to obtain sobriety. Topiramate tends to show a greater beneficial effect in subjects who experience cravings characterized by drinking obsessions and automaticity of drinking.

In treating obesity and weight gain, there are several types of medications that are often utilized:

1) Stimulant/Appetite Suppressants

MECHANISM OF ACTION

Phentermine (Adipex), topiramate/phentermine combination (Qsymia), bupropion/naltrexone combination (Contrave)

- Phentermine and bupropion likely serve to increase noradrenergic tone to dampen and curb appetite and general caloric intake.
- Topiramate may actually be a sugar analogue with similar properties to diabetes medications and liraglutide, where it may improve insulin sensitivity, lower glucagon secretion, and enhance carbohydrate metabolism instead of storage.
- Naltrexone dampens opioid reward pathways and makes eating less enjoyable. This likely lowers the positive reward to excessive or comfort maladaptive eating.

2) Lipase Blockers

MECHANISM OF ACTION

Orlistat (Xenical)

- This drug works within the intestinal lumen.
- It inhibits gastric lipases making it difficult to digest fats that are naturally occurring in meals and likely creates a mild to moderate malabsorption scenario.
- Patients may need to take vitamins D, E, A, and K supplements, as they are fat soluble and may not be absorbed.
- This is similar to a patient going on a low-fat diet where fatty food intake and storage is lowered.

3) Serotonin Receptor Agonists

MECHANISM OF ACTION

Lorcaserin (Belviq)

- This drug stimulates serotonin 5HT-2c receptors.
- Psychotropics with affinity for blocking or antagonizing the 5HT-2c receptor have greater risks for weight gain side effects.
- In human and animal models, 5HT-2c blockade may increase appetite and adipose tissue volume, and may decrease leptin sensitivity.
- This agent provides the exact opposite and possibly a reversal mechanism by agonizing the 5HT-2c receptor.

4) GLP-1 Agonists

MECHANISM OF ACTION

Liraglutide (Saxenda)

- This is a relatively new drug used for weight gain treatment. It stimulates the glucagon-like-peptide-1 receptors in the brain and lowers appetite, caloric craving, and intake.
- This drug improves insulin secretion and lowers glucagon secretion. This may improve carbohydrate management and storage metabolism.

In treating weight gain and obesity, there are other types of medications that may be utilized in an off-label manner, as there is an evidence base to support their use. All the following drugs are either used to treat type 2 diabetes or share mechanisms similar to those noted above for topiramate. Topiramate has been used alone to promote weight loss clinically and was first investigated for AAWG. Zonisamide (Zonegran) is a very similar AED mechanistically but has a minimum of supportive data. Metformin (Glucophage) likely has the greatest evidence base to either prophylactically avoid AAWG, halt it, or reverse it. This may have become a standard of care when using metabolically unfriendly second-generation antipsychotics (SGA). Exenatide (Byetta) is an injectable diabetes medication well known to cosmetically lower weight, and acts similarly to that of liraglutide noted above.

Table 9.1 Prescribing Table for Substance Misuse and Weight Management

Drugs listed in BOLD are approved agents. Dosing is based upon clinical application. Approved dosing guidelines should be further referenced by the prescriber.

Brand	Generic	Indication (Bold for FDA Approved)	Drug Mechanism	Dosing Tips	Monitoring Tips	Medicolegal Tips
Nicotine Use Disorder (NUD) Medications						
Nicotrol (inhaler) Nicorette (gum/ lozenge) Nicoderm (patch)	**Nicotine Replacement Therapy**	• **Cigarette cessation**	• 100% full nicotine agonist reducing withdrawal symptoms and cravings	• >10 cigarettes a day: 21mg/day patch for 6 weeks, 14mg/day patch for 2 weeks, and 7mg/day patch for 2 weeks • <10 cigarettes a day: 14mg/day patch for 6 weeks, then 7mg/day patch for 2 weeks • Gum, lozenges, etc. per packaging directions	• Common side effects: nausea, headache, sleep disturbance	• Instruct not to smoke while using
Zyban	**Bupropion SR**	• Same as above	• Norepinephrine and dopamine reuptake inhibitor which allows for CNS activation in the absence of nicotine	• Start at 150mg once daily 7 days prior to cigarette quit-date • Increase to 150mg twice daily on quit-date • Use for 2–3 months after cessation is successful	• Common side effects include dry mouth, constipation, nausea, anorexia, sweating, insomnia, tremor, headache • Serious side effects include seizures, induction of mania, and suicidality	• Do not use in patients with eating disorders or history of seizures

Chantix	**Varenicline**	• **Same as above**	• Partial agonist at alpha 4 beta 2 nicotinic receptor, activating these receptors but not the extent of nicotine full agonism	• Start titration 7 days prior to quit-date as follows: 0.5mg/day x3 days, then increase to 0.5mg twice daily x4 days • On quit date increase to 1mg twice daily • Treat for 3 months after cessation is successful	• Common side effects include nausea, vomiting, insomnia, headache, abnormal dreams • Serious side effects include rare induction of depression and suicidality or other mental state changes	• Clearly explain life-threatening or serious side effects (e.g., activation of suicidal ideation)
Pamelor	Nortriptyline	• Same as above	• Norepinephrine reuptake inhibitor which allows for CNS activation in the absence of nicotine	• No standard dosing for smoking cessation exists • For dosing related to depression, refer to the Depression Chapter	• Common side effects include sedation, weight gain, anticholinergic side effects, alpha adrenergic side effects (dizziness, orthostasis) • Serious side effects include QTc prolongation, activation of mania, and suicidality	• Use in limited doses in those with suicidal symptoms • Use with caution in cardiac patients • Obtain EKG prior to and periodically during use • Obtain blood levels prior to and during use

(*Continued*)

Table 9.1 (Continued)

Brand	Generic	Indication (Bold for FDA Approved)	Drug Mechanism	Dosing Tips	Monitoring Tips	Medicolegal Tips
Alcohol Use Disorder (AUD) Medications						
Campral	**Acamprosate**	• **Alcohol dependence and maintenance of alcohol abstinence**	• Dampens excitatory glutamate transmission and enhances inhibitory GABA neurotransmission	• Usual dose is 666mg 3 times a day without titration • Started as soon as possible after achieving sobriety (ex. when safely sober and not in withdrawal)	• Common side effects include GI side effects, insomnia, weakness, fatigue, dry mouth, emergence of depression/anxiety	• None
ReVia Vivitrol Injection	**Naltrexone**	• **Same as above**	• Blocks mu-opioid receptors preventing exogenous opioids from binding there and thereby preventing euphoria (positive reward) from alcohol opioid consumption	• Oral: usual dose is 50mg/day • Start 25mg/day on day 1 and increase to 50mg/day on day 2 • Injection: usual dose is 380mg every 4 weeks • Patients should be opioid free for 7–10 days prior to initiating treatment	• Common side effects include GI side effects, dizziness, dysphoria, anxiety, injection site reactions • Serious side effects include rare eosinophilic pneumonia, hepatotoxicity, severe injection site reaction, severe opioid withdrawal if patient taking legal or illegal opioids • Monitoring should consider LFT and urine drug screen	• Clearly explain life-threatening or serious side effects (e.g., fatality with overdose when attempting to override naltrexone with large amount of opioids, hepatotoxicity)

Antabuse	**Disulfiram**	• **Same as above**	• Irreversibly inhibits aldehyde dehydrogenase causing acetaldehyde build up/toxicity and aversive side effects	• Usual dose is 250–500mg/day for 1 year duration • Patient should not take disulfiram until at least 12 hours after drinking • Start 250–500mg/day	• Common side effects include metallic taste, rash, sedation, headache, acne • Common side effects when alcohol consumed: flushing, headache, tachycardia, nausea, vomiting • Serious side effects include hepatotoxicity, neuropathy • Monitor LFTs	• Clearly explain life-threatening or serious side effects (e.g., hepatotoxicity, alcohol toxicity when alcohol is consumed)
Topamax	Topiramate	• Off-label for alcohol use disorder (AUD)	• Blocks voltage sensitive sodium channels and dampens excessive neuronal firing • May dampen glutamate receptor activity	• No standard dosing for alcohol use disorder exists • Usual dose is 25–200mg twice daily • Start at 25mg/day and may increase to 25mg twice daily after 1 week • Increase by 25–50mg/day every 7 days through accepted dosing range	• Common initial side effects include sedation, dizziness, GI side effects, weight loss, psychomotor impairment • Serious side effects include metabolic acidosis, kidney stone formation, secondary angle closure glaucoma, activation of suicidality and excessive weight loss, oligohydrosis • Monitor blood at baseline and annually with a BMP. Check weight routinely	• Clearly explain life-threatening or serious side effects (e.g., metabolic acidosis, weight loss, oligohydrosis, glaucoma)

(Continued)

Table 9.1 (Continued)

Brand	Generic	Indication (Bold for FDA Approved)	Drug Mechanism	Dosing Tips	Monitoring Tips	Medicolegal Tips
Opiate Use Disorder (AUD) Medications						
Dolophine	**Methadone**	• **Maintenance treatment of opioid dependence**	• Agonizes mu-opioid with slow absorption and long half-life pharmacokinetics and provides less addicting opioid for maintenance against illegal opioid use	• Abstinence maintenance: 15–30mg/day for first day of treatment. Add 5–10mg every 2–4 hrs to a max of 40mg/day • Increase or decrease dose to avoid withdrawal or over sedation	• Common side effects include headache, sedation, lightheadedness, diaphoresis, constipation, nausea • Serious side effects include respiratory suppression, and hepatotoxicity, QTc prolongation • Monitor possibly with EKG, urine drug screens, and LFT	• Clearly explain life-threatening or serious side effects (e.g., fatality with overdose, dependence potential) • Do not use with alcohol or MAO inhibitors

Subutex	**Buprenorphine**	• **Same as above**	• Partially agonizes mu-opioid receptor preventing withdrawal from illegally taken opioids and theoretically lowers the risk of euphoria like effects	• Patient must be off illegal opioids and in withdrawal • Usual dose is 8–32 mg/day • Patients must be in mild withdrawal state prior to starting • Initiation (7 days): on day 1 give 2–8mg SL, then 8–16mg/day • On days 3–7 may increase in increments of 4mg. Maximum dose is 32mg • Observe patient for at least 2 hrs with initial dose and schedule 1–2 visits in the first week • Titrate to lowest dose that rids of withdrawal symptoms and illicit opioid dependence • During stabilization (up to 2 months) patients should be seen once a month • Maintenance dose is generally 8–24mg	• Common side effects include headache, constipation, nausea, orthostatic hypotension, bradycardia • Serious side effects include resppiratory suppression	• Clearly explain life-threatening or serious side effects (e.g., fatality with overdose, dependence potential)

(*Continued*)

Table 9.1 (Continued)

Suboxone	**Buprenorphine-naloxone combination**	• **Same as above**	• Same as above for buprenorphine • Addition of naloxone prevents euphoria that may be caused by intravenous abuse of buprenorphine as it has poor sublingual bioavailability but excellent parenteral bioavailability	• Patient must be off illegal opioids and in withdrawal • Start 2mg/0.5mg to 4mg/1mg SL on day 1 • May increase by 2mg/0.5mg–4mg/mg every 2 hrs up to 8mg/2mg on day 1. Titrate until resolution of withdrawal symptoms • May give up to 16mg/4mg SL on day 2	• Same as above	• Same as above
Catapres	Clonidine	• ADHD • Hypertension • Substance withdrawal, including opioid	• Stimulates alpha 2 adrenergic receptors reducing sympathetic outflow from CNS, lowering withdrawal symptoms	• Usual dose is 0.1mg 3 times daily. Usually titrated from twice daily dose to a thrice daily regimen • Maximum for hypertension is 2.4mg/day	• Common side effects include dry mouth, dizziness, sedation • Serious side effects include sinus bradycardia, AV block, and rare withdrawal hypertensive crisis • Monitor vital signs	• Abrupt discontinuation may lead to rare hypertensive crisis, encephalopathy, stroke, and death • Taper over 2–4 days or longer to avoid rebound in blood pressure

Brand	Generic	Indication (Bold for FDA Approved)	Drug Mechanism	Dosing Tips	Monitoring Tips	Medicolegal Tips
Obesity Medications						
Xenical	**Orlistat**	• **Weight loss and weight management**	• Reversible inhibitor of GI lipase that blocks absorption of fats	• Take 60–120mg 3 times daily with meals containing fat • Take with multivitamin	• Common side effects include fatty stool, marked flatulence, diarrhea, fecal incontinence • Serious side effects include rare hepatotoxicity • Monitoring of LFTs is suggested	• Clearly explain life-threatening or serious side effects
Belviq	**Lorcaserin**	• **Chronic weight management in adults with initial BMI of at least 30 (obese) or at least 27 (overweight) in the presence of at least 1 weight-related comorbidity**	• Selective serotonin 2C receptor agonist causing activation of anorexigenic neurons in the hypothalamus	• Usual dose is 10mg twice a day without titration	• Common side effects include GI side effects, fatigue, headache • Serious side effects may include serotonin syndrome or change in emotional states	• Clearly explain life-threatening or serious side effects

(*Continued*)

Table 9.1 (Continued)

Adipex	**Phentermine**	• **Same as above**	• Dopamine and norepinephrine reuptake inhibitor which activates POMC neurons involved in appetite-suppressing effects	• Usual dose is 15mg–30mg/day • Start 15mg and increase over several weeks to 30mg or 37.5mg	• Common side effects include anxiety, insomnia, weight loss, nausea, palpitations, dry mouth, or diaphoresis • Serious side effects include psychosis, seizures, hypertension, rare activation of (hypo)mania and suicidal ideation, and cardiovascular adverse events, including sudden death	• Stimulants carry classic warning of drug dependency and in younger adults activation of suicidal ideation • Avoid stimulants in those with cardiac structural abnormalities
Qsymia	**Phentermine-topiramate combination**	• **Same as above**	• Dopamine and norepinephrine reuptake inhibitor which activates POMC neurons involved in appetite-suppressing effects • Topiramate may increase insulin sensitivity and improve carbohydrate metabolism	• Dosing is 3.75/23mg/day–15/92mg/day • Dose range is 7.5mg/45mg/day to 15mg/92mg/day • After starting low dose, may increase to 7.5mg/46mg/day after 14 days • If at least 3% weight loss not achieved after 12 weeks, increase to 11.25mg/69mg per day Increase to 15mg/92mg per day after 14 days • Discontinue if at least 5% weight loss is not achieved after 12 weeks on 15mg/92mg per day	• Same as above for phentermine • For topiramate, common initial side effects include sedation, dizziness, GI side effects, weight loss, psychomotor impairment • Serious side effects include metabolic acidosis, kidney stone formation, secondary angle closure glaucoma, activation of suicidality, excessive weight loss, oligohydrosis • Monitor blood at baseline and annually with a BMP. Check weight routinely	• Clearly explain life-threatening or serious side effects (e.g., metabolic acidosis, weight loss, oligohydrosis, glaucoma)

Contrave	**Naltrexone-Bupropion combination**	• **Same as above**	• Naltrexone may dampen endogenous opioid rewards and lower drive to eat, and bupropion may curb appetite via NRI activity	• Dosing is 8mg/90mg–16mg/90mg/day • Start 8mg/90mg in the morning for 1 week, increase to 8mg/90mg twice daily for week 2, increase to 16mg/90mg in the morning and 8mg/90mg at night for week 3, and increase to 16mg/90mg twice daily from week 4 onward	• Common side effects include GI side effects, dizziness, insomnia, dry mouth, diarrhea, anxiety, tremors • Serious side effects include rare seizures, hypertension, hepatotoxicity, induction of suicidal thoughts • Consider monitoring LFT	• Clearly explain life-threatening or serious side effects • Avoid in patients with seizures or chronic opioid use
Topamax	Topiramate	• Chronic weight management	• Blocks voltage sensitive sodium channels and dampens excessive neuronal firing, and may improve insulin sensitivity and carbohydrate metabolism	• No standard dosing for weight management exists • Usual dose is 25–200mg twice daily • Start at 25mg/day and may increase to 25mg twice daily after 1 week • Increase by 25–50mg/day every 7 days through accepted dosing range	• Common initial side effects include sedation, dizziness, GI side effects, weight loss, psychomotor retardation, cognitive dulling • Serious side effects include metabolic acidosis, kidney stone formation, secondary angle closure glaucoma, activation of suicidality, excessive weight loss, oligohydrosis • Monitor blood at baseline and annually with basic metabolic panel for renal function and acidosis. Check weights routinely	• Clearly explain life-threatening or serious side effects (e.g., metabolic acidosis, weight loss, oligohydrosis, glaucoma)

(*Continued*)

Table 9.1 (Continued)

Zonegran	Zonisamide	• Weight management	• Blocks voltage sensitive sodium channels, T-type calcium channels, and dampens excessive neuronal firing. May improve insulin sensitivity and carbohydrate metabolism	• No standard dosing exists for weight management. • Usual dose is 100–400mg/day • Start at 100mg/day and increase by 100mg every 2 weeks as needed	• Common initial side effects include sedation, depression, GI side effects, headache, weight loss, psychomotor retardation, cognitive dulling • Serious side effects include rare Stevens-Johnson syndrome, oligohydrosis, blood dyscrasias, liver failure, sudden death, induction of suicidal ideation	• Clearly explain life-threatening or serious side effects (e.g., Stevens-Johnson syndrome)
Glucophage	Metformin	• **Type 2 diabetes** • Weight management	• Decreases hepatic glucose production • Decreases intestinal absorption of glucose • Improves peripheral insulin sensitivity • Does not produce hypoglycemia or hyperinsulinemia	• Dosing is 500–1000mg twice daily • May increase after 2 weeks	• Common initial side effects include GI distress (diarrhea, nausea, flatulence), headache • Serious side effects include rare bicarbonate wasting acidosis (in those with renal, liver, or heart failure) • Monitor with baseline and annual BMP	• Clearly explain life-threatening or serious side effects (e.g., lactic acidosis in those with end-organ diseases)

Byetta	Exenatide	• **Type 2 diabetes** • Weight management	• Glucagon-like peptide-1 (GLP-1) receptor agonist that leads to increased insulin synthesis and secretion in a dose-dependent manner with glucose	• Start 5μg per dose administered twice daily for a month. Increase to 10μg per dose twice daily as needed • Administer as a subcutaneous injection in the thigh, abdomen, or upper arm within the 60-minute period before the morning and evening meals	• Common initial side effects include GI distress, injection site reactions • Serious side effects include risk of hypoglycemia (when used with sulfonylurea), bleeding (with concomitant use with warfarin), rare renal failure, pancreatitis	• Clearly explain life-threatening or serious side effects (e.g., serious hypoglycemia, rare pancreatitis)
Saxenda	**Liraglutide**	• **Type 2 diabetes**	• GLP-1 receptor agonist similar to exenatide	• 3mg SC injection/day • May increase by 0.6mg every 7 days	• Common initial side effects include GI distress, headache, fatigue, dizziness, injection site reactions • Serious side effects include risk of rare thyroid cancers, hypoglycemia, pancreatitis • Monitoring of thyroid necessity is unclear	• Clearly explain life-threatening or serious side effects (e.g., serious hypoglycemia, rare pancreatitis, and thyroid cancer)

Good Polypharmacy for Reaching Remission in Resistant Patients

DO

For smoking cessation:

- **Start low dose prior to quit date for all but NRT.**
- **Escalate dosing within full range for optimal effectiveness on quit date.**
- **Combine any of the three classes of agents for effective polypharmacy.**

For alcohol sobriety maintenance:

- **Start low dose and escalate through full dose range.**
- **Combine acamprosate and naltrexone as needed.**

For opioid maintenance:

- **Titrate methadone or buprenorphine for effect to halt withdrawal symptoms.**
- **Most states require extra training and licensing to issue these medications.**
- **Combine clonidine for additional hyperarousal-based (anxiety, insomnia, etc.) withdrawal symptoms.**

For obesity management

- Start low dose and escalate through full dose range.
- Combine agents with different mechanisms into polypharmacy if needed.

Good Polypharmacy for Reaching Remission in Comorbid Patients

NUD + Major Depressive Disorder or ADHD

- **Use of NDRI:** bupropion SR (Zyban) monotherapy.
- **Use of TCA:** nortriptyline (Pamelor) monotherapy.

AUD and OUD

- **Use of naltrexone (ReVia/Vivitrol)** products may help both conditions.

Obesity + Major Depressive Disorder

- **Use of NDRI:** bupropion (Wellbutrin XL) monotherapy.

Obesity + ADHD

- **Use of NDRI:** bupropion XL (Wellbutrin XL) monotherapy.
- **Use of stimulants:** d/l mixed amphetamine (Adderall XR), methylphenidate ER (Concerta).

Bibliography

American Psychiatric Association. (2013) *Diagnostic and Statistical Manual of Mental Disorders: DSM-5* (5th ed.). Washington, D.C.: American Psychiatric Association.

Apovian, C. M., et al. (2015) "Pharmacological management of obesity: an endocrine society clinical practice guideline." *The Journal of Clinical Endocrinology & Metabolism* 100(2), 342–362.

Bauer, I. E., Soares, J. C., & Nielsen, D. A. (2015) "The role of opioidergic genes in the treatment outcome of drug addiction pharmacotherapy: a systematic review." *The American Journal on Addictions* 24(1), 15–23.

Center for Substance Abuse Treatment. (2005) *Medication-Assisted Treatment for Opioid Addiction in Pioid Treatment Programs.* Rockville, MD: Substance Abuse and Mental Health Services Administration. http://store.samhsa.gov/shin/content//SMA12-4214/SMA12-4214.pdf, Accessed 4/12/16.

Conway, K. P., Swendsen, J., Husky, M. M., He, J. P., & Merikangas, K. R. (2016) "Association of Lifetime Mental Disorders and Subsequent Alcohol and Illicit Drug Use: results from the National Comorbidity Survey–Adolescent Supplement." *Journal of the American Academy of Child & Adolescent Psychiatry* 55(4), 280–288.

Evins, A. E., et al. (2014) "Maintenance treatment with varenicline for smoking cessation in patients with schizophrenia and bipolar disorder: a randomized clinical trial." *JAMA* 311(2), 145–154.

Ewing, J.A. (1984) "Detecting alcoholism: The CAGE Questionnaire." *JAMA* 252, 1905–1907 1984.

Fenton, M. C., et al. (2012) "Psychiatric comorbidity and the persistence of drug use disorders in the United States." *Addiction* 107(3), 599–609.

Global Adult Tobacco Survey Collaborative Group. (2011) *Tobacco Questions for Surveys: A Subset of Key Questions from the Global Adult Tobacco Survey (GATS),* (2nd ed.). Atlanta, GA: Centers for Disease Control and Prevention. www.who.int/tobacco/surveillance/en_tfi_tqs.pdf, Accessed 9/13/16.

Grant, B. F., Dawson, D. A., Stinson, F. S., Chou, S. P., Dufour, M. C., & Pickering, R. P. (2004) "The 12-month prevalence and trends in DSM-IV alcohol abuse and dependence: United States, 1991–1992 and 2001–2002." *Drug and Alcohol Dependence* 74(3), 223–234.

Grant, B. F., et al. (2015) "Epidemiology of DSM-5 alcohol use disorder: results from the National Epidemiologic Survey on Alcohol and Related Conditions III." *JAMA Psychiatry* 72(8), 757–766.

Guglielmo, R., Martinotti, G., Quatrale, M., Ioime, L., Kadilli, I., Nicola, M., & Janiri, L. (2015) "Topiramate in alcohol use disorders: review and update." *CNS Drugs* 29(5), 383–395.

Hartz, S. M., et al. (2014) "Comorbidity of severe psychotic disorders with measures of substance use. *JAMA Psychiatry* 71(3), 248–254.

Haworth, C., Carnell, S., Meaburn, E. L., Davis, O. S., Plomin, R., & Wardle, J. (2008) "Increasing heritability of BMI and stronger associations with the FTO gene over childhood." *Obesity* 16(12), 2663–2668.

"Instrument: Drug Abuse Screening Test (DAST-10)," NIDA CTN Common Data Elements website. https://cde.drugabuse.gov/instrument/e9053390-ee9c-9140-e040-bb89ad433d69, Accessed 9/13/16.

Jamal, A., et al. (2015) "Current cigarette smoking among adults—United States, 2005–2014." *Morbidity and Mortality Weekly Report* 64(44), 1233–1240.

Johnson, B., & Faraone, S. V. (2013) "Outpatient detoxification completion and one-month outcomes for opioid dependence: a preliminary study of a neuropsychoanalytic treatment in pain patients and addicted patients." *Neuropsychoanalysis* 15(2), 145–160.

Kerridge, B. T., et al. (2015) "Gender and nonmedical prescription opioid use and DSM-5 nonmedical prescription opioid use disorder: results from the National Epidemiologic Survey on Alcohol and Related Conditions–III." *Drug and Alcohol Dependence* 156, 47–56.

Lancaster, T., & Cahill, K. (2015) "Review: varenicline does not differ from placebo for adverse neuropsychiatric events." *Annals of Internal Medicine 163*(2), JC6–JC6.

Love, T., Laier, C., Brand, M., Hatch, L., & Hajela, R. (2015) "Neuroscience of Internet pornography addiction: a review and update." *Behavioral Sciences* 5(3), 388–433.

Mbarek, H., et al. (2015) "The genetics of alcohol dependence: twin and SNP-based heritability, and genome-wide association study based on AUDIT scores." *American Journal of Medical Genetics Part B: Neuropsychiatric Genetics* 168(8), 739–748.

Meule, A. (2011) "How prevalent is 'food addiction.'" *Front Psychiatry* 2(61), 1–4.

Meyers, J. L., et al. (2015) "Frequency of alcohol consumption in humans: the role of metabotropic glutamate receptors and downstream signaling pathways." *Translational Psychiatry* 5(6), e586.

Mistry, C. J., Bawor, M., Desai, D., Marsh, D. C., & Samaan, Z. (2014) "Genetics of opioid dependence: a review of the genetic contribution to opioid dependence." *Current Psychiatry Reviews* 10(2), 156.

Mizuno, Y., Suzuki, T., Nakagawa, A., Yoshida, K., Mimura, M., Fleischhacker, W. W., & Uchida, H. (2014) "Pharmacological strategies to counteract antipsychotic-induced weight gain and metabolic adverse effects in schizophrenia: a systematic review and meta-analysis." *Schizophrenia Bulletin*, sbu030.

Nice Pathway. (2008) "Stop Smoking Service." Retrieved from https://www.nice.org.uk/guidance/ph10/chapter/4-Recommendations.

Noor, F., et al. (2014) "A 24-week multicentre, randomised, double-blind study to evaluate the efficacy and safety of varenicline in combination with nicotine replacement therapy vs. varenicline alone for smoking cessation." *Hospital* 1(2), 3–4.

Potenza, M. N. (2013) "Neurobiology of gambling behaviors." *Current Opinion in Neurobiology* 23(4), 660–667.

Prochaska, J. J., & Hilton, J. F. (2012) "Risk of cardiovascular serious adverse events associated with varenicline use for tobacco cessation: systematic review and meta-analysis." *The BMJ* 344, e2856.

Reynolds, G. P., Zhang, Z. J., & Zhang, X. B. (2002) "Association of antipsychotic drug induced weight gain with a 5-HT2C receptor gene polymorphism." *The Lancet* 359(9323), 2086–2087.

Schulte, E. M., Grilo, C. M., & Gearhardt, A. N. (2016) "Shared and unique mechanisms underlying binge eating disorder and addictive disorders." *Clinical Psychology Review* 44, 125–139.

Skinner, H. A. (1982) "The Drug Abuse Screening Test." *Addictive Behavior* 7(4), 363–371.

Sobieraj, D. M., White, W. B., & Baker, W. L. (2013) "Cardiovascular effects of pharmacologic therapies for smoking cessation." *Journal of the American Society of Hypertension* 7(1), 61–67.

Substance Abuse and Mental Health Services Administration and National Institute on Alcohol Abuse and Alcoholism. (2015) *Medication for the Treatment of Alcohol Use Disorder: A Brief Guide.* Rockville, MD: Substance Abuse and Mental Health Services Administration. http://store.samhsa.gov/shin/content//SMA15-4907/SMA15-4907.pdf, Accessed 4/12/16.

Taber, K. H., Black, D. N., Porrino, L. J., & Hurley, R. A. (2012) "Neuroanatomy of dopamine: reward and addiction." *The Journal of Neuropsychiatry and Clinical Neurosciences* 24(1), 1–4.

Vink, J. M., & Boomsma, D. I. (2011) "Interplay between heritability of smoking and environmental conditions? A comparison of two birth cohorts." *BMC Public Health 11*(1), 1.
Vink, J. M., Willemsen, G., & Boomsma, D. I. (2005) "Heritability of smoking initiation and nicotine dependence." *Behavior Genetics* 35(4), 397–406.
Yanovski, S. Z., & Yanovski, J. A. (2014) "Long-term drug treatment for obesity: a systematic and clinical review." *JAMA* 311(1), 74–86.

Index

Note: bold page numbers indicate figures and tables.

Printed in the United States
by Baker & Taylor Publisher Services